Cardiology and Angiology

Cardiology and Angiology

Edited by **Janice Hunter**

hayle
medical

New York

Published by Hayle Medical,
30 West, 37th Street, Suite 612,
New York, NY 10018, USA
www.haylemedical.com

Cardiology and Angiology
Edited by Janice Hunter

© 2016 Hayle Medical

International Standard Book Number: 978-1-63241-388-8 (Hardback)

Printed in the United States of America.

Contents

Preface

This book was inspired by the evolution of our times; to answer the curiosity of inquisitive minds. Many developments have occurred across the globe in the recent past which has transformed the progress in the field.

This book is a compilation of chapters that discuss the most vital concepts and emerging trends in the fields of cardiology and angiology. Cardiology is the branch of medical science that deals with heart related diseases while angiology studies the diseases of lymphatic system and blood vessels. These are interrelated fields as angiology tries to prevent diseases related to cardiovascular systems such as heart attack and strokes. Diagnostic procedures include auscultation, echocardiography, cardiac stress test, sphygmomanometer, cardiovascular magnetic resonance imaging, cardiac marker, optical coherence tomography, etc. Cardiology and angiology are upcoming branches of medical science that have undergone rapid development over the past few decades. This book covers in detail some existent theories and innovative concepts revolving around these disciplines. It will provide comprehensive knowledge to all the readers including researchers, doctors and students.

This book was developed from a mere concept to drafts to chapters and finally compiled together as a complete text to benefit the readers across all nations. To ensure the quality of the content we instilled two significant steps in our procedure. The first was to appoint an editorial team that would verify the data and statistics provided in the book and also select the most appropriate and valuable contributions from the plentiful contributions we received from authors worldwide. The next step was to appoint an expert of the topic as the Editor-in-Chief, who would head the project and finally make the necessary amendments and modifications to make the text reader-friendly. I was then commissioned to examine all the material to present the topics in the most comprehensible and productive format.

I would like to take this opportunity to thank all the contributing authors who were supportive enough to contribute their time and knowledge to this project. I also wish to convey my regards to my family who have been extremely supportive during the entire project.

Editor

Role of Hs-CRP and Exercise Stress Echocardiography in Cardiovascular Risk Stratification of Asymptomatic Type 2 Diabetic Patients

Puneet Aggarwal[1*], Tilak Raj Khurana[1], Ranjeet Nath[2] and Swati Yadav[3]

[1]*Department of Internal Medicine, PGIMER & Dr RML Hospital, Baba Kharag Singh Marg, New Delhi, India.*
[2]*Department of Cardiology, PGIMER & Dr RML Hospital, Baba Kharag Singh Marg, New Delhi, India.*
[3]*Department of Pathology, AIMSR, Bhathinda, Punjab, India.*

Authors' contributions

This work was carried out in collaboration between all authors. Author PA designed the study, wrote the protocol, wrote the first draft of the manuscript and searched the literature. Author TRK managed the proof reading and correction of manuscript. Author RN managed the experimental process with exercise stress echocardiography and angiography and author SY analyzed the study. All authors read and approved the final manuscript.

Editor(s):
(1) Francesco Pelliccia, Department of Heart and Great Vessels University La Sapienza, Rome, Italy.
(2) Gen-Min Lin, Division of Cardiology, Hualien-Armed Forces General Hospital, National Defense Medical Center, Taiwan.
Reviewers:
(1) Adrie J. M. Verhoeven, Cardiovascular Research School COEUR, Erasmus MC, The Netherlands.
(2) Anonymous, University of Bari, Italy.
(3) Radha Acharya Pandey, Kathmandu University School of Medical Sciences, Nepal.

ABSTRACT

Background: Silent ischaemia is a well known cause of mortality and morbidity in type-2 diabetic patients; however the role of high-sensitive C-Reactive Protein (hs-CRP) and exercise stress echocardiography in early detection of silent ischaemia is still less understood.
Methods: Seventy three asymptomatic diabetic patients were enrolled from Dr Ram Manohar Lohia Hospital, Delhi in year 2013-15 and the baseline characteristics of the patients were studied.

---

*Corresponding author: E-mail: puneetaggarwal4u@gmail.com, drpuneetaggarwal@outlook.com

All the patients underwent exercise stress echocardiography for screening of coronary artery disease (CAD). All the patients with positive exercise stress echocardiography underwent angiography for confirmation of coronary artery disease. The patients were divided into two groups on basis of exercise stress echocardiography result as positive and negative and the baseline characteristics and risk factors including high-sensitivity C-reactive protein (hs-CRP) concentrations were compared between two groups in cross sectional study.

Results: Silent ischaemia was found in 17.81% in asymptomatic diabetic patients. The positive predictive value of exercise stress echocardiography taking angiography as gold standard was found to be 84.6%. Sensitivity of hs-CRP >3 mg/L in predicting a positive exercise stress echocardiography is 53.8% and specificity is 90%. Negative predictive value of hs-CRP ≤3 mg/L in ruling out CAD is 90.0% and positive predictive value in detecting positive exercise stress echocardiography was 53.8%. Positive exercise stress echocardiography was found to be significantly associated with hypertension (HTN) (P=0.048), smoking (P=0.018), family history of CAD (P=0.002), total cholesterol (P=0.031), serum low-density lipoprotein (LDL) concentrations (P=0.041), serum hs-CRP (P=0.001), strict glycaemic control (glycated haemoglobin <7%) (P=0.028) and final ejection fraction after exercise stress (P=0.01).

Conclusion: hs-CRP and exercise stress echocardiography can be used as simple screening tool for coronary artery disease in asymptomatic diabetic patients.

Keywords: Diabetes; stress echocardiography; hs CRP; silent ischaemia.

1. INTRODUCTION

Diabetes Mellitus (DM) is a major source of cardiovascular morbidity and mortality in developed and developing countries. According to the World Health Organization (WHO) estimates (2004), India had 32 million diabetic subjects in the year 2000 and this number would increase to 80 million by the year 2030 [1]. The International Diabetes Mellitus Federation (2006) also reported that the total number of diabetic subjects in India was 41 million in 2006 and that this would rise to 70 million by the year 2025 [2]. This means by that time India will contribute to more than one fifth (20%) of the total diabetic population of the world [2].

There is a close relationship between type-2 DM and the development of coronary artery disease (CAD) [3]. Cardiovascular complications are a major cause of mortality, accounting for 65% to 85% deaths in the diabetic population [3]. Accordingly, both the American Heart Association and American College of Cardiology defined DM as an equivalent to previous CAD for cardiovascular risk [4]. Type-2 diabetics are also prone to silent myocardial ischaemia even before the development of overt CAD [5].

Exercise echocardiography is a valuable method for diagnosis, risk stratification and prognosis of CAD [6-10]. C-reactive protein (CRP) has emerged as the most exquisitely sensitive systemic marker of inflammation and a powerful predictive marker of future cardiovascular risk [11].

As the early diagnosis of silent ischaemia would help in reducing the mortality and morbidity, it becomes all the more important to identify these patients in Indian population who are genetically prone to develop DM and CAD.

Our study was planned to establish the role of stress echocardiography and hs-CRP as a significant tool to screen these asymptomatic diabetic patients for silent ischaemia.

2. MATERIALS AND METHODS

The study was conducted on 73 type 2 diabetic patients (diagnosed by WHO criteria) attending various clinic in Dr Ram Manohar Lohia Hospital, New Delhi over a period of 2 year. The cases of DM (WHO criteria) that were being treated by dietary restrictions and /or oral hypoglycemic agents and / or insulin for at least 6 months were included in this study. Patients with signs and symptoms of overt CAD (patients with history suggestive of angina, baseline Electrocardiogram (ECG) or Echocardiography with any regional wall motion abnormality suggestive of CAD), past history of CAD, clinically significant valvular heart disease or cardiomyopathy, any systemic disease with poor prognosis or severe incapacitation, severe respiratory disease, renal disease were excluded from the study. Prior approval from hospital ethical committee and written consent from the patients were taken before enrolment into the study.

Seventy-three patients (53 male and 20 female) of type-2 DM above the age of 35 were included in the study. Patients were evaluated by detailed history regarding DM, history of angina, CAD, family history, HTN, smoking, alcohol intake. Clinical examination included blood pressure, body mass index (BMI), waist hip ratio and fundoscopy for retinopathy. Laboratory investigation included blood urea, serum creatinine, lipid profile (total cholesterol, High-Density Lipoprotein (HDL), Low-Density Lipoprotein (LDL), Very Low Density Lipoprotein (VLDL) and triglyceride (TG) concentrations), glycated haemoglobin (HbA1C), hs-CRP concentration and urine examination for albuminuria. Patients with macroalbuminuria were not included in the study.

The patients were subjected to exercise stress echocardiography. The baseline echocardiogram performed at the time of stress echocardiography contained a screening assessment of ventricular function, chamber sizes, wall-motion thicknesses, aortic root, and valves. Patients underwent symptom-limited treadmill exercise testing according to the standard Bruce protocol. Wall motion at rest and with exercise was scored from 1 through 4 (1, normal; 2, hypokinesis; 3, akinesis; 4, dyskinesis) according to a 16-segment model. Wall motion score index (WMSI), was determined at rest and peak exercise as the sum of the segmental scores divided by the number of visualized segments. The diabetics were sub- grouped, according to the presence or absence of CAD into two groups by subjecting these cases to exercise stress echocardiography.

- Non – CAD – exercise stress echocardiography negative
- CAD – exercise stress echocardiography positive

2.1 Statistical Analysis

The analysis was carried out in SPSS software version 17. Mean values and frequencies of various risk factors (variables) were studied in the group as a whole and individually in the two subgroups, namely those with silent CAD and those without CAD. Risk factors for CAD were used as variables and CAD as outcome.

Statistical significance of outcomes with different variables was determined by chi-square/ Mann Whitney U test. A p-value of ≤0.05 was taken as level of statistical significance.

3. RESULTS

A total of 73 patients (53 male and 20 female) fulfilled the inclusion criteria were analyzed. The clinical, anthropometrical and biochemical parameter of the patients are shown in Tables 1, 2, 3 respectively.

Table 1. Cardiovascular risk factors in asymptomatic Type-2 DM study population (History based)

Variable	Male (n=53)	Female (n=20)	Total (n=73)
Age(years)	54.0±8.94	54.95±8.76	54.41±8.65
Duration of DM (years)	8.60±9.26	7.70±6.86	8.36±6.38
HTN	31(58.49%)	13(65%)	46(63.13%)
History of smoking	17(32.07%)	3(15%)	14(19.18%)
History of alcohol	9(16.99%)	2(10%)	11(15.07%)
Family history of CAD	7(13.21%)	2(10%)	9(12.33%)
Family history of DM	9(16.99%)	2(10%)	11(15.07%)
Family history of HTN	5(9.43%)	2(10%)	7(9.59%)

Table 2. Anthropometric parameters in asymptomatic Type-2 DM study group

Variable	Male (n=53)	Female (n=20)	Total (n=73)
BMI (kg/m^2)	24.27±1.18	24.05±1.04	24.2±1.15
Waist hip ratio	0.95±0.59	0.94±0.48	0.95±.05

All the patients were subjected to exercise stress echocardiography. 13 patients were found to have positive exercise stress echocardiography with prevalence of 17.81%. The prevalence of silent ischaemia was found to be higher In female group than male group (male-15.09%, female-25%) however it was not statistically significant. Patients with stress echocardiography positive were compared with stress echocardiography negative patients (Tables 4, 5).

In the positive exercise stress echocardiography group, the prevalence of HTN, smoking, family history of CAD was significantly higher as compared to negative exercise stress echocardiography group.

Table 3. Biochemical parameters in asymptomatic Type-2 DM study group

Variables	Male (n=53)	Female (n=20)	Total (n=73)
Blood urea (mg/dl)	27.92±9.98	27.60±13.15	27.84±1.84
Serum creatinine (mg/dl)	0.74±0.272	0.67±0.28	0.72±0.27
Uric acid (mg/dl)	5.25±1.716	5.64±1.944	5.36±1.78
HbA1c (%)	8.09±1.55	8.38±2.24	8.17±1.76
Total Cholesterol (mg/dl)	147.4±32.02	164.2±33.92	152.01±33.18
HDL (mg/dl)	41.94±5.78	40.35±7.2	41.51±6.19
LDL (mg/dl)	79.96±33.45	96.45±32.94	84.48±33.91
VLDL (mg/dl)	25.91±12.43	27.30±9.57	26.29±11.67
TG (mg/dl)	129.08±82.47	137.35±52.20	131.34±59.59
hs-CRP (mg/L)	1.70±1.38	1.59±1.34	1.67±1.35
Urinary albumin excretion (mg/24 hr urine)	23.32±27.71	28.30±18.82	24.68±25.55

Table 4. Comparison of risk factors in exercise stress negative & exercise stress positive asymptomatic Type-2 DM patients

Variables	Exercise stress echocardiography negative (n=60)	Exercise stress echocardiography positive (n=13)	P value
Age (Years)	54.5±8.6	54±9.3	0.554
Duration of DM (Years)	7.9±6.1	10.5±7.5	0.227
HTN (%)	33(55%)	11(84.62%)	0.048
Smoking (%)	13(21.67%)	7(53.85%)	0.018
Family history of CAD	1(1.67%)	4(30.77%)	0.002
BMI (kg/m^2)	24.1±1.2	24.5±1	0.209
Waist hip ratio	0.9±0.1	1±0.03	0.133
Fundus abnormality (%)	6(10%)	3(23.08%)	0.194
HbA1c (%)	8.1±1.8	8.5±1.6	0.296
<8.5	40	8	
8.5-9.5	10	2	
>9.5	10	3	
Total Cholestrol (mg/dl)	148.3±32.8	169.2±30.5	0.031
HDL (mg/dl)	41.1±6.3	43.5±5.3	0.150
LDL (mg/dl)	80.9±33.9	100.8±29.8	0.041
VLDL (mg/dl)	26.6±12.3	24.9±8.3	0.994
TG (mg/dl)	133.1±62.9	123.4±42	0.971
hs-CRP (mg/L)	1.4±1.2	2.9±1.5	0.001
≤3	54	6	
>3	6	7	
Urinary albumin excretion (mg/24-hour urine)	23.5±26.6	30.3±20.1	0.103
Ejection Fraction (EF) (%)	60.7±3.6	58.5±5.4	0.07
Post stress EF (EF2) (%)	75.2±5	71.2±6.1	0.032
EF2-EF (%)	14.5±5.6	12.6±5.4	0.460
Wall Motion Score Index(WMSI)	1±0	1.2±0.1	

Table 5. Comparison of HbA1c with exercise stress echocardiography in Type-2 DM patients

HbA1c (%)	Exercise stress echocardiography		P value
	Negative	Positive	
<7	17	0	0.028
≥7	43	13	

Anthropometric parameters were found to be similar in two subgroups. In the biochemical parameters total cholesterol, LDL and hs-CRP were found to be significantly higher in positive exercise stress echocardiography group.

During the baseline echocardiography the ejection fraction of negative exercise stress echocardiography group was higher as compared to positive exercise stress echocardiography group (60.7±3.6 & 58.5±5.4 respectively) but the different was not significant. Ejection fraction of negative exercise stress echocardiography group after exercise was significantly higher than the positive exercise stress echocardiography group (75.2±5 & 71.2±6.1 respectively).

All exercise stress echocardiography positive patients underwent angiography. Out of 13 patients 11 had stenosis of one or more coronary arteries and only 2 patients (15.4%) had normal angiographic findings.

6 out of 13 (46.1%) had single vessel disease, 4 (30.8%) had double vessel disease and just 1 (7.7%) had triple vessel disease in angiography. This data gave the positive predictive value of 84.6% to exercise stress echocardiography to detect silent ischaemia in asymptomatic type-2 diabetic patients.

hs-CRP values ≤3 mg/L were seen in 54 patients with negative exercise stress echocardiography and those >3 mg/L were seen in 6 patients with negative exercise stress echocardiography while 6 patients with positive exercise stress echocardiography had hs-CRP ≤3 mg/L and 7 had values of >3 mg/L. Sensitivity of hs-CRP >3 mg/L in predicting positive exercise stress echocardiography was 53.8% and specificity is 90%. Negative predictive value of hs-CRP ≤3 mg/L in ruling out CAD by exercise stress echocardiography is 90.0% and positive predictive value for positive exercise stress echocardiography was 53.8%.

Wall motion score index in exercise stress echocardiography patients increased with the number of vessel stenosis on angiography. WMSI in single vessel disease was lesser than WMSI in double vessel disease which in turn was lesser than WMSI in triple vessel disease.

4. DISCUSSION

DM is a heterogeneous group of disorder of intermediary metabolism characterized by absolute or relative lack of insulin mediated glucose utilization and the resultant vascular complications. The diabetic condition contributes to the progression of micro and macro complications [12]. Of all, cardiovascular complications are the leading cause of mortality and morbidity in DM.

Type-2 DM person are also prone to silent myocardial ischaemia even before the development of overt CAD [5]. The overall prevalence of silent myocardial ischaemia in type-2 diabetics ranges from 9 to 57 % [13-16].

This broad range is probably due to difference in the populations studied (e.g., age of patients, duration of DM, inclusion or exclusion criteria of patients with high risk factors or symptoms of CAD, and definition of silent myocardial ischaemia), screening technique used (e.g., resting ECG, exercise testing, stress ultrasound, schintigraphy, or coronary angiography) and the diagnostic criteria (e.g., definition of positive exercise tests and confirmation by coronary angiography).

In our study, 13 out of 73 patients were found to have positive exercise stress echocardiography with prevalence of 17.81%. The prevalence of silent ischaemia was found to be higher in female group than male group (male-15.09%, female-25%) however the difference was not statistically significant.

Exercise echocardiography is a valuable method for diagnosis, risk stratification and prognosis of CAD [6-10]. Sensitivity has ranged from a low of 71% to a high of 97% [17,18]. As the threshold level of wall motion abnormality required to define a positive study has varied, there has been the expected inverse relationship between sensitivity and specificity, with specificity ranging from 64% in the studies reporting the highest sensitivity to over 90% in studies with lower sensitivity [17,18]. As with all other imaging modalities, the sensitivity for detection of patients with single-vessel disease has been lower (59% to 94%) than sensitivity for detection of patients with multivessel disease (85% to 100%). In studies by Armstrong et al. Crouse et al. Marwick et al. (1995), Quinone et al. the positive predictive value of exercise stress echocardiography was found to be 88%, 89%, 81%, 78% respectively [18-21].

Positive predictive value of exercise stress echocardiography to detect silent ischaemia in asymptomatic type-2 diabetic patients in our study was found to be 84.6%.

CRP has emerged as the most exquisitely sensitive systemic marker of inflammation and a powerful predictive marker of future cardiovascular risk [11].

In present study, Sensitivity of hs-CRP >3 mg/L in detecting positive exercise stress echocardiography is 53.8% and specificity is 90%. Negative predictive value of hs-CRP ≤3 mg/L in ruling out CAD by exercise stress echocardiography is 90.0% and positive predictive value in detecting positive exercise stress echocardiography was 53.8%. So, hs-CRP can be used as an important tool to rule out CAD.

After statistical analysis, it was observed that there was a difference in the prevalence of various risk factors between the two subgroups (CAD versus non-CAD) in our study.

HTN is a well known risk factor for CAD in both diabetics and non diabetics. In study group, the prevalence of HTN was higher in positive exercise stress echocardiography group as compared to negative exercise stress echocardiography group (85% vs. 55%). Prevalence of HTN was also found to be significantly associated with silent ischaemia (P=0.048).

History of smoking in the present study was not widely prevalent. There were more smokers in positive exercise stress echocardiography group (53.9%) than negative exercise stress echocardiography group (21.7%). History of smoking shows significant statistical association with positive exercise stress echocardiography (P=0.018).

The glycaemic control in both groups of present study was comparable. More patients in negative exercise stress echocardiography group had a good glycaemic control (HbA1c <8.5) than in positive exercise stress echocardiography group (66.6% vs. 61.5%) however, strict glycaemic control was seen only in negative exercise stress echocardiography group (P=0.028). This suggests that strict glycaemic control may be important to prevent further complications of DM, contributing to occurrence of silent myocardial ischaemia.

In our study the amount of total cholesterol and LDL were significantly higher in positive exercise stress echocardiography group (P= 0.031 and P=0.041 respectively).

Microalbuminuria/ albuminuria were not found to be significantly associated with silent myocardial ischaemia. In positive exercise stress echocardiography group, prevalence of microalbuminuria was 23.3%, more in females 30% as compared to 20.75% in males. Mean value of 24 hour urinary microalbumin excretion is 24.68±25.55 mg/ 24 hour of urine (male-23.32±27.71 mg vs. female-28.30±18.81 mg). Since the patients with macroalbuminuria were not included in the study the amount of albuminuria was found to be lesser than several other studies.

5. CONCLUSION

As the epidemic of DM is spreading, there will be larger population that will be at risk for CAD and its related morbidity and mortality. Therefore, there is an urgent need for realization that there is high prevalence of silent CAD in asymptomatic type-2 DM and these patients should be put to regular screening to detect the same so as to prevent the morbidity and mortality associated with silent ischaemia. hs-CRP concentrations and exercise stress echocardiography can be useful tools to predict individuals at risk for silent ischaemia and subsequent damage to myocardium, leading to compromise in the quality of patient's life.

6. LIMITATION OF STUDY

1. The sample size used in the study was small.
2. The study population did not considered some risk factors of CAD like Obstructive sleep Apnea, other CAD equivalents like carotid artery disease, peripheral artery disease in evaluation.
3. Multivariate regression model in order to evaluate the role of confounding factors on results was not done due to small sample size.

ACKNOWLEDGEMENTS

The author would like to thank Dr Ritu Gupta, Dr Shalabh Jain, Dr Siddharth Yadav for their support in formulation of manuscript.

COMPETING INTERESTS

Authors have declared that no competing interests exist.

REFERENCES

1. Wild S, Roglic G, Green A, Sicree R, King H. Global prevalence of diabetes mellitus:

Estimates for the year 2000 and projections for 2030. Diabetes Mellitus Care. 2004;27:1047-53.

2. Sicree R, Shaw J, Zimmet P. Diabetes mellitus and impaired glucose tolerance. Diabetes Mellitus Atlas. International Diabetes Mellitus Federation. 2006;3:15-103.

3. Beller Ga. Non-invasive screening for coronary atherosclerosis and silent ischaemia in asymptomatic type-2 diabetic patients: Is it appropriate and cost-effective? J Am Coll Cardiol. 2007;49: 1918-23.

4. Heller GV. Evaluation of the patient with diabetes mellitus and suspected coronary artery disease. Am J Med. 2005; 118(Suppl 2):9S-14S.

5. Weiner DA, Ryan TJ, Parsons L, Fisher LD, Chaitman BR, Sheffield LT, Tristani FE. Significance of silent myocardial ischaemia during exercise testing in patients with diabetes mellitus: A report from Coronary Artery Surgery Study (CASS) registry. Am J Cardiol. 1991;68: 729-734.

6. Elhendy A, Arruda AM, Mahoney DW, Pellikka PA. Prognostic stratification of diabetic patients by exercise echocardiography. J Am Coll Cardiol. 2001;37:1551-1557.

7. Garrido IP, Peteiro J, Garcia Lara J, Montserrat L, Aldama G, Vazquez-Rodriguez JM, et al. Prognostic value of exercise echocardiography in patients with Diabetes Mellitus and known or suspected coronary artery disease. Am J Cardiol. 2005;96:9-12.

8. Marwick TH, Mehta R, Arheart K, Lauer MS. Use of exercise echocardiography for prognostic evaluation of patients with known or suspected coronary artery disease. J Am Coll Cardiol. 1997;30:83-90.

9. Yao SS, Qureshi E, Syed A, Chaudhry FA. Novel stress echocardiographic model incorporating the extent and severity of wall motion abnormality for risk stratification and prognosis. Am J Cardiol. 2004;94:715-719.

10. Arruda-Oslon AM, Juracan EM, Mahoney DW, McCully RB, Roger VL, Pellikka PA. Prognostic value of exercise echocardiography in 5,798 patients: Is there a gender difference? J Am Coll Cardiol. 2002;39:625-631.

11. Nyandak T, Gogna A, Bansal S, Deb M. High sensitive C - reactive protein (hs-CRP) and its correlation with angiographic severity of coronary artery disease (CAD) JIACM. 2007;8:217-21.

12. Ramachandran A, Snehalatha C, Satyavani K, Latha E, Sasikala R, Vijay V. Prevalence of vascular complications and their risk factors in type-2 diabetes mellitus. J. Assoc. Phys. India. 1999;47: 1152-6.

13. Koistinen MJ. Prevalence of asymptomatic myocardial ischaemia in diabetic subjects. BMJ. 1990;301:92-5.

14. Milan Study on Atherosclerosis and Diabetes Mellitus (MiSAD) Group: Prevalence of recognized silent myocardial ischaemia and its association with atherosclerotic risk factors in non insulin-dependent diabetes mellitus. Am J Cardiol. 1997;79:134-9.

15. Nesto PW, Watson FS, Kowalchuk GJ, Zarich SW, Hill T, Lewis SM, et al. Silent myocardial ischaemia and infarction in diabetics with peripheral vascular disease: assessment by dipyridamole thallium-201 scintigraphy. Am Heart J. 1990;120:1073-7.

16. Holley J, Fenton A, Arthur RS. Thallium stress testing does not predict cardiovascular risk in diabetic patient with end stage renal disease undergoing cadaveric renal transplantation. Am J Med. 1991;90:563-70.

17. Marwick TH, Torelli J, Harjai K, Haluska B, Pashkow FJ, Stewart WJ, et al. Influence of left ventricular hypertrophy on detection of coronary artery disease using exercise echocardiography. J Am Coll Cardiol. 1995;26:1180–6.

18. Crouse LJ, Harbrecht JJ, Vacek JL, Rosamond TL, Kramer PH. Exercise echocardiography as a screening test for coronary artery disease and correlation with coronary arteriography. Am J Cardiol. 1991;67:1213–8.

19. Armstrong WF, O'Donnell J, Ryan T, Feigenbaum H. Effect of prior myocardial infarction and extent and location of coronary disease on accuracy of exercise echocardiography. J Am Coll Cardiol. 1987;10:531–8.

20. Marwick TH, Anderson T, Williams MJ, Haluska B, Melin JA, Pashkow F, et al. Exercise echocardiography is an accurate

and cost-efficient technique for detection of coronary artery disease in women. J Am Coll Cardiol. 1995;26:335–41.

21. Quinones MA, Verani MS, Haichin RM, Mahmarian JJ, Suarez J, Zoghbi WA. Exercise echocardiography versus 201Tl single-photon emission computed tomography in evaluation of coronary artery disease: Analysis of 292 patients. Circulation. 1992;85:1026–31.

2

Infantile Cardiac Rhabdomyoma–Pearls Inside the Heart

Prem Krishna Anandan[1*], Basavaraj Baligar[1], J. S. Patel[1], Prabhavathi Bhatt[1], Cholenahally Nanjappa Manjunath[2] and C. Dhanalakshmi[3]

[1]Resident in Cardiology, Sri Jayadeva Institute of Cardiovascular Science and Research, Bengaluru, Karnataka, India.
[2]Department of Cardiology, Sri Jayadeva Institute of Cardiovascular Science and Research, Bengaluru, Karnataka, India.
[3]Department of Echocardiography, Sri Jayadeva Institute of Cardiovascular Science and Research, Bengaluru, Karnataka, India.

Authors' contributions

This work was carried out in collaboration between all authors. Author PKA designed the study, Author CNM wrote the protocol, and author PB wrote the first draft of the manuscript. Author BB managed the literature searches. Author CDL recorded the echocardiogram. All authors read and approved the final manuscript.

Editor(s):
(1) Francesco Pelliccia, Department of Heart and Great Vessels University La Sapienza, Rome, Italy.
(2) Gen-Min Lin, Division of Cardiology, Hualien-Armed Forces General Hospital, National Defense Medical Center, Taiwan.
Reviewers:
(1) Andrea Borghini, Institute of Clinical Physiology- CNR, Pisa, Italy.
(2) Anonymous, University of São Paulo, Brazil.
(3) Anonymous, Dicle University, Turkey.
(4) Anonymous, University of Bari, Italy.

ABSTRACT

Cardiac rhabdomyoma is the most common primary pediatric tumor of the heart. We report a 1-month old male infant who presented to our institute for routine cardiac evaluation since he was diagnosed to have a cardiac mass in the right ventricle (RV) in utero. After he was born, an echocardiogram showed two large cardiac masses occupying entire RV cavity and origin of right ventricular outflow tract (RVOT). Although our patient was asymptomatic, surgical removal of these two masses was done due to its proximity to RVOT and also because it was almost obliterating the entire RV cavity.

*Corresponding author: E-mail: premkrishna2k1@gmail.com

Keywords: Cardiac tumor; rhabdomyoma; right ventricular mass.

1. INTRODUCTION

Cardiac tumors were first described by Boneti [1]. Cardiac rhabdomyoma usually occurs as multiple masses, and arises from ventricular free wall and septal wall. 50-80% of these patients had associated tuberous sclerosis. Although cardiac rhabdomyoma has benign prognosis and is known to undergo spontaneous regression, some may require surgical removal if the location was near or in the right ventricular outflow tract (RVOT), left ventricular outflow tract (LVOT), or when they produce intractable arrhythmias.

2. CASE REPORT

A 1-month-old male infant presented to our institute for routine cardiac evaluation. Fetal echo had showed intracardiac mass at 30 weeks of gestation. The baby was born to non-consanguineous parents. Tuberous sclerosis (TCS) screening was negative. The baby was asymptomatic at the time of evaluation. A routine echocardiogram (Fig. 1) showed a large 3 x 1.2 cm mass occupying entire RV cavity and another 0.9 x 0.7 cm mass at the origin of RVOT causing mild obstruction. In view of the size and location, despite being asymptomatic, the infant underwent successful surgical removal of the masses (Fig. 2) and was discharged uneventfully.

3. DISCUSSION

The prevalence of cardiac tumor is extremely rare in infants and children (0.027 to 0.17%). Cardiac rhabdomyoma is the most common type of cardiac tumor. More than 60% of antenatally diagnosed cardiac tumors are rhabdomyomas and are often associated with tuberous sclerosis [2]. Cardiac rhabdomyoma is seen in 30-80% of patients with tuberous sclerosis and usually regresses spontaneously over time [3]. In addition, 50–60% of patients with tuberous sclerosis will develop cardiac rhabdo-myoma [4,5].

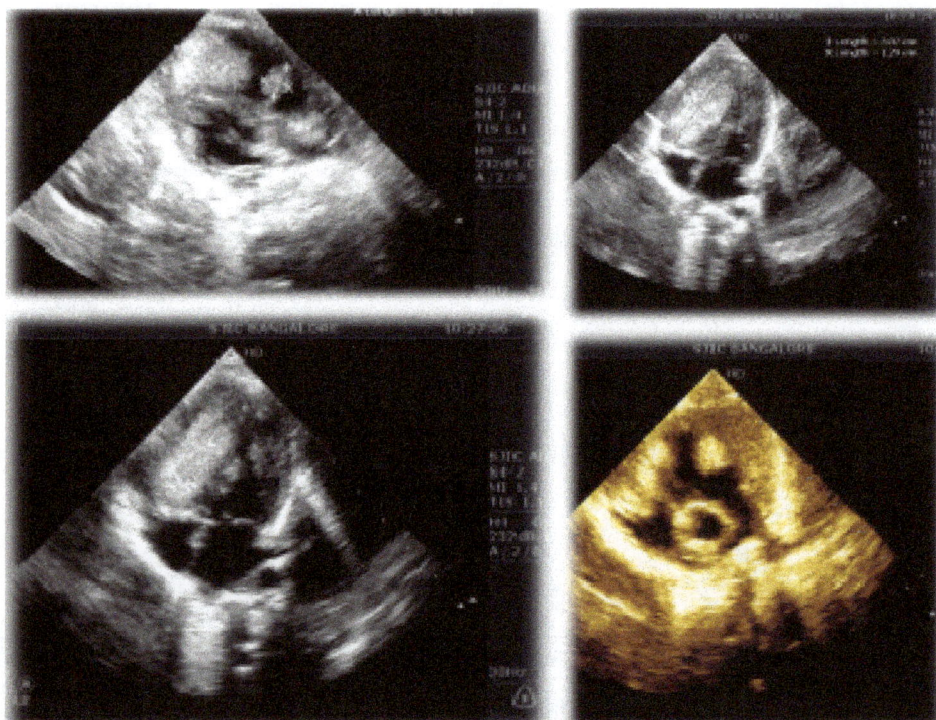

Fig. 1. Trans thoracic echo (TTE) showing rhabdomyoma in right ventricular (RV) cavity and origin of right ventricular outflow tract (RVOT).

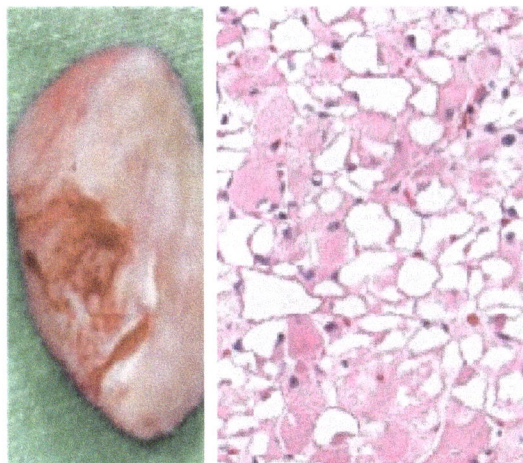

Fig. 2. Gross and histopathological specimen showing rhabdomyoma extracted from RV cavity

A meta-analysis showed that most rhabdomyomas associated with tuberous sclerosis are non-obstructive [6]. The natural history of cardiac rhabdomyoma in infants and children has been well studied [7]. The younger the age at diagnosis, the higher the chance for spontaneous regression, and complete regression being more common in the first 4 years of life. In 2D echocardiogram, they appear as round, homogenous masses [8]. Indications for surgery included life-threatening arrhythmias, and outflow tract obstructions [9]. If complete surgical resection is not possible because of the location of the tumor, a partial resection can be done and the residual tumor usually regresses. The mortality from surgery for cardiac tumor in children is about 5% [10].

A serial echocardiography may help in selecting patients who are at risk of developing ventricular outflow obstruction and who need early surgery. All cases of cardiac rhabdomyoma must be followed up closely for the future developed tuberous sclerosis.

4. CONCLUSION

Although watchful waiting is the general strategy for cardiac rhabdomyomas, certain clinical situations like intractable arrhythmias and locations near outflow tract causing obstruction warrant early surgical intervention. Our patient underwent surgery empirically due to its location near the RVOT and the tumor occupying almost the entire RV cavity. Because rhabdomyoma is known to undergo spontaneous regression, general agreement was indicated for surgical treatment, which should be individualized and considered only in the presence of significant hemodynamic obstruction to the ventricular inflow or the outflow tract.

CONSENT

All authors declare that 'written informed consent was obtained from the patient (or other approved parties) for publication of this case report and accompanying images.

ETHICAL APPROVAL

It is not applicable.

COMPETING INTERESTS

Authors have declared that no competing interests exist.

REFERENCES

1. Perlstein, et al. Sarcoma of the heart. Am. J. M. SC. 1918;156:214.

2. Isaacs H Jr. Fetal and neonatal cardiac tumors. Pediatr Cardiol. 2004;25(3):252-273.

3. Smythe JF, Dyck JD, Smallhorn JF, Freedom RM. Natural history of cardiac rhabdomyoma in infancy and childhood. Am J Cardiol. 1990;66:1247-1249.

4. Webb DW, Thomas RD, Osborne JP. Cardiac rhabdomyomas and their association with tuberous sclerosis. Arch Dis Child. 1993;68(3):367-370.

5. Harding CO, Pagon RA. Incidence of tuberous sclerosis in patients with cardiac rhabdomyoma. Am J Med Genet. 1990;37(4):443-446.

6. Verhaaren H A, Vanakker O, De Wolf D, Suys B, Francois K, Matthys D. Left Ventricular outflow tract obstruction in rhabdomyoma of infancy: Meta-analysis of the literature. J Pediatr. 2003;143:258-263.

7. Bosi G, Lintermans JP, Pellegrino PA, Svaluto-Moreolo G, Vliers A.The natural history of cardiac rhabdomyoma with and without tuberous sclerosis. Acta Paediatr. 1996; 85(8):928-931.

8. Chao AS, Chao A, Wang TH, Chang YC, Chang YL, Hsieh CC, Lien R, et al.

Outcome of antenatally diagnosed cardiac rhabdomyoma: case series and a meta-analysis. Ultrasound Obstet Gynecol. 2008;31(3):289-295.

9. Stiller B, Hetzer R, Meyer R, Dittrich S, Pees C, Alexi-Meskishvili V, Lange P. Primary cardiac tumours: When is surgery necessary? Eur J of Cardio-thoracic surgery. 2001;20:1002-06.

10. Takach TJ, Reul GJ, Ott DA, Cooley DA. Primary cardiac tumors in infants and children: immediate and long term operative results. Ann Thorac Surg. 1996; 62(2):559-564.

3

Sex Hormones and Their Relationship with Leptin and Cardiovascular Risk Factors in Pre and Post-Menopausal Nigerian Women with Metabolic Syndrome

U. A. Fabian[1], M. A. Charles-Davies[1*], A. A. Fasanmade[2], J. A. Olaniyi[3],
O. E. Oyewole[4], M. O. Owolabi[2], J. R. Adebusuyi[5], O. Hassan[5], B.M. Ajobo[6],
M. O. Ebesunun[7], K. Adigun[8], K. S. Akinlade[1], O. G. Arinola[1]
and E. O Agbedana[1]

[1]*Department of Chemical Pathology, College of Medicine, University of Ibadan, Ibadan 200284, Nigeria.*
[2]*Department of Medicine, College of Medicine, University of Ibadan, Ibadan 200284, Nigeria.*
[3]*Department of Haematology, College of Medicine, University of Ibadan, Ibadan 200284, Nigeria.*
[4]*Department of Health Promotion and Education, College of Medicine, University of Ibadan, Ibadan 200284, Nigeria.*
[5]*Medical Social Services Department, University College Hospital, Ibadan 200212, Nigeria.*
[6]*Dietetics Department, University College Hospital, Ibadan 200212, Nigeria.*
[7]*Department of Chemical Pathology, College of Health Sciences, Olabisi Onabanjo University, Ago-Iwoye 120005, Nigeria.*
[8]*General Out Patient Unit, University College Hospital, Ibadan 200212, Nigeria.*

Authors' contributions

The authors contributed to the intellectual content of this paper and have met the following requirements: a) Significant contributions to the concept and design, data acquisition, analysis and interpretation; b) Drafting and reviewing the article for intellectual content; c) Final approval of the article for publication.

Editor(s):
(1) Francesco Pelliccia, Department of Heart and Great Vessels, University La Sapienza, Rome, Italy.
Reviewers:
(1) A. Papazafiropoulou, Department of Internal Medicine and Diabetes Center, Tzaneio General Hospital of Piraeus, Greece.
(2) Mario Bernardo-Filho, Departamento de Biofísica e Biometria, Universidade do Estado do Rio de Janeiro, Brazil.
(3) Ronald Wang, Obstetrics & Gynaecology, The Chinese University of Hong Kong, Hong Kong, China.
(4) Pietro Scicchitano, Cardiology Department, San Giacomo Hospital, Monopoli, Italy.

*Corresponding author: E-mail: mcharlesdavies@yahoo.com

ABSTRACT

Metabolic Syndrome (MS), which affects 33.1% of Nigerians, predisposing them to cardiovascular disease (CVD) risk, has been associated with the female gender. The cardioprotective effect of oestradiol against CVD is now controversial and was investigated in premenopausal with MS (PRMMS) and postmenopausal women with MS (POMMS).

A total of 191 women (44 PRMMS, 126 POMMS and 21 premenopausal women without MS (PRM) (controls) with mean (s.d) age of 40.0 (6.9), 57.0 (8.8), 29.0 (6.8) years were participants of this study. Demography, blood pressure (BP), anthropometry, hormones, fasting plasma glucose (FPG) and lipids were obtained by standard methods. Data were significant at ($P<.05$).

Age, parity, all anthropometric measures, FPG, leptin, ET ratio and FSH were significantly higher while HDLC, testosterone and prolactin were significantly lower in PRMMS compared with controls ($P<.03$). In comparison of POMMS with PRMMS, age, parity, WHR, systolic BP, TG, FSH and LH were significantly higher while body weight, HC, and leptin were lower in POMMS compared with PRMMS ($P<.05$). DBP positively predicted oestradiol in PRM only ($P=.044$) while oestradiol positively predicted testosterone in PRMMS only ($P<.001$). In POMMS only, DBP positively predicted testosterone; testosterone, ET ratio and FSH positively predicted oestradiol while LDLC and oestradiol positively predicted the ET ratio ($P<.03$).

Metabolic syndrome may predispose both pre and postmenopausal women to the risk cardiovascular disease and type 2 diabetes mellitus. Oestradiol may protect against cardiovascular diseases in women without metabolic syndrome only.

Keywords: Sex hormones; metabolic syndrome; cardiovascular disease; menopause; leptin.

1. INTRODUCTION

Cardiovascular disease (CVD) is a major cause of morbidity and mortality worldwide especially in women and the elderly in Western countries [1,2]. The negative cardiovascular profile observed in MS, which has also been associated with the female gender, may be determined by its main features- abdominal obesity and insulin resistance [3,4]. Contrary to observations in other regions of the world, elevated waist circumference (WC), reduced high density lipoprotein cholesterol (HDLC) and high blood pressure (BP) are prevalent MS components in the Nigerian with gender differences. Elevated WC was more frequent in females while reduced HDLC was more frequent in males [5]. These observations may be important in the management of CVD in the Nigerian, the most populous sub-Sahara African country as hormonal signaling has been implicated in the regulation of cardio-protective mechanisms [1].

Oestrogen is a female sex hormone produced by the ovaries and known to have several cardio-protective mechanisms that change the vascular tone by increasing nitrous oxide production, stabilize the endothelial cells and enhance antioxidant effects. These mechanisms get lost with the onset of menopause [6,7], when the ovaries cease to produce significant amounts of oestrogen. The loss of ovarian follicular activity due to falling follicle stimulating hormone levels explains the decline in oestrogen at menopause [8,9].

Menopause is the permanent cessation of menstruation for a period of one year and marks the transition from reproductive (premenopausal) to non-reproductive (postmenopausal) status, occurring at a mean age of 51 years [7,10]. This transition is associated with increased susceptibility to cardiovascular events possibly due to the protective effect of oestrogen in premenopausal women without MS (PRM) [2,7,11,12]. It is postulated that abdominal tissue redistribution in menopause could be related to a relative deficit in circulating oestrogens [12,13]. It is not clear whether such effects could manifest in women with MS.

Menopause has been reported to have a negative impact on plasma lipoprotein-lipid levels, adverse changes in glucose and insulin metabolism and body fat distribution [7,14]. Though controversial, recent evidence suggests that oestrogen may not be cardio-protective [5]. Studies on cardioprotective effects of sex hormones in PRM women with MS are sparse in our geographical region. Thus, the association of sex hormones with cardiovascular risk factors was investigated in PRM, premenopausal and postmenopausal Nigerian women with MS (PRMMS and POMMS respectively).

2. METHODOLOGY

2.1 Study Design

The study was a cohort study conducted over a period of 6 months. Ethical approval was obtained from the University of Ibadan/University College Hospital (UI/UCH) Joint Ethical Committee.

2.2 Participants

A total of 191 apparently healthy women consisting of 44 PRMMS, 126 POMMS of >1 year duration and 21 PRM women (controls)] with mean (standard deviation) ages of 40.0 (6.9), 57.0 (8.8), 29.0 (6.8) years respectively from Bodija and University College Hospital, Ibadan community, and environs; enrolled in this study at the Department of Chemical Pathology, University of Ibadan, Ibadan, after written informed consent. They were part of the cohort of 784 participants in the study on Risk Assessment of Type 2 Diabetes Mellitus in Individuals with MS, in Ibadan, South West Nigeria. All the participants were non-diabetic (from their pretest questionnaire) and were not aware of their metabolic status. Those on antihypertensive, lipid lowering and hormonal medications or hormonal contraceptives, cardiovascular diseases like stroke and those who did not give consent were excluded from the study. Diagnosis of MS was made using the International Diabetes Federation diagnostic criteria [15]. The criteria include central obesity measured as WC (≥80 cm) and any two of raised triglycerides (TG): ≥150 mg/dL(1.7 mmol/L), reduced HDLC (females: <50 mg/dL, raised BP (≥130/ ≥85 mmHg) or raised fasting plasma glucose (FPG) (≥100 mg/dL).

2.3 Sample Collection

Ten ml of venous blood sample was aseptically obtained by venepuncture from the participants during the follicular phase of their menstrual cycle, after an overnight fast (10-14 h). 4 ml was dispensed into potassium ethylene diamine tetra acetic acid (K_3EDTA) tube for the determination of lipid profile (total cholesterol (TC), triglyceride (TG) and HDLC). Two ml was dispensed into fluoride oxalate tube for FPG estimation while 4 ml was dispensed into plain tubes for the estimation of hormones. All samples were centrifuged at 500 g for 5 min after which plasma/serum were aspirated in small aliquots

into clean vials and stored at -20ºC until analyses were done [16].

2.4 Anthropometric and Blood Pressure Measurements

Reproductive history was obtained through semi structured pretest questionnaire administered to participants. Adiposity measures (body weight, height, body mass index (BMI), waist circumference (WC), hip circumference (HC), waist hip ratio (WHR), percentage body fat (PBF)) and blood pressure (BP) (systolic and diastolic) were obtained from the participants by standard methods described elsewhere [3,17].

2.5 Biochemical Estimations

TG, TC, HDLC and FPG were estimated by enzymatic methods while low density lipoprotein cholesterol (LDLC) was calculated using Friedwald's formula as described by Charles-Davies et al. [3]. Leptin was estimated by enzyme-linked immunosorbent assay (Diagnostic Automation, Inc., CA). Oestradiol, testosterone, luteinizing hormone (LH), follicle stimulating hormone (FSH) and prolactin were determined by enzyme immunoassay {Immunometrics (UK) Ltd.} while oestradiol-testosterone ratio (ET ratio) was calculated.

2.6 Statistical Analysis

Data obtained were analysed statistically using Student's t-test for comparison of variables. Stepwise Multiple Regression model was used to identify specific determinants of dependent variables. $P < .05$ was considered significant.

3. RESULTS AND DISCUSSION

3.1 Results

Table 1 shows comparisons of mean (s.e) age, parity, blood pressure, anthropometric measures and biochemical parameters among PRMMS, POMMS and PRM. All parameters except, TG, TC, LDLC, LH, oestradiol were significantly different when PRMMS was compared with PRM ($P > .05$). Age, parity, all anthropometric measures, FPG, leptin, ET ratio and FSH were significantly higher while HDLC, testosterone and prolactin were significantly lower in PRMMS compared with controls ($P < .03$). In comparison of POMMS with PRMMS, age, parity, WHR, systolic BP, TG, FSH and LH were significantly higher while body weight, HC, and leptin were lower in POMMS compared with PRMMS (P<.05).

All CVD risk factors, LH, FSH and prolactin with dependent variables- testosterone, oestradiol, and testosterone oestradiol ratio, in a stepwise multiple regression model showed the following relationships: DBP positively predicted oestradiol in PRM only (P=.044) while oestradiol positively predicted testosterone in PRMMS only (P<.001). In POMMS only, DBP positively predicted testosterone; testosterone, ET ratio and FSH positively predicted oestradiol while LDLC and oestradiol positively predicted the ET ratio (P<.03) (Table 2.)

3.2 Discussion

Metabolic syndrome predisposes individuals to the development of CVD. Nigerians with MS have shown higher levels of cardiovascular risk factors than those without MS. Interestingly, MS appears more common in females than males and differences in MS components have been observed between males and females [5].

Protecting the myocardium against the deleterious consequences of myocardial ischaemia may reduce the high mortality of the disease particularly in females. Age, parity, blood pressure and all anthropometric measures were significantly higher in PRMMS compared with controls (P<.05) (Table 1). These findings are consistent with our earlier observations in the general population [5,18] and suggest that PRMMS are at high risk of CVD.

Oestrogen is a female hormone and is thought to prevent the development of atherosclerosis [19]. All steroid hormones (including oestradiol) are derived from cholesterol, mainly circulated in blood as low density lipoprotein. Comparisons of TG, TC, LDLC (known atherogenic risk factors), LH and oestradiol were not significantly different between PRMMS and controls (P>.05) suggesting that these indices may have limited role in CVD risk in PRMMS. Moreover, DBP positively predicted oestradiol only in PRM only (P<.05) (Table 2). Additionally, leptin, ET ratio, FSH and FPG were significantly higher while HDLC and testosterone were significantly lower in PRMMS when compared with controls (Table 1). In our previous study, elevated leptin levels were associated with increased adiposity and might be involved in compensatory mechanisms aimed at maintaining normal blood pressure in individuals with MS [16].

In PRM, oestradiol level is controlled by FSH through negative feedback mechanism. It appears that this control may be reduced or lost in MS implicating oestradiol synthesis in adipose tissue. The increase in ET ratio and reduced testosterone levels in PRMMS compared with controls (P<.001) suggests that aromatase enzyme in increased adipose mass (non-gonadal site) in MS increases conversion of testosterone to oestradiol. Oestadiol predicted testosterone positively in PRMMS only (P<.001) (Table 2). There may also be the compensatory effect of FSH, which is raised in PRMMS compared with controls to maintain oestradiol levels due to possible loss of feedback mechanism. It is also possible that this process might be due to the older age of the PRMMS compared with PRM as a result of aging follicles. However, the observed reduction of HDLC and elevated FBG levels in PRMMS compared with the PRM group may implicate mechanisms of MS. Reduced HDLC and elevated FBG are components of metabolic syndrome [15]. Reduction in HDLC and testosterone, and increase in FPG levels were observed in males with MS and type 2 diabetes mellitus in an earlier study [17]. Over 80% of Nigerian males and females with type 2 diabetes mellitus had MS [20]. Moreover, age did not predict any of the sex hormones or their ratio in any of the groups in our present study (Table 2).

Hip circumference measures subcutaneous adipose tissue while WHR together with WC and WHT measure abdominal fat. WHR correlates with all metabolic risk factors and its increase may reflect either a relative abundance of abdominal fat (increased WC) or a relative lack of gluteal muscle (decreased HC) [5]. WHR is positively and independently related to the occurrence of arterial HTN [21]. Abdominal tissue redistribution in menopause could be related to a relative deficit in circulating oestrogens [12,13]. Age, parity, WHR and systolic BP were significantly higher while body weight and HC were lower in POMMS compared with PRMMS (P<.05) (Table 1).

Menopause is associated with ovarian failure and removal of feedback inhibition as observed by other studies [9,10]. We observed significantly higher levels of TG, LH and FSH lower leptin level in POMMS compared with PRMMS (P<.05) (Table 1). In POMMS only, DBP positively predicted testosterone; testosterone, ET ratio and FSH positively predicted oestradiol while LDLC and oestradiol predicted ET ratio (P< .05)

(Table 2). These findings may be attributed to menopause since MS is common to both groups. However, the similarity of levels of oestradiol in POMMS and PRMMS, implicate non-gonadal oestrogen synthesis from testosterone particularly from increased adipose tissue mass. Elevated triglyceride level is a component of MS [15]. Our earlier report showed TG as the least component of MS observed the general population [15]. Although, similar level of TG was observed in both PRM and PRMMS, TG was significantly higher in POMMS than PRMMS in this present study (P<.05). Our findings suggest that CVD risk is exaggerated in menopause. Menopause has been epidemiologically linked with increased CVD risk [1]. During the menopausal transition, there is an emergence of the characteristics of the metabolic syndrome which increases cardiovascular risk [11,12].

Menopause has been reported to have a negative impact on plasma lipoprotein-lipid levels, adverse changes in glucose and insulin metabolism and body fat distribution [7,14]. The menopausal transition has been associated with an accelerated increase of total cholesterol and triglyceride concentrations [22]. Systolic and diastolic BP have been shown to correlate inversely with age at menopause and positively to the length of the postmenopausal period. These reports are partially contrary to our observations, which we attribute to MS and not menopause. Although low level of female steroids has been reported as a major factor for blood pressure elevation [23], In this present study, increase in elevation of BP was observed in both pre and postmenopausal women in association with normal oestrogen levels (Table 1). Only one (0.8%) of the 127 postmenopausal

Table 1. Comparison of age, parity, blood pressure, anthropometric measures and biochemical parameters in premenopausal women with metabolic syndrome, postmenopausal women with metabolic syndrome and premenopausal women without metabolic syndrome (controls)

Index	PRMMS n=44	PRM (Control) n =21	POMMS n = 126	P_1	P_2
Age (years)	40.0 (1.0)	29.0 (1.5)	57.0 (0.8)	<.001*	<.001*
Parity	4.3 (0.2)	2.9 (0.6)	6.3 (0.2)	.016*	<.001*
Height (m)	1.60 (0.0)	1.57 (0.0)	1.59 (0.0)	.011*	0.112
Body weight (kg)	77.8 (2.3)	53.2 (1.3)	72.5 (1.2)	<.001*	0.029*
Body mass index (kg/m^2)	29.9 (0.8)	21.5 (0.4)	28.6 (0.4)	<.001*	0.124
Waist circumference (cm)	101.3 (1.6)	75.8 (1.0)	102.5 (1.0)	<.001*	0.545
Hip circumference (cm)	110.8 (1.5)	92.6 (1.2)	104.9 (0.8)	<.001*	0.001*
Waist Hip Ratio	0.9 (0.0)	0.8 (0.0)	1.0 (0.0)	<.001*	<0.001*
Systolic BP (mmHg)	142.7 (3.8)	112.4 (1.5)	154.3 (2.3)	<.001*	0.010*
Diastolic Blood Pressure(mmHg)	89.3 (1.9)	71.9 (0.9)	90.2 (1.3)	<.001*	0.714
Percentage body fat	42.3 (0.9)	28.4 (1.1)	40.9 (0.6)	<.001*	0.218
FPG (mmol/L)	5.7 (0.4)	4.4 (0.1)	5.1 (0.2)	.021*	0.123
Triglyceride (mmol/L)	0.8 (0.1)	0.6 (0.1)	0.9 (0.0)	.170	0.020*
Total Cholesterol (mmol/L)	3.6 (0.2)	3.8 (0.2)	3.9 (0.1)	.546	0.112
HDLC(mmol/L)	0.9 (0.0)	1.5 (0.1)	0.9 (0.0)	<.001*	0.735
LDLC (mmol/L)	2.4 (0.1)	2.0 (0.2)	2.6 (0.1)	.161	0.232
Leptin (µg/L)	33.6 (5.0)	12.6 (2.0)	18.7 (2.2)	.006*	0.003*
Testosterone (nmol/L)	5.9 (1.0)	16.1 (2.0)	8.0 (0.8)	<.001*	0.155
Oestradiol (nmol/L)	2.1 (0.7)	0.3 (0.1)	1.4 (0.3)	.055	0.283
ET ratio	0.29 (0.1)	0.02 (0.1)	0.2 (0.0)	.025*	0.265
LH (IU/L)	19.8 (2.8)	14.0 (1.9)	26.7 (1.3)	.180	0.014*
FSH (IU/L)	25.1 (4.3)	10.4 (2.8)	54.3 (2.5)	.027*	<0.001*
Prolactin (mIU/L)	453.8(58.3)	945.6 (286.1)	328.9(33.8)	.025*	0.063

values are in mean (s.e), PRM=premenopausal women without metabolic syndrome (controls), PRMMS= premenopausal women with metabolic syndrome, POMMS=postmenopausal women with MS, t=student's t-test, P_1=probability between PRMMS & PRM (controls), *=significant, n=number of participants, P_2=probability between PRMMS & POMMS, FPG=fasting plasma glucose, HDLC=high density lipoprotein cholesterol, LDLC=low density lipoprotein cholesterol, ET ratio=estrogen-testosterone ratio, LH=luteinizing hormone, FSH=follicle stimulating hormone, n=number of participants, n for leptin is PRMMS=23, PRM=14, POMMS=50; n for parity is PRMMS=42, PRM=10; POMMS=111; n for percentage body fat is PRM=20.

Table 2. Multiple regression analyses in premenopausal women without metabolic syndrome (Controls), premenopausal and postmenopausal women with metabolic syndrome

Groups	Dependent parameter	Predictors	β	T	P
PRM					
R^2=.196, F=4.630, P=.044	Oestradiol	Diastolic BP	.443	2.152	.044*
PRMMS					
R^2=.567, F=54.998, P= <.001	Testosterone	Oestradiol	.753	7.416	<.001*
POMMS					
R^2=.107, F=5.768, P=.020	Testosterone	Diastolic BP	.328	2.402	.02*
R^2=.299, F=52.507, P=<.001	Oestradiol	Testosterone	.456	6.469	<.001*
R^2=.447, F=49.378, P=<.001	Oestradiol	ET ratio	.342	5.242	<.001*
R^2=.503, F=40.751, P=<.001	Oestradiol	FSH	.261	3.665	<.001*
R^2=.132, F=18.733, P=<.001	ET ratio	Oestradiol	.369	4.490	<.001
R^2=.177, F=13.145, P=<.001	ET ratio	LDLC	.212	2.587	.011

PRM=premenopausal women without metabolic syndrome (controls), PRMMS= premenopausal women with metabolic syndrome, POMMS=postmenopausal women with MS, t=Student's t-test, P=probability, *=significant, β=beta coefficient, F=F statistics, BP=blood pressure, ET ratio=oestradiol-testosterone ratio, FSH=Follicle Stimulating Hormone, LDLC=low density lipoprotein cholesterol

participants did not have MS and was excluded from the study, which is the limitation in this study. It is possible that mechanisms involving leptin may be involved in maintaining oestrogen levels in MS in both stages in an attempt to normalize blood pressure [16]. Leptin level, though significantly lower in POMMS than PRMMS, was higher in POMMS than PRM (Table 1).

Cardioprotection of oestrogen and the use of hormone replacement therapy (HRT) on postmenopausal women are controversial. It is thought that HRT may actually increase the risk of cardiovascular events. Patients and clinicians are therefore reluctant in continuing the use of HRT regimes [1]. Contrarily, Ciccone et al. [24] showed improvement in CVD risk on oestradiol administration in postmenopausal women. Both general and central obesity were associated with MS in our previous studies [3,5]. This is confirmed by our present findings of significant and negative alterations of these indices in PRMMS compared with PRM, which were aggravated in POMMS. Our observations suggest association of MS with CVD risk in pre and postmenopausal women irrespective of oestradiol levels. The observed elevated FPG and reduction of HDLC and testosterone levels in addition to increase in adipose tissue mass both in PRMMS and POMMS may be important in CVD and type 2 diabetes mellitus risk. Short-term dietary modulation and the use of carotenoids have been shown to improve cardiovascular risk, inflammation and oxidative stress associated with MS [25,26]. We postulate

that postmenopausal women without MS may benefit from oestrogen replacement therapy because of expected menopause induced reduction of oestradiol levels. However, testosterone replacement therapy may benefit individuals with MS. DBP predicted testosterone in POMMS only in this present study (Table 2). Functional androgen receptors are present in the heart and testosterone acts directly at the myocardium suggesting that testosterone confers cardio protection by direct action on the myocardium. Moreover, low testosterone in patients with ischemic disease and alleviation of observed symptoms with testosterone treatment have been reported [27]. Further studies possibly in younger MS and non-MS premenopausal women as well as MS and non-MS postmenopausal women may be necessary to elucidate these findings.

4. CONCLUSION

Observations from our present study suggest that oestradiol may protect against cardiovascular risk in premenopausal women without MS only. This protection diminishes as these women develop MS, which worsens as women attain menopause, with redistribution of abdominal tissue. Hormone replacement therapy may take MS status into consideration in the management of postmenopausal women with CVD risk. Dietary modulation and the use of carotenoids may improve cardiovascular risk, inflammation and oxidative stress associated with MS.

ACKNOWLEDGEMENTS

This study was partly funded by the University of Ibadan MacArthur Foundation grant. The authors appreciate the financial contributions of Unyime A. Fabian for the analyses of pituitary and gonadal hormones in the study.

COMPETING INTERESTS

Authors have declared that no competing interests exist.

REFERENCES

1. Ballard VL, Edelberg JM. Harnessing hormonal signaling for cardio protection. Sci Aging Knowledge Environ. 2005; 51:re6.

2. Bhupathy P, Haines CD, Leinwand LA. Influence of sex hormones and phytoestrogens on heart disease in men and women. Womens Health (LondEngl). 2010;6(1):77–95. DOI:10.2217/whe.09.80.

3. Charles-Davies MA, Arinola OG, FasanmadeAA, Olaniyi JA, Oyewole OE, Owolabi MO, et al. Indices of metabolic syndrome in 534 apparently healthy traders in a local market in Ibadan, Nigeria. Journal of US China Medical Science. 2012;9(2):91–100.

4. Faloia E, Michetti G, De Robertis M, Luconi MP, Furlani Giorgio, Boscaro M. Inflammation as a link between obesity and metabolic syndrome. J Nutr and Metab; 2012. Article ID 476380, 7 pages. DOI:10.1155/2012/476380.Epub 2012 Mar 1.

5. Charles-Davies MA, Fasanmade AA, Olaniyi JA, Oyewole OE, Owolabi MO, Adebusuyi JR, et al. Prevalent components of metabolic syndrome and their correlates in apparently healthy individuals in Sub-Saharan Africa. International Journal of Tropical Disease & Health. 2014;4(2):740-52.

6. Igweh JC. The effects of menopause on the serum lipid profile of normal females of south east Nigeria. Niger J of Physiol Sci. 2005;20(1-2):48–53.

7. Kilim SR, Chandala SR. A comparative study of lipid profile and oestradiol in Pre- and Post-Menopausal Women. J Clin Diagn Res. 2013;7(8):1596–98.

8. Burger HG, Dudley EC, Robertson DM, Dennerstein L. Hormonal changes in the menopause transition. Recent ProgHorm Res. 2002;57:257–75.

9. Collins P, Rosano G, Casey C, Daly C, Gambacciani M., Hadji P, et al. Management of cardiovascular risk in the peri-menopausal woman: A consensus statement of European cardiologists and gynaecologists. European Heart Journal. 2007;28:2028–40.

10. Turky K, Elnahas N, Ramadhan O. Effects of Exercise Training on Postmenopausal Hypertension: Implications on Nitric Oxide Levels. Med J Malaysia. 2013;68(6):459-64.

11. Lobo RA. Metabolic syndrome after menopause and the role of hormones. Maturitas 2008;60:10-8.

12. Perez-Lopez F R, Chedraui P, Gilbert JJ, Perez-Roncero G. Cardiovascular risk in menopausal women and prevalent related co-morbid conditions: facing the post-women's health initiative era. Fertil Steril. 2009;92:1171-86.

13. Tchernof A, Desmeules A, Richard C, LaBerge P, Daris M, Mailloux J, et al. Ovarian hormone status and abdominal visceral adipose tissue metabolism. J Clin Endocrinol Metab. 2004;89:3425-30.

14. Saha KR, Rahman MM, Paul AR,Das S, Haque S, Jafrin W, et al. Changes in lipid profile of postmenopausal women. Mymensingh Med J. 2013;22(4):706-11.

15. International Diabetes Federation. The IDF consensus worldwide definition of the metabolic syndrome. Brussels: IDF.2005. Available:http://www.idf.org/webdata/docs/I DF Metasyndrome definition.pdf

16. Fabian UA, Charles-Davies MA, Adebusuyi JR, Ebesunun MO, Ajobo BM, Hassan OO, et al. Leptin Concentrations in African Blacks with Metabolic Syndrome and Type 2 diabetes Mellitus. Journal of the US-China Medical Science. 2011;8(8)493-500.

17. Umoh U, Charles-Davies MA, Adeleye J. Serum Testosterone and Lipids in Relation to Sexual Dysfunction in Males with Metabolic Syndrome and Type2 diabetes Mellitus. International Journal of Medicine and Medical Sciences. 2009;2(12):402-12.

18. Charles-Davies MA, Fasanmade AA, Olaniyi JA, Oyewole OE, Owolabi MO, Adebusuyi JR, et al. Metabolic alterations in different stages of hypertension in an apparently healthy Nigerian population. International Journal of Hypertension; 2013. Article ID 351357, 6 pages.

Available:http://dx.doi.org/10.1155/2013/35 1357

19. Moolman JA. Unravelling the cardio protective mechanism of action of estrogens. Cardiovasc Res. 2006;69:777-80.

20. Ogbera AO. Prevalence and gender distribution of the metabolic syndrome. Diabetol Metab Syndr. 2010;2:402-12.

21. Syed S, Hingorjo MR, Charania A. Qureshi MA. Anthropometric and metabolic indicators in hypertensive patients. J Coll Physicians Surg Pak. 2009;19(7):421-27.

22. Graff-Iversen S1, Thelle DS, Hammar N. Serum lipids, blood pressure and body weight around the age of the menopause. Eur J Cardiovasc Prev Rehabil. 2008;15(1):83-8.

23. Izumi Y1, Matsumoto K, Ozawa Y, Kasamaki Y, Shinndo A, Ohta M, et al. Effect of age at menopause on blood pressure in postmenopausal women. Am J Hypertens. 2007;20(10):1045-50.

24. Ciccone MM, Scicchitano P, Gesualdo M, Fornarelli F, Pinto V, Farinola G, et al.

Systemic vascular hemodynamic changes due to 17-β-estradiol intranasal administration. J Cardiovasc Pharmacol Ther. 2013;18(4):354-8.

25. Ciccone MM, Cortese F, Gesualdo M, Carbonara S, Zito A, Ricci G, et al. Dietary intake of Carotenoids and their antioxidant and anti- inflammatory effects in cardiovascular care. Mediators Inflamm; 2013; Article ID782137, 11 pages. Available:http://dx.doi.org/10.1155/2013/78 2137.Epub 2013 Dec 31.

26. Rahamon SA, Charles-Davies MA, Akinlade KS, Olaniyi JA, Fasanmade AA, Oyewole OE, et al. Impact of dietary intervention on selected biochemical indices of inflammation and oxidative stress in Nigerians with Metabolic Syndrome: A pilot study. European Journal of Nutrition & Food Safety. 2014;4(2):137-49.

27. Tsang S, Liu J, Ming Wong T. Testosterone and cardio protection against myocardial ischemia. Cardiovasc Hematol Disord Drug Targets. 2007;7(2):119-25.

4

Nstemi "But" Stemi-De Winters Sign

Prem Krishna Anandan[1*], **Subramanyam K**[1], **Shivananda Patil**[1], **R. Rangaraj**[1]
and **Cholenahally Nanjappa Manjunath**[1]

[1]*Department of cardiology, Sri Jayadeva Institute of Caridovascular Science & Research, Bengaluru, Karnataka, India.*

Authors' contributions

This work was carried out in collaboration between all authors. Author PKA designed the study, wrote the protocol, and wrote the first draft of the manuscript. Author RR managed the literature searches, analyses of the study. All authors read and approved the final manuscript.

<u>Editor(s):</u>
(1) Anonymous.
<u>Reviewers:</u>
(1) Alexander Berezin, Internal Medicine, Medical University, Zaporozhye, Ukraine.
(2) Pietro Scicchitano, Cardiology, University of Bari, Italy.

ABSTRACT

Anterior ST elevation myocardial infarction can present with a specific electrocardiographic (ECG) pattern without ST segment elevations, known as De Winter sign. Recognizing this ECG pattern is important since it is considered an equivalent to ST elevation myocardial infarction (STEMI), hence may require thrombolysis when primary PCI facilities are not available or delayed. We report a28 year old male who presented to us with de winters ecg pattern. Subsequent coronary angiogram showed Proxmial left anterior descending (LAD) artery occlusion.

Keywords: De winters sign; proximal left anterior descending artery; STEMI; STEMI equivalent.

1. INTRODUCTION

De winters sign on ECG is a specific pattern equivalent of an anterior STEMI, but presents like an NSTEMI. Approximately 2% of such patients have proximal LAD occlusion. Like wellness pattern recognizing this sign is of utmost importance since it should be managed like any STEMI.

2. CASE REPORT

A 28 year old male patient presented to our institute with typical angina since 2 hours

---

Corresponding author: E-mail: premkrishna2k1@gmail.com

duration. He had no significant past history of diabetes, hypertension, dyslipidemia nor any family history of coronary artery disease (CAD). The patient was a non smoker. Admission ECG [Figs. 1,2] showed up sloping ST depression with up Wright T waves in the anterior precordial leads, with 1mm ST elevation in lead aVR. Troponin T was within normal limits since the window period of presentation was early. His hemodynamics was stable. With a provitional diagnosis of acute coronary syndrome-Unstable angina/NSTEMI he was taken for primary percutaneous coronary intervention (PCI) immediately. Coronary angiogram [Fig. 3] showed 95% thrombus filled lesion in the Proxmial left anterior descending (LAD) artery. The patient underwent successful angioplasty [Fig.4] with a 4 x 25 mm second generation Drug eluting stent. Post procedure ecg showed a pattern of typical evolved anterior wall myocardial infarction [Fig. 5].

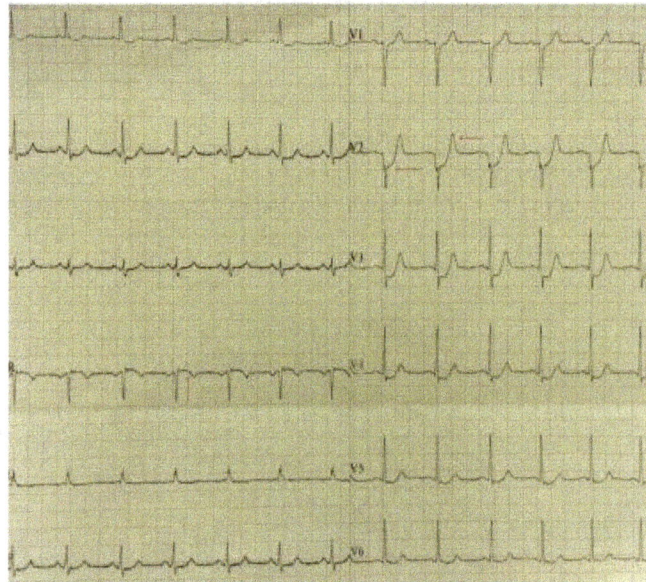

Fig. 1. ECG-upsloping ST depression with upwright T waves in the anterior precordial leads, with 1mm ST elevation in lead aVR

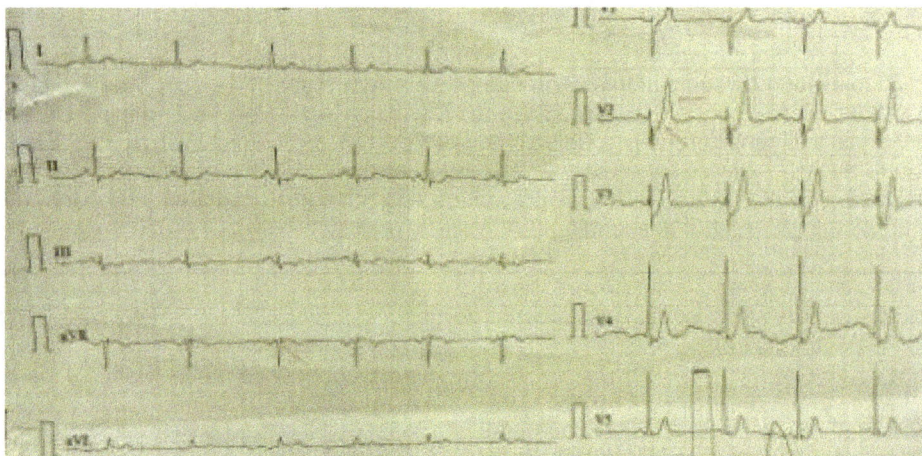

Fig. 2. Ecg 15 mins after admission showing classical de winters pattern

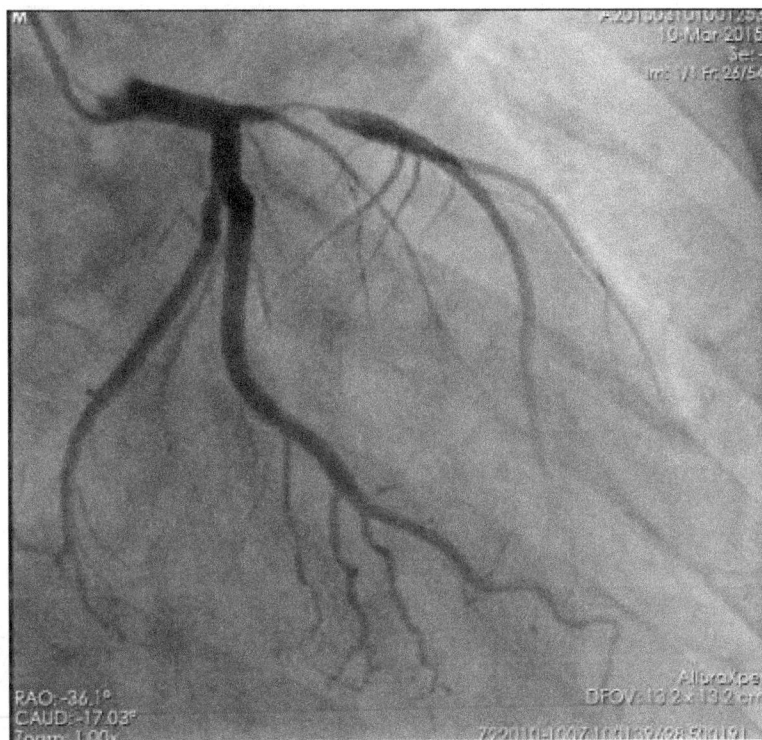

Fig. 3. Coronary angiogram showing proximal LAD lesion with thrombus

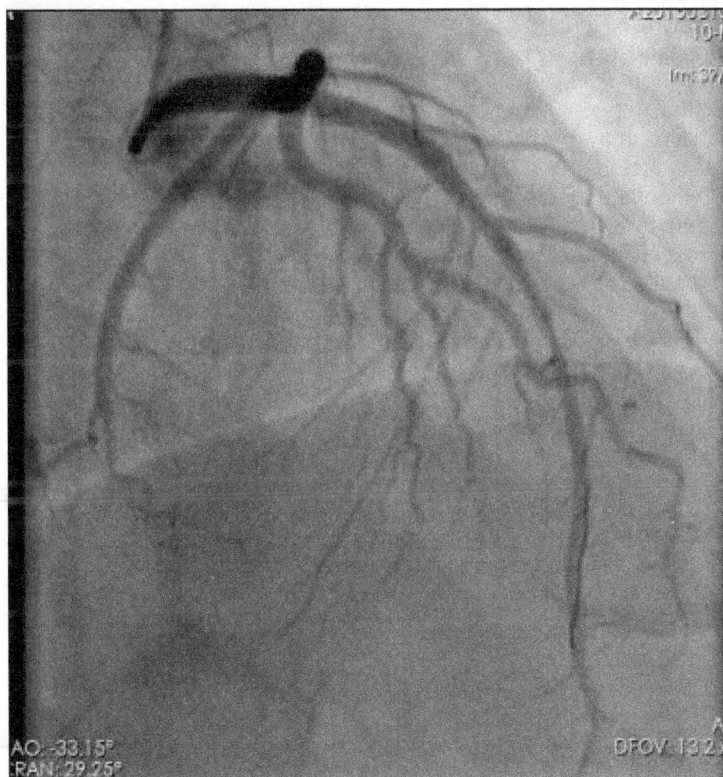

Fig. 4. Coronary angiogram post PTCA to LAD showing TIMI 3 flow

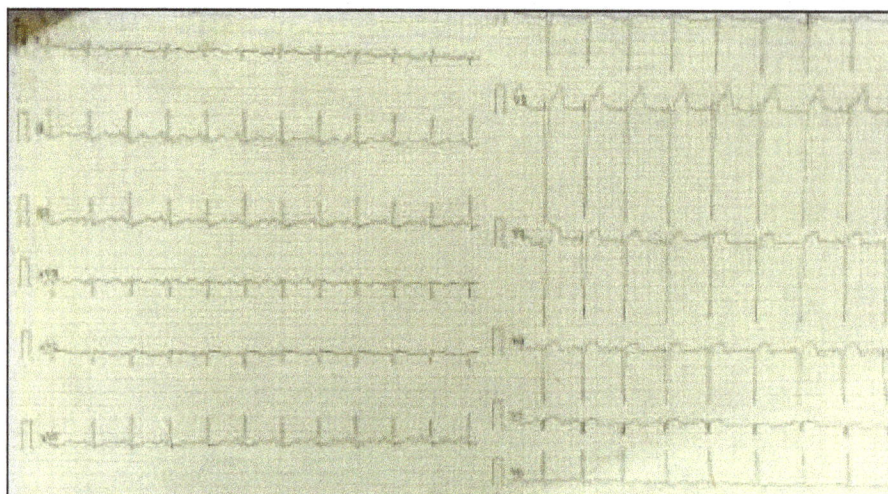

Fig. 5. Post PTCA ecg showing Evolved anterior wall MI changes

3. DISCUSSION

The de Winter ECG pattern is an equivalent of anterior STEMI. Recognizing it is clinically important since it presents without obvious ST segment elevation and may lead to under treatment [1]. ST depression and peaked T waves in the precordial leads is the usual presentation. Mechanism of these ecg changes that have been proposed are, theoretically, an anatomical variant of the Purkinje fibers, with endocardial conduction delay. Alternatively, the absence of ST elevation may be related to the lack of activation of sarcolemmal ATP sensitive potassium (KATP) channels by ischemic ATP depletion, as has been shown in KATP knockout animal models of acute ischemia [2]. This pattern is seen in ~2% of acute LAD occlusions. This was first reported by De Winter and Wellens, in 30 / 1532 patients with acute LAD occlusions [3]. Verounden et al. [4] also reported similar pattern in 35 / 1890 patients requiring PCI to the LAD. The profiles of such patients were usually younger males with a higher incidence of hypercholesterolemia compared to patients with a classic STEMI pattern. Knowledge about pattern of changes in an ECG that are associated with acute occlusion of a coronary artery helps us to plan an immediate invasive stratergy [5-7]. De Winter ECG pattern is highly predictive of acute LAD occlusion. Some consider it a "STEMI equivalent" similar to wellens pattern, ST elevation in lead aVR [8]. Prompt recognition is a must and such patients should receive emergent reperfusion therapy with PCI or thrombolysis.

Diagnostic Criteria for De winters sign:-

1) Tall, prominent, symmetric T waves in the precordial leads
2) Upsloping ST segment depression >1 mm at the J-point in the precordial leads
3) Absence of ST elevation in the precordial leads
4) ST segment elevation (0.5 mm-1 mm) in aVR
5) Normal STEMI morphology may precede or follow the deWinter pattern

4. CONCLUSION

Knowledge about this specific ecg pattern is important for physicians since it may be mistaken for NSTEMI and treatment with thrombolysis would be delayed or missed.

CONSENT

Informed and written consent was taken from the patient regarding this case report.

ETHICAL APPROVAL

It is not applicable.

COMPETING INTERESTS

Authors have declared that no competing interests exist.

REFERENCES

1. Goebel M, Bledsoe J, Orford JL, Mattu A, Brady WJ. A new ST-segment elevation myocardial infarction equivalent pattern? Prominent T wave and J-point depression in the precordial leads associated with ST-segment elevation in lead aVr. Am J Emerg Med. 2014;32(3):287.

2. Li RA, Leppo M, Miki T, Seino S, Marban E. Molecular basisof electrocardiographic ST-segment elevation. Circ Res. 2000;87:837-9.

3. de Winter R, Verouden N, Wellens H, Wilde A. A new ECG sign of proximal LAD occlusion. N Engl J Med. 2008;359:2071–3.

4. Verouden NJ, Koch KT, Peters RJ, et al. Persistent precordial "hyperacute" T-waves signify proximal left anterior descending artery occlusion. Heart. 2009;95:1701–6.

5. Engelen DJ, Gorgels AP, Cheriex EC, et al. Value of the electrocardiogram in localizing the occlusion site in the left anterior descending coronary artery in acute anterior myocardial infarction. J Am Coll Cardiol. 1999;34:389-95.

6. Zimetbaum PJ, Josephson ME. Use of the electrocardiogram in acute myocardial infarction. N Engl J Med. 2003;348:933-40.

7. Wang K, Asinger RW, Marriott HJ. ST-segment elevation in conditions other than acute myocardial infarction. N Engl J Med. 2003;349:2128-35.

8. Yan AT, Yan RT, Kennelly BM, Anderson FA Jr, Budaj A, et al. Relationship of ST elevation in lead aVR with angiographic findings and outcome in non–ST elevation acute coronary syndromes. Am Heart J. 2007;154(1):71-8.

5

Polyarteritis Nodosa in Infancy – Generalized Vascular Problem Diagnosed after Initial Cardiac Manifestation in Emergency Cardiovascular Catheterization

Ireneusz Haponiuk[1,2*], Maciej Chojnicki[1], Konrad Paczkowski[1], Radosław Jaworski[1], Mariusz Steffens[1] and Katarzyna Gierat-Haponiuk[3]

[1]Department of Pediatric Cardiac Surgery, Mikolaj Kopernik Hospital in Gdańsk, Poland.
[2]Department of Physiotherapy, Gdańsk University of Physical Education and Sport, Poland.
[3]Department of Rehabilitation, Medical University of Gdańsk, Poland.

Authors' contributions

This work was carried out in collaboration between all authors. All authors read and approved the final manuscript.

Editor(s):
(1) Francesco Pelliccia, Department of Heart and Great Vessels University La Sapienza, Rome, Italy.
Reviewers:
(1) Paul Schoenhagen, Cleveland Clinic Foundation, Ohio, USA.
(2) Kim Hyun Jung, Eulji University Hospital, South Korea.

ABSTRACT

Aim: Coronary artery diseases in children are uncommon, but in selected cases general vascular problems also affect the heart.

Case: We present the case of 4-month old girl admitted to Pediatric Intensive Care Unit after the incident of cardiac arrest and ventricular tachycardia, who underwent diagnostic catheterization due to cardiac ischemia. Coronary angiography showed changes in coronary arteries in the form of disseminated aneurysms, mixed with severely stenosed segments. General angiography discovered also changes in the number of peripheral arteries, with the most significant right subclavian and left iliac artery aneurysms.

Results: Upon angiographic images and a history of untreated infection, polyarteritis nodosa (PAN) was diagnosed, with an appropriate administration of intensive treatment.

Corresponding author: E-mail: konradpaczkowski@gmail.com

> **Conclusion:** The case prove the significance of invasive cardiovascular diagnostics (cardiac catheterization) in every unclear clinical course.

Keywords: Cardiovascular imaging; emergency; interventional cardiology.

1. INTRODUCTION

An isolated coronary artery disease in children is uncommon and its essential reason is usually congenital or infectious. As well as there is lack of typical atherosclerotic injury. In selected cases generalized vascular non-cardiac problems in childhood affect also the heart. The diagnosis of general vascular disorder with cardiac manifestation is more difficult if the symptoms appear in a small child in life-threatening condition. Initial sequelae of various forms of coronary insufficiency and severe heart dysfunction usually accompany different disorders that easily lead to cardiorespiratory insufficiency in small babies.

In critical condition routinely performed noninvasive emergency diagnostics remains unclear, especially in patients without previous cardiovascular problems and comorbidities. The differential diagnostics in children suffering from coronary circulation emergencies should consider anomalous origin of left coronary artery from pulmonary artery (ALCAPA), Kawasaki disease (KD), polyarteritis nodosa (PAN) and nonspecific organ vascular reactions [1]. An adequate diagnosis is important because of the need to prevent small babies from the most dangerous severe arrhythmias that can cause sudden cardiopulmonary arrest.

In unclear clinical course of severely ill babies nothing but an aggressive diagnostics path including coronary and peripheral angiography could provide an appropriate diagnosis, and become respective treatment on immediately. Here we present the case of an infant after the incident of cardiac arrest and ventricular tachycardia, who underwent an emergency diagnostic catheterization due to cardiac ischemia.

2. PRESENTATION OF THE CASE

We present the case of 4-month-old girl admitted to pediatric intensive care after the incident of cardiac arrest and ventricular tachycardia.

The indications for emergency angiography were established after meticulous analysis of risk-to-benefit ratio. Finally, despite the risk of invasive catheterization in decompensated child, the baby was referred to cardiac catheterization. Initial transthoracic echocardiography (TTE) performed on admission showed significant akinesia of the apex, lateral wall of the left ventricle (LV) and interventricular septum, with dilated LV (Fig. 1 D). There were no alarming patterns of coronary or pulmonary fistula, the heart muscle showed no signs of non-compaction. Coronary angiography showed changes in coronary arteries in the form of disseminated aneurysms, mixed with severely stenosed segments (Fig. 1 A). Simultaneously performed general angiography discovered also the injuries in the number of peripheral arteries, with the most significant right subclavian and left iliac artery aneurysms. The aorta showed no angiographic thickening or stenosis, while there were findings of vasculitis-related changes in aortic arch branches, significantly present in cervical, subclavian and brain arteries (Fig. 1 B). Thoracic descending and abdominal aorta were affected with visceral, renal and the most evident left common iliac aneurysms (Fig. 1 C). Finally upon her angiographic images and a history of untreated infection, the PAN was diagnosed. Intensive treatment was administrated immediately.

3. DISCUSSION

Although polyarteritis nodosa still remains rare disease in childhood, diagnosis of this disease should be kept in mind, especially in infancy. There is no single pattern of clinical presentation of PAN, but abdominal pain, central or peripheral nervous system disease, arthritis, myalgia and skin lesions occur during the course of the illness. The symptoms listed above remain unspecific, thus an advanced diagnostics is necessary to establish the correct diagnosis and appropriate treatment.

Angiographic view of polyarteritis nodosa mainly affects the bifurcation areas of medium-sized muscular arteries and intravisceral small arteries of the testis, spermatic cord, nerves, muscles, skin, kidneys, gastrointestinal tract and joints [2]. Disseminated vascular disease cause severe clinical manifestations with life-threatening conditions in groups of every age, including

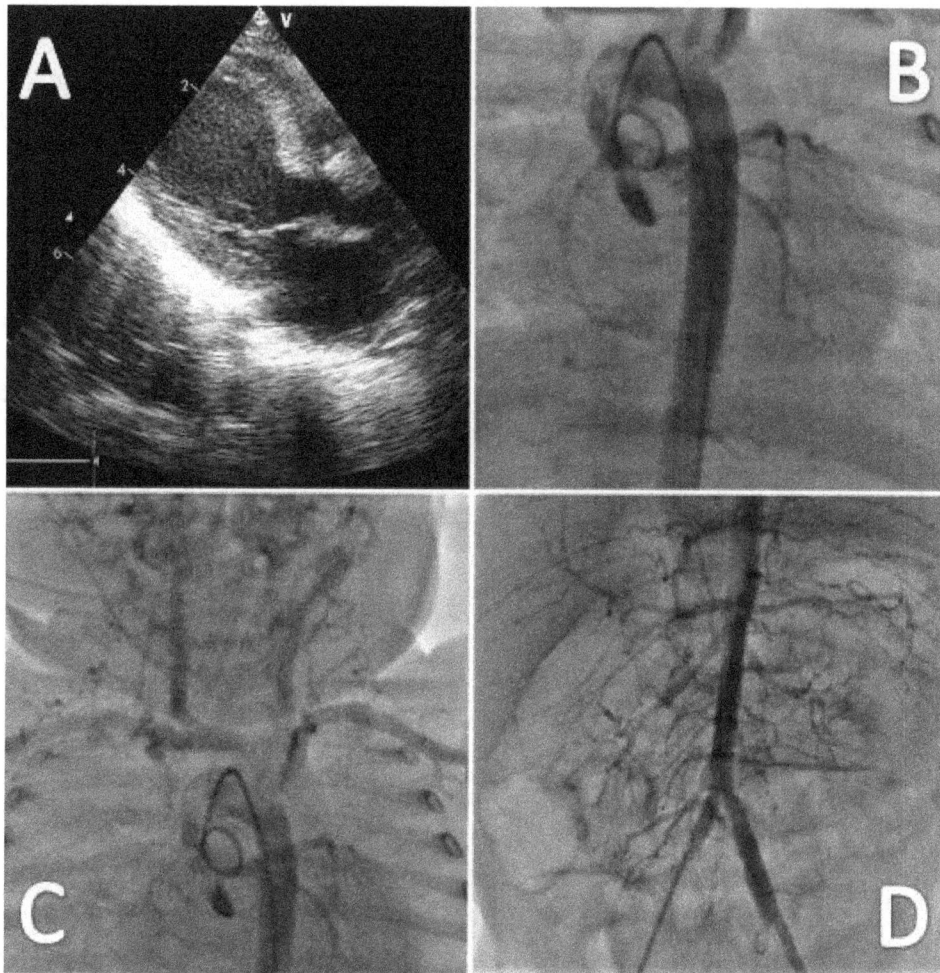

Fig. 1. 1 A – Dilated, sphere shaped left ventricle, 1 B – Dilatation of left main and circumflex coronary arteries, 1 C - Right subclavian artery aneurysm, 1 D – Left common iliac artery aneurysm

infants [1]. The clinical course of PAN with initial critical cardiac and respiratory insufficiency is uncommon. Nevertheless in small babies, like in the presented case, life-threatening cardiopulmonary emergencies could be caused by various reasons, including PAN.

The diagnosis of PAN is based on central and peripheral cardiovascular catheterization. Following the 2012 Revised International Chapel Hill Consensus Conference Nomenclature of Vasculitides (CHCC) classifies vasculitides into three types primarily according to the predominant type of vessel involved: large vessel vasculitis, medium vessel vasculitis, and small vessel vasculitis [3]. Large vessels are defined as the aorta and its major branches. Medium vessels include major extravisceral arteries and their branches. Small vessels include

intravisceral arteries, arterioles, capillaries, venules and veins [2].

We finally diagnosed three above mentioned CHCC vasculitis types in the presented infant girl suffering from PAN, nevertheless in differential diagnostics KD was considered as well. In our infant peripheral vessels affected in the pathology were relatively smaller in caliber than those usually observed in KD, although we keep in mind that these two conditions can overlap [4,5].

Following our patient's history we highly appreciate contemporary technical advances in emergency cardiovascular imaging, what enabled complete diagnosis. That had utmost importance for the child in her real critical condition. In summary we carefully considered well-defined risk of infant emergency cardiac catheterization procedures, although taking into consideration the potential to establish life-saving final diagnosis we became convinced to follow our strategy in forthcoming cases.

4. CONCLUSIONS

The images obtained while emergency catheterization of an infant after cardiac arrest enabled an appropriate diagnosis and effective treatment with no wasted time, thus the case prove the significance of invasive cardiovascular diagnostics in every unclear clinical course.

CONSENT

All authors declare that written informed consent was obtained from the patient for publication of this case report and accompanying images.

ETHICAL APPROVAL

It is not applicable.

COMPETING INTERESTS

Authors have declared that no competing interests exist.

REFERENCES

1. Shields LBE, Burge M, Hunsaker III JC. Sudden death due to polyarteritis nodosa. Forensic Sci Med Pathol. 2012;8(3):290-5.

2. Takahashi S, Takada A, Saito K, Hara M, Yoneyama K, Nakanishi H, Takahashi K, Moriya T, Funayama M: Sudden death of a child from myocardial infarction due to arteritis of the left coronary trunk. Legal Medicine. 2015;17(1):39-42.

3. Jennette JC, Falk RJ, Bacon PA, Basu N, Cid MC, Ferrario F, et al. 2012 revised international Chapel Hill consensus conference nomenclature of vasculitides. Arthritis Rheum. 2013;65(1):1-11.

4. Senzaki H. Long-term outcome of Kawasaki disease. Circulation. 2008; 118(25):2763-72.

5. Obersztyn A, Baranowska A, Rycaj J, Haponiuk I, Banaszak P, Kocyba-Mateja K, Szkutnik M. Changes in the coronary arteries during early and long-term follow-up of Kawasaki syndrome: a single centre experience. Folia Cardiologica. 2006;13: 584-590.

6

Treatment of ST Elevation Myocardial Infarction from Fibrinolysis to Primary PCI: In Terms of Risks and Benefits

Hadi A. R. Hadi Khafaji[1*] and Jassim M. Al-Suwaidi[2]

[1]*Department of Cardiology, Saint Michael's Hospital, Toronto University, Canada.*
[2]*Qatar Cardiovascular Research Center and Adult Cardiology, Heart Hospital, Hamad Medical Corporation, Doha, Qatar.*

Authors' contributions

This work was carried out in collaboration between all authors. Author HARK managed the literature searches designed the study, wrote the manuscript, and wrote the first draft of the manuscript. Author JAIS assisted in literature searches and in writing the manuscript. All authors read and approved the final manuscript.

Editor(s):
(1) Francesco Pelliccia, Department of Heart and Great Vessels University La Sapienza, Rome, Italy.
(2) Anonymous Editor.
Reviewers:
(1) Anonymous, Laval University, Canada.
(2) Ana Christina Vellozo Caluza, Cardiology Department, UNIFESP-Federal University of Sao Paulo - Brazil.
(3) Anonymous, Venezuelan Institute for Scientific Research, Venezuela.
(4) Anonymous, Ankara Numune Research and Education Hospital, Turkey.
(5) Anonymous, Prince Sultan Cardiac Center, Saudi Arabia.
(6) Anonymous, Pernambuco University, Brazil.
(7) Pedro Beraldo de Andrade, Invasive Cardiology, Santa Casa de Marília and Faculdade de Medicina de Marília, São Paulo, Brazil.

ABSTRACT

The treatment of ST elevation myocardial infarction (STEMI) has undergone significant advances over the past three decades. Current practice guidelines raise the importance of promptly restoring normal coronary blood flow and myocardial perfusion in the infarct zone after the onset of chest pain, through either pharmacologic or mechanical reperfusion strategies.
Fibrinolytic therapy remains the most widely used reperfusion strategy worldwide. With the development of newer fibrinolytic agents and adjuvant potent anti-platelets therapies, this approach carries an increased risk of bleeding complications. The current research present up-date review of

*Corresponding author: E-mail: hadi968@hotmail.com

the use of reperfusion strategies for the treatment of STEMI, using data through the search of MEDLINE, PubMed, EMBASE, as well as related extracts from the annual report of the American Heart Association, the American College of Cardiology, and the European Society of Cardiology. We summarized data from the available studies conducted over the past last 30 years in relation to pharmacologic reperfusion therapy in regards to risks and benefits.

Conclusion: Fibrinolytic therapy remains the main reperfusion strategy used for the treatment of STMI worldwide. In the current era, there is a lack of fibrinolytic therapy trials, mainly because of increased focus in mechanical reperfusion therapies' studies in the developed world. Clinical trials on the use of the fibrinolytics with newer platelet agents are urgently needed.

Keywords: Fibrinolytic agents; streptokinase; retaplase; alteplase; tenecteplase; acute myocardial infarction; patency rate; bleeding; intracranial hemorrhage.

ABBREVIATIONS

SK; streptokinase, t-PA; Alteplase, r-PA; Reteplase, AMI: Acute Myocardial infarction, iv.Intravenous, sc.; subcutaneous, CHF: Congestive heart failure, STEMI; ST elevation Myocardial infarction, (GISSI-1) trail: Gruppo Italiano per lo Studio Streptokinasi nell'Infarto Miocardico trail, ISAM study: The Intravenous Streptokinase in Acute Myocardial infarction study, ISIS trail: Second International Study of Infarct Survival trail. EMERAS: Estudio Multicentrico Estreptoquinasa Republicas de America del Sur, GUSTO: Global Use of Strategies to Open Occluded Coronary Arteries, PRIMI Trial: Randomised double-blind trial of recombinant pro-urokinase against streptokinase in acute myocardial infarction trial, TIMI trail; Thrombolysis in Myocardial infarction trail, PAIMS: Plasminogen Activator Italian Multicenter Study, COBALT: comparison of continuous infusion of alteplase with double-bolus administration for acute myocardial infarction, INJECTtrial: International Joint Efficacy Comparison of Thrombolytics trial, COBALT: Continuous Infusion versus Double-Bolus Administration of Alteplase, RAPID: More rapid, complete, and stable coronary thrombolysis with bolus administration of reteplase compared with alteplase infusion in acute myocardial infarction, RAPID-2: Randomized Comparison Of Coronary Thrombolysis Achieved With Double-Bolus Reteplase And Front-Loaded, Accelerated Alteplase, ASSENT-1; The Assessment of the Safety and Efficacy of a New Thrombolytic Agent, ENTIRE-TIMI 23: Enoxaparin as Adjunctive Anti-thrombin Therapy for ST-Elevation Myocardial Infarction, INTEGRITI: integrilin and tenecteplase in acute myocardial infarction, EXTRACT-TIMI 25 trial: Enoxaparin versus Unfractionated Heparin with Fibrinolysis for ST-Elevation Myocardial Infarction, CAPITAL AMI: Combined angioplasty and pharmacological intervention versus thrombolysis alone in acute myocardial infarction, WEST: Which Early ST-elevation myocardial infarction Therapy study, GRACIA-2: Groupo de Análisis de Cardiopatía Isquémica Aguda) Investigators, SESAM Study; the Study in Europe with Saruplase and Alteplase in Myocardial Infarction, COMASS trial: Comparison Trial of Saruplase and Streptokinase trial, GREAT trial: Grampian Region Early Anistreplase Trial, CLARITY trial: Addition of clopidogrel to aspirin and fibrinolytic therapy for myocardial infarction with ST-segment elevation, COMMIT study: ClOpidogrel and Metoprolol in Myocardial Infarction Trial, PLATO study; The Study of Platelet Inhibition and Patient Outcomes, SPEED study: Patency Enhancement in the Emergency Department study, PARADIGM trial: Platelet Aggregation Receptor Antagonist Dose Investigation and Reperfusion Gain in Myocardial Infarction trail, IMPACT-AMI: Combined accelerated tissue-plasminogen activator and platelet glycoprotein IIb/IIIa integrin receptor blockade with integrilin in acute myocardial infarction, INTRO AMI trial: Integrilin and Low-Dose Thrombolysis in Myocardial Infarction trial; INTEGRITI trial: Integrilin and Tenecteplase in Acute Myocardial Infarction, HART II: second trial of Heparin and Aspirin Reperfusion Therapy, BIOMACS II: biochemical markers in acute coronary syndromes, OASIS-6: trial: Organization for the Assessment of Strategies for Ischemic Syndromes 6, FRAMI trial: Fragmin in Acute Myocardial Infarction, HIT-III study: the Hirudin for the Improvement of Thrombolysis-3 trial, HERO trial: Hirulog Early Reperfusion/ Occlusion.

1. INTRODUCTION

Thrombolytic (fibrinolytic) therapy is a major advance in the management of AMI; it acts by lysing thrombi and attaining reperfusion therapy, reducing infarct size, upholding left ventricular function, and improving survival. Several techniques and regimens are used in which reperfusion rates increase and accordingly result in improvement of clinical outcome. These techniques include the followings; different dosing regimens of established agents; combinations of different agents; use with adjunctive agents such as direct anti-thrombin (AT) agents, low-molecular-weight heparin (LMWH), or glycoprotein IIb/IIIa receptor antagonists and the development of novel thrombolytic agents with enhanced fibrin specificity, resistance to native inhibitors, or prolonged half-lives permitting bolus administration. The term thrombolytic agent is ambiguous when applied to plasminogen activators (convert plasminogen to plasmin) that degrades fibrin, a major structural component of the thrombus and hence; the more correct term is *fibrinolytic therapy*. The field of thrombo-cardiology deals with the frail equilibrium between thrombotic complications and bleeding risk which is an important part of clinical cardiology [1-4].

We identified studies via MEDLINE, PubMed, EMBASE, and Current Contents searches and by reviewing reference lists. Pertinent abstracts from the annual meetings of the American Heart Association, the American College of Cardiology, and the European Society of Cardiology were reviewed. We selected for review studies that evaluated the pharmacokinetics and pharmacodynamics of the various fibrinolytic agents including streptokinase, alteplase, reteplase and tenecteplase, and assessed the effects of these fibrinolytic drugs in clinical and angiographic perspective in terms of benefits, risks and long-term clinical outcomes. We also reviewed publications of observational studies of fibrinolytic therapy use among AMI patients in registries from around the world. The current review summarizes the findings from studies published over the last 30 years in this field. Studies are categorized into two subgroups; clinical or angiographic studies.

2. HISTORICAL BACKGROUND OF FIBRINOLYSIS

Fletcher and colleagues in 1958 were the first to report the use of fibrinolytic therapy in patients with AMI [5]. Early in the 1960s and 70s up to 24 trials evaluated the efficacy of intravenous streptokinase [6], but without established theoretical basis for the administration of thrombolytic therapy, together with the lack of evidence of efficacy in a single trial, led to the desertion of further investigation into this mode of treatment. In 1969, Chazov was the first who administered intracoronary streptokinase in Russia and it is now nearly 35 years since Rentrop et al. [7,8] reported its use, thereby invigorating interest in reperfusion as a treatment modality for the management of AMI. Since then, several newer fibrinolytic agents were developed, including tissue plasminogen activators, TPA (alteplase or reteplase). Furthermore, the development in fibrinolytic agents was accompanied by significant advances in adjunctive therapies including antiplatelet agents as well as the emergence of newer antithrombotic regimens, which are outlined in the current review.

3. CLINICAL TRIALS

3.1 Streptokinase (SK) (Table1)

In 1958, SK was first used in AMI patients, which has revolted the treatment of AMI. SK had not been exposed to a true form of dose ranging angiographic trial only until 1980s [9]. Nevertheless, the placebo-controlled trials of this agent were very influential in terms of significant mortality reduction with intravenous SK for AMI. Several trials [10-27] have reported patency of the infarct related artery (IRA) at different time points among patients not receiving fibrinolytic therapy. Most patients did receive aspirin and heparin, although aspirin was not standard therapy for AMI until the International Study of Infarct Survival *(ISIS)-2* trial [28] results in 1988. Several angiographic trials also were done to discover the patency and recanalization rates with intravenous SK.

The efficacy of SK with regard to mortality reduction was evaluated in 4 large, placebo-controlled trials (Table 1) [28-31]. The first true mortality trial for SK [the *Gruppo Italiano per lo Studio Streptokinasi nell'Infarto Miocardico (GISSI-1)* trial]; an open label, randomized trial of 11,806 patients. In this trial 14% of patients received aspirin and only 62% received any heparin (adjunctive therapies were at the investigator's discretion). SK use resulted in 18% reduction in-hospital mortality compared with standard therapy. This benefit was time dependent, mortality reduction decreasing from a 47% reduction in patients treated within 1 h, to 23% for those treated within 3 h, and to 17% for those treated within 6 h of symptom's onset. The reduction in mortality was maintained at 12 months (17.2% with SK vs. 19.0% for control subjects; p=0.008). SK treatment was comparable to placebo in regards to the rate of intra-cranial hemorrhage (ICH) and other major bleeding complications (Table1) [29].

The Intravenous Streptokinase in Acute Myocardial infarction study (ISAM) [30]: a double blind randomized trial of SK vs. placebo in 1,741 patients with ST elevation AMI (STEMI), there was 11% reduction in 21-day mortality, although not of statistical significance, but in harmony with the GISSI-1 conclusions. Significantly more bleeding is seen in SK group vs. placebo group (p=0.0001) (Table1); cerebral hemorrhage occurred in 4 patients in the SK group resulting in 2 deaths. Brady and tachy-arrhythmias occurred more frequently in patient treated with SK.

The 2nd ISIS trial; a large double blind placebo-controlled study of IV SK in patients with suspected MI, (17,187 patients enrolled up to 24 h of symptoms' onset, but the majority were enrolled within 12 h of symptoms' onset) in 417 hospitals worldwide. The study's aim was testing aspirin alone (162.5 mg/d for 1 month), SK alone (1.5 MU. 1 h), both, or neither; SK resulted in a 25% reduction in 35-day vascular mortality vs. placebo. Aspirin alone resulted in relative mortality reduction by 23%. Combination of SK and aspirin significantly reduced re-infarctions, strokes and deaths. The differences in vascular and in all-cause mortality produced by SK and by aspirin remained highly significant after 15 months of follow-up. Aspirin also reduced re-infarction rates, cardiac arrest, rupture and stroke. Again, as in GISSI-1 trail, the benefit was is time dependent; treatment within 6 h of symptoms resulted in improved survival and this benefit persisted for treatment within up to 12 h after symptom's onset. SK resulted in excess bleeding requiring transfusion and of confirmed ICH, but with fewer other strokes. Aspirin did not result in increased risk of ICH or in bleeding requiring transfusion. An excess of non-fatal re-infarction was observed in the SK only group [28].

A smaller, South American trial (Estudio Multicentrico Estreptoquinasa Republicas de America del Sur); a double-blind, placebo-controlled trial of SK strictly which included patients presenting at least 6 h after but within 24 h of symptom's onset. The 35 days mortality did not differ significantly in the 3,568 studied patients, a conclusion was contradictory with the other 3 major trials (Table 1) [31].

A clear conclusion can be drawn from all the above trials in terms of the benefits; treatment value witnessed in the first 21 - 42 days was maintained up to 1 year. The overall benefit was perceived among patients with ST-segment elevation or bundle-branch block regardless of age, sex, blood pressure, heart rate, prior MI, or diabetic status. Into the bargain; the earlier treatment commenced the greater benefit. In the term of risks: SK therapy was associated with about 4/1000 extra strokes occurred within 2 days. Approximately 50% were associated with an early death, accounted for in the overall mortality reduction, 25% are moderately to severely disabled and the other 25% were not [32].

3.2 Alteplase (t-PA) Table (2)

Alteplase (t-PA), historically was the second fibrinolytic agent studied after SK in many trials. The accelerated infusion of t-PA for AMI (most common used protocol in AMI) is 15 mg IV bolus, followed by 0.75 mg/kg (up to 50 mg) IV/30 minutes, then 0.5 mg/kg (up to 35 mg) IV/60 minutes. The maximum total dose is 100 mg for patients weighing >67 kg.

The hypothesis of early reperfusion improves survival was strongly supported by the results of GUSTO-1 trial (41,021 AMI patients) with 30-day mortality as primary end point [33,34]. It involved 4 groups; the reference two groups both used SK, one with subcutaneous heparin and one with IV heparin. Third arm used front-loaded t-PA and IV heparin. The fourth arm: used combination fibrinolytic therapy, which involved about 2/3 of the typical doses of t-PA and SK with IV heparin. All patients received aspirin, 325 mg/d. There was significant reduction in 30 days mortality rate in the accelerated t-PA arm when compared with each of the 3 other groups. The mortality improvement was evident as early as 24 h after treatment was initiated; with t-PA treated patients having a significantly lower mortality rate, cardiogenic shock, CHF and ventricular arrhythmias [33]. Overall thrombolysis resulted in 25% relative (2% absolute) improvement in mortality rates compared with placebo. Accelerated t-PA benefit was seen in almost every subgroup: patients with anterior or inferior

MI, in all age groups. The absolute benefit was greater in higher-risk patients ICH occurred only rarely in GUSTO-1 despite the aggressive regimens of thrombolysis, aspirin, and heparin. For each of the SK arms, ICH occurred in 0.5% compared with 0.7% of patients treated with accelerated t-PA and 0.9% of patients treated with combination fibrinolytics [33].

The *TIMI-4 trial*; a double-blind trial comparing accelerated t-PA, anistreplase and their combinations, in addition to aspirin and IV heparin.60 minutes patency rate was seen in 78% with accelerated t-PA vs. 60% for anistreplase or combination fibrinolytics [35]. At 90 min, patency and TIMI grade 3 flow rates significantly better in the accelerated t-PA arm. Superior overall clinical outcomes and 1-year survival was observed with t-PA. This result was consistent with that of the GUSTO-1 trial. The *GISSI-2* and *ISIS-3* trials used the slower infusion of t-PA or duteplase and delayed sc. heparin, which did not elevate the APTT level until approximately 24 h after the start of treatment during which re-occlusion of IRA frequently occurred resulting in 3 folds higher mortality. The benefits of accelerated t-PA seen in the GUSTO-1 and TIMI-4 trials compared to the lack of benefit seen in GISSI-2 and ISIS-3 in a pooled analysis of coronary arterial patency and LV function after IV thrombolysis for AMI can be explained by the t-PA regimen used and heparin dosing. GUSTO-1 and TIMI-4 used the accelerated t-PA regimen, which begets higher rates of IRA patency and early IV heparin use enhanced late IRA patency. This link between early reperfusion i.e. TIMI grade 3 flow and improved survival was established in the GUSTO-1 angiographic sub study [27,36-39].

The attentiveness of a double bolus regimen of t-PA was derived from a series of patients to whom two 50-mg boluses of t-PA were given 30 min apart which achieved TIMI grade 3 flow in 88% of patients. [40]. *COBALT trial* (7169 patients) compared double-bolus vs. accelerated t-PA. This study was terminated early with the concern about the safety of the double-bolus regimen. 30-day mortality rates tended to be higher in the double-bolus group than in the accelerated-infusion group. The rates of hemorrhagic stroke = 1.12% after double-bolus t-PA vs. 0.81% after accelerated infusion of t-PA [41] in a later randomized trial, however, double-bolus t-PA resulted in TIMI grade 3 flow in only 58% of patients compared with a 66% rate in patients treated with the accelerated 90-min

infusion of t-PA [42]. Other studies in the term of the risks and benefits are summarized in Table 2.

3.3 Reteplase (r-PA)

The r-PA was one of the first mutant t-PA molecules which had undergone extensive clinical testing with best therapeutic efficacy resulted when r-PA was divided into two boluses (10 U/10 U) given 30 min apart (Table 3) [43].

The *INJECT* study compared the use of double-bolus r-PA to SK (Table 3). 35-day mortality rate with r-PA = 9% vs. 9.5% with SK. In-hospital stroke rates were 1.23% for r-PA vs. 1% for SK, with similar bleeding rates in the both groups (0.7% 1.0% respectively) and similar incidence of recurrent MI, but significantly fewer cases of atrial fibrillation, asystole, cardiac shock, heart failure and hypotension in the r-PA group. The study suggested that r-PA was at least equivalent to SK [44].

The *GUSTO-3 study*: a superiority trial, (15,059AMI patients within 6 h of symptom's onset), compared double-bolus r-PA with accelerated t-PA and tested whether the reported 16% increase in TIMI grade 3 flow with r-PA compared with t-PA would result into improved 30-day mortality, primary end point of 30-day mortality rates reached in 7.47% of r-PA vs. 7.24% of t-PA. The 95% CI for the absolute mortality difference of 0.23% ranged from 1.11% in favor of t-PA to 0.66% in favor of r-PA. The mortality rates were comparable when patients were sorted into subgroups by; age, infarct location, and enrolling region. There was an interaction between symptom duration and outcomes with r-PA vs. t-PA with borderline significance (p= 0.05). No significant difference in the rates of stroke, bleeding, and ICH [45].

3.4 Clinical (Mortality) Trials with Tenecteplase (TNKase) (Table 4)

TNKase: A highly fibrin specific. The TNKase conformational change reduces its elimination and prolongs its plasma half-life. Nitrates do not appear to affect TNKase levels, additionally, it is less to inhibit PAI-1 by 80 times, with more intense antiplatelet properties both in vitro and in vivo compared with those of t-PA. In experimental models the thrombolytic potency of TNKase is 3-fold higher than that of t-PA [46-49].

Several trails have evaluated TNKase for the treatment of STEMI (Table 4). *TIMI-10A trial*: 113 patients presenting within 12 hours treated with a single bolus of TNK-TPA over 5 to 10 seconds with doses ranging from 5 to 50 mg. TIMI grade 3 flow at 90 minutes in the IRA appeared to be higher with the 30- to 50-mg doses compared to lower doses with a 30 days mortality of 3.5%. Patency (TIMI grade II-III flow) of the IRA was seen 85%in overall with no differ across the full range of doses tested. Serious bleeding occurred in 6.2% at the vascular access sites. No strokes or ICH reported. Re-infarction spotted in 4.4% of patients, pulmonary edema in 2.7%. No immune reaction to TNK-TPA detected t at 30 days (Table 4) [50].

The *TIMI 10B*, 886 patients presented within 12 hours of symptoms' onset were randomized to receive either a single bolus of 30 or 50 mg TNK-t-PA or front-loaded t-PA and underwent immediate coronary angiograph, both agents result in similar TIMI grade 3 flow rates at 90 minutes (62.8% vs. 62.7%, respectively, P=NS); with lower rate for the 30-mg dose (54.3% vs. 65.8%) for the 50-mg dose. A pre-specified analysis of weight-based TNK-t-PA dosing using median TIMI frame count demonstrated a dose response (P=0.001). *In terms of risk*; dose responses for serious bleeding and ICH has been reported, but significantly lower rates were observed for both TNK-t-PA and t-PA after the heparin doses were lowered and titration of the heparin was started at 6 hours in this trial. The 50-mg dose discontinued early because of ICH and replaced by a 40-mg dose, with lower heparin doses (Table 4) [51].

In the *ASSENT-1 trial*:safety assessment was made of 3235 patients receiving either 30 or 40 or 50 mg TNKase as a bolus injection or front-loaded t-PA. At 30 days: total stroke rate =1.5% and ICH rate = 0.8% reported without significant differences between groups. Serious bleeding, requiring transfusion, occurred in 1.4% in the TNKase group vs. 7% with front-loaded t-PA [52]. Importantly, TIMI-10B and ASSENT-1 displayed the magnitude of reducing the heparin dose in conjunction with TNKase to lessen ICH risk [53].

In *ASSENT-2 trial*, an equivalence trial (16,949 patients presented within 6 hours of symptoms' onset) received either weight-adjusted TNKase over 5 to 10 seconds or front-loaded t-PA, in addition to aspirin and reduced-dose UFH with the primary end points of all-cause mortality at 30 days. No difference in mortality (6.18% vs.

6.15%) and stroke rates, including ICH was observed. Moreover, the TNKase group had fewer rates of non-cerebral bleeding major bleeding (4.68% vs. 5.94%, p = 0.0002) and blood transfusion. Female above 75 years who weighed <67 kg had less ICH. ASSENT-2 trial's results confirmed the benefits in all major subgroups regardless of age, gender, infarct location, Killip class or diabetes status. TNKase reduced the rate of CHF. In summary, ASSENT-2 trial indicated that single-bolus TNKase is equivalent to the more complex accelerated t-PA infusion, in terms of mortality and mortality/stroke combination, with decreased major bleeding rate. Such results persist after 1 year [54-56].

In the *ASSENT-3 trial*, anefficacy plus safety trial (6095 STEMI patients) treated with full-dose TNKase + UFH, full-dose TNKase + enoxaparin, or half-dose TNKase + UFH and the GPIIb-IIIa inhibitor abciximab. The study also compared enoxaparin with UFH; the primary end-point (30-day mortality plus in-hospital re-infarction and in-hospital refractory ischemia) was reduced by enoxaparin and by the combination of UFH + abciximab. Significant reduction (14.2%, p = 0.01416) was observed in the enoxaparin group and in the UFH + abciximab group; on adding the in-hospital ICH or major bleeds to the primary end-point (efficacy plus safety end-point). Higher rate of thrombocytopenia with Abciximab vs. enoxaparin and UFH (3.2% vs. 1.2% and 1.3% respectively, p = 0.0001) with higher treatment cost [57,58].

The *ENTIRE-TIMI- 23trial* [59], the design was similar to that of ASSENT-3, with the additional group receiving enoxaparin in combination with abciximab and half-dose TNKase. Enoxaparin with TNKase, compared to UFH resulted in reduction in the combined incidence of death/MI at 30 days. Abciximab did not decrease events and was associated with increased risk of major bleeding. Major bleeding increased when half-dose TNKase was combined with eptifibatide, a small-molecule GP IIB-IIIA inhibitor in the *INTEGRITI* study [60]. In conjunction with the GUSTO-V data [61], ASSENT-3, ENTIRE-TIMI-23 and INTEGRITI (see below) indicate that GP IIB-IIIA agents should not be coupled with thrombolytic drugs.

The *ASSENT-3-PLUS* study evaluated the pre-hospital phase of STEMI treatment. With electrocardiographic confirmation obtained in the field in 1639 patients treated with TNKase and randomly allocated to enoxaparin or UFH adjunctive treatment. Enoxaparin reduced the composite of 30-day mortality or in-hospital re-infarction, or in-hospital refractory ischemia to 14.2% vs. 17.4% for UFH (P=0.080), no difference for composite end point plus in-hospital ICH or major bleeding was observed. There were reductions in in-hospital re-infarction and refractory ischemia but increases in total stroke and ICH (> 75 years) were observed in this study (Table 4) [62].

Data analysis of ASSENT-3 and ASSENT-3-PLUS trials essentially confirmed the usefulness of using enoxaparin as an alternative to UFH in combination with TNKase in reducing the primary efficacy end-point from and the primary efficacy plus safety (ICH or major bleeding) end-point. This advantage was greater in the urgent revascularization setting (15.4% vs. 10.1%, p = 0.013). The high stroke rates observed with enoxaparin (1.3% vs. 0.9%, P=NS), was mainly due to excess in ICH among women of more than 75 years old in *ASSENT-3-PLUS*[63]. In the *EXTRACT-TIMI 25 trial*, treatment with enoxaparin as additive to fibrinolysis for STEMI throughout the index hospitalization was superior to the treatment with UFH for 48 hours but on the expense of increased major bleeding episodes [64].

4. TRIALS ON OTHER FIBRINOLYTICS

4.1 Staphylokinase

Undergone limited testing in humans. In a randomized angiographic trial, 48 patients received staphylokinase (double bolus of either 10 mg or 20 mg), dose dependent TIMI grade 3 flow rate of 62% vs. 58% for 52 patients given t-PAwere observed. No excess mortality, hemorrhagic, mechanical or allergic complications were reported, however, anti-staphylokise antibodies were observed after the second week of treatment [65,66]. In conflicting study of 82 patients, a bolus and infusion dose tested (15 mg, 30 mg, or 45 mg). 90-min TIMI grade 3 flow rates showed no evidence of a dose response [67].

4.2 Urokinase

Studied in sparse clinical trials. A number of smaller angiographic trials were carried out in the 1980s [68-71]. These collectively showed angiographic patency and TIMI grade 3 flow rates that were superior to SK and similar to those observed with t-PA, particularly with higher dose (3 million units). Urokinase was tested in a trial of 2,201 patients with a dose of 2 million units of urokinase plus heparin vs. heparin alone achieved 16 days mortality rate 8% vs. 8.3% respectively [72]. An angiographic trial with saruplase (scu-PA), achieve higher 60 min patency rate vs. SK alone. Such effect was modest at 90-min. Saruplase had less bleeding complications (p<0.01) [73]. *SESAM* Study; an angiographic trial compared saruplase against 3 h of t-PA (473 patients). 60 min patency rates were similar with similar safety data [74]. Consequently *COMPASS trial*; a randomized equivalence trial compared saruplase to SK (3,089 patients randomized to 80 mg of scu-PA or 1.5 million units of SK with IV heparin in both groups) [75]. 30-day mortality rates were 5.7% for saruplase and 6.7% for SK. Significantly higher rate of ICH with scu-PA (0.9%) vs. with SK (0.3%; p=0.038), mistrust the validity of the SESAM Study [76,77].

4.3 Lanoteplase (n-PA)

Modified single-bolus agent t-PA molecule with longer half-life tested in an angiographic trial (602 patients with AMI, doses of 15-120 KU/kg), at the highest dose, the patency rate was higher with n-PA vs. accelerated t-PA. There was a trend toward higher TIMI grade 3 flow rates (57% vs. 46%, respectively). Lanoteplase was well tolerated at all doses with safety comparable to that of t- PA [77]. In a large phase-III randomized equivalence trial; The *In TIME-II*. A (15,078 patients treated with n-PA (120- KU/kg) vs. accelerated t-PA.30-day mortality was similar between the two agents (n-PA, 6.7% vs. t-PA, 6.6%; p<0.05 for equivalence). Though, n-PA resulted in higher ICH (1.13% vs. ·0.62%; p<0.003) [78].

4.4 Anistreplase

The *GREAT Trial*; a randomized double-blind parallel-group clinical trial; 311 patients received anistreplase (30 UIV) either at home or in hospital. The median time saved by domiciliary thrombolysis about 130 min. after 1-year lower mortality rates were seen in patients who received anistreplase at home (10.4% vs. 21.6%, p = 0.007) [79].

Table1. Clinical trials with streptokinase (SK)

Author/year	Study	Patient included	Benefits	Risk
GISSI-1 investigator [29] 1986	GISSI-1	11,806 STEMI patients/1.5 IU SK	Overall hospital mortality = 10.7% in SK recipients vs. 13% in controls, 18% RRR (p = 0.0002, 0.81).	▼Incidence major bleeds (>2 U of blood) &anaphylactic shock. Cerebrovascular events (ischemic+ Hemorrhagic episodes) in the SK & control groups:<1%)
ISAM investigator 1986 [30]	ISAM	1741 STEMI patients/1.5 IU SK	21 days mortality = 6.3 % in the SK group &7.1% in the placebo group. SK group had↑global EF (56.8 vs. 53.9 %, P<0.005)	Bleeding occurred in 5.6% in SK group vs. 1.5% in the Placebo group (p=0.0001) ICH occurs in 4 patients in SK group result in 2 deaths.
ISIS-2 investigator 1988 [28]	ISIS-2	17,187 STEMI patients	Significant ▼ in 5-week vascularmortality 9 2% in SK treated pt. vs. 12.0% placebo treated patient (OR: 25% SD 4; 2p<0.00001); 9.4% vascular deaths in aspirin treated patients vs. 11.8%√in placebo group (OR: 23% p<0.00001).	▲bleeds requiring transfusion (0.5% vs. 0.2%), ICH= (0.1% vs. 0.0%) in SK treated pt., but with fewer other strokes (0.6% vs. 0.8%). No ▲ in total strokes (0.7% SK vs. 0.8% placebo infusion)
EMERAS investigator 1993 [31]	EMERAS	4534 patients admitted up to 24 h after the onset of suspected AMI	No significant difference in in- hospital mortality (11.9% in SK group vs. 12.4% in controls). Patients presented 7-12 h have ▼ deaths with SK (11.7% SK vs. 13.2% control). Slight difference among the 1791 patients presenting after 13-24 h (11.4% vs.10.7%)	- Significant trend for ▲ bleeding with heparin addition -No significant difference in the incidence if stoke between treatment groups

▼ =Decrease; ▲ = Increase; STEMI = ST elevation myocardial infarction, SK =streptokinase, EF= Ejection fraction, RRR=relative risk reduction, ICH =intracranial hemorrhage

Table 2. Clinical trials with alteplase (t-PA)

Author/year	Study	Patient included	Benefits	Risks
No Author listed 1993 [33]	GUSTO-1	41,021 patients with evolving MI	The mortality rates in the 4 treatment groups: SK &subcutaneous heparin, 7.2% ; SK& IV heparin, 7.4 %; accelerated t-PA & IV heparin, 6.3 %, & The combination SK &tPA with IV heparin, 7.0 %. With 14 % ▼ (95 % CI, 5.9 to 21.3 %) in mortality for accelerated t-PA vs. 2 SK -only strategies (P=0.001).	Hemorrhagic stroke=0.49 %, 0.54 %, 0.72 %, & 0.94%in the 4 grps, respectively, with significant ↑of hemorrhagic strokes for accelerated t-PA (P = 0.03)& for the combination strategy (P< 0.001 vs.SK only. ▲combined end point of death or disabling stroke in the accelerated-tPA grp. vs. SK-only grp. (6.9 % vs. 7.8 %, P = 0.006).
Cannon CP et al. 1994 [35]/USA	TIMI 4	382 patients with STEMI	IRAP atency [TIMI] grade 2-3 flow) at 60 min after the start of thrombolysis significantly ▲ inrt-PA (77.8% vs. 59.5% for APSAC-treated pts. & 59.3% for combination-treated [r-PA vs. APSAC, p = 0.02; rt-PA vs. combination, p = 0.03). At 90 min, the incidence IRA patency &TIMI grade 3 flow significantly ▲ in rt-PA (60.2% had TIMI grade 3 flow vs. 42.9% & 44.8% of APSAC- & combination; respectively [rt-PA vs. APSAC, p < 0.01; rt-PA vs. combination, p = 0.02]).	The incidence of unsatisfactory outcome = 41.3% for rt-PA vs. 49% for APSAC &53.6% for the combination (rt-PA vs. APSAC, p = 0.19; rt-PA vs. combination, p = 0.06).
No authors listed 1990 [36]	GISSI-2	12,490 AMI pts. randomized to 4treatment gps (SK, SK +heparin, tPA alone, tPA+ heparin).	No specific differences between 2 thrombolytic agents in regards the combined end-point (tPA 23.1%; SK 22.5%; relative risk 1.04, 95% CI 0.95-1.13), nor after the addition of heparin to the aspirin treatment (heparin 22.7%, no heparin 22.9%; RR 0.99, 95% CI 0.91-1.08).	→major in-hospital cardiac complications (reinfarction, post-infarction angina). The incidence of major bleeds significantly ▲ in SK + heparin treated patients (respectively, tPA 0.5%, SK 1.0%, RR 0.57, 95% CI 0.38-0.85; hep 1.0%, no hep 0.6%, RR 1.64, 95% CI 1.09-2.45). -similar overall incidence of stroke in all groups.
No authors listed 1992 [37]	ISIS-3	41 299 AMI patients up to 24 h (median 4 h) after the onset	Randomized: SK: 1.5 MU tPA, duteplase: 0.60 MU/kg (APSAC), anistreplase: 30 U over about 3 min). No significant difference in the pre-specified endpoint of 35-day mortality (10.3%) aspirin+ heparin vs. 2189 [10.6%] aspirin alone). , slightly fewer deaths in the aspirin + heparin group (days 0-7 in hospital: 7.4% vs.7.9%; 2 p = 0.06) with a slight convergence by day 35 (598 further deaths [3.1% of survivors] vs. 556 [2.9%]).	Heparin+ aspirin was associated with ▲transfused or major non-cerebral bleeds (1.0% aspirin + heparin vs. 0.8% aspirin alone; 2p<0.01) & of definite or probable ICH (0.56% vs. 0.40%; 2p<0.05), no significant differences in total stroke (1.28% vs. 1.18%). Re-infarctions were slightly less common among those allocated aspirin plus heparin (3.16% vs. 3.47%; 2p = 0.09).
Purvis JA et al. 1994 [40] UK	Prospective study	84 patients with AMI	IRA patency of TIMI flow grade 3 in 86%pts (95% [CI] 75%-93%) TIMI flow grade 2 or 3 in 91%pts (95% CI 81% to 97%). At 90 min IRA patency of TIMI flow grade 3 achieved in 88%pts(95% CI 79% to 94%)& TIMI flow grade 2 or 3 in 93% pts (95% CI 85% - 97%).	Minor bleeding episodes reported. No cerebrovascular bleeding. - One month mortality=6 %. - Early angiographic re-occlusion=2.4% -Late reinfection=11.9%
No Author listed 1993 [41]	COBALTst udy	7169 patients with AMI	30-days mortality ▲ in the double-bolus group than in the accelerated-infusion group: 7.98 % vs. 7.53%.	The respective rates of any stroke &of hemorrhagic stroke = 1.92 & 1.12 % after double-bolus t-PA vs. 1.53 & 0.81% after an accelerated infusion of t-PA (P=0.24 & P=0.23, respectively).
Bleich SD et al. 1998 [42]	multicente r, randomize d, open-label trial,	461 patients with AMI	The 90-minute angiographic patency rates = 74.5% in the double-bolus group & 81.4% in the infusion group (p = 0.08). Patency rates were comparable for the 2 groups at 60 minutes (76.8% vs. 77.5%) & 24 hrs (95.5% vs. 93.5%) after initiation of treatment.	In-hospital mortality rates = 4.5% in the bolus group & 1.3% in the infusion group (p = 0.04); 30-day mortality rates = 4.5% & 1.7%, respectively (p = NS)with comparable frequency of all other adverse events in both group.

▼ = Decrease; ▲ = Increase,→ = no difference/ similar, AMI = acute myocardial infarction, IRA = infarct related artery. SK =streptokinase, t-PA = alteplase, grp = group. IV = intravenous

Table 3. Clinical trials with reteplase (r-PA)

Study	Patients, no.	Fibrinolytic agent	Benefits:Mortality at 30–35 d, %	Risks comment
INJECT trial 1995 [44]	3,004 3,006	r-PA 10 U +10 U SK. 1.5 MU	Mortality at 30–35 d, = 9.02 % Mortality at 30–35 d, = 9.53%	In-hospital stroke rates = 1.23% for rPA & 1.00% for SK. Bleeding events = 0.7% in rPA, 1.0% SK. ICH= 0.77% for r-PA&0.37% SK.
GUSTO-III 1997 [45]	10,138 4,921	r-PA 10 U + 10 U Accelerated t-PA	Mortality at 30–35 d, = 7.47% Mortality at 30–35 d, = 7.24%	Stroke rate: 1.64% of patients treated with r-PA & in 1.79 % of those treated with t-PA (P= 0.50).ICH=0.91% in r-PA group vs.0.87% in t-PA group The respective rates of the combined end point of death ornon-fatal, disabling stroke =7.89 %& 7.91 % (P=0.97; OR, 1.0; 95 %CI, 0.88 to 1.13).

Table 4. Clinical trials with tenecteplase (TNKase)

Trial (year)	Patients no.	Comparison	Benefits	Risks
Cannon CP 1997 [50] TIMI 10A	113patients STEMI presenting within 12 hrs	a single bolus of TNK-t-PA /5– 10 seconds / 5 to 50 mg. doses	TIMI grade 3 flow at 90 minutes = 57% - 64% of pts. at the 30- 50-mg doses. Mortality at 30 days =3.5%	Serious bleeding =6.2% at a vascular access site in 6 patients & after CABG in 1 patient. There were no strokes or ICH.
TIMI 10B 1998 [51]	886patients with AMI	a single bolus 30 or 50 mg TNK-t-PAvs. Front loaded t-PA	TNK-t-PA, as a single 40-mg bolus, achieved rates of TIMI grade 3 flow = 90-minute bolus & infusion of t-PA	The 50-mg dose discontinued early because of ▲ I CH &replaced by a 40-mg dose, heparin doses decreased. A prespecified analysis of weight-based TNK-t-PA dosing using median TIMI frame count showed a dose response (P=0.001). Similar dose responses observed for serious bleeding &ICH but significantly ▼rates observed for both TNK-t-PA & t-PA after the heparin doses ▼& titration of the heparin started at 6 hours.
ASSENT-1 1999 [52]	3235patients with AMI	TNKase as a bolus vs. front loaded t-PA	This is safety trail	Total stroke rate at 30 days = 1.5%. ICH rates=0.77%): (0.94%)in the 30-mg group &0.62%). the 40-mg group No strokes occurred in the 73 patients treated with 50 mg TNK-t-PA. In patients treated within 6hrsafter symptom onset the rates of ICH= 0.56% (30 mg TNK-t-PA) & 0.58 (40 mg TNK-t-PA). Death, death or nonfatal stroke, or severe bleeding complications: 6.4%, 7.4%, and 2.8%, respectively, without significant differences among treatment groups.
ASSENT-2 1999 [54]	16,949patients with AMI	TNKase vs. r-PA	-Identical covariate-adjusted 30-day mortality rates for the two groups--6.18% for TNKase= 6.15% & for t-PA. -The 95% one-sided upper boundaries of the absolute & relative differences in 30-day mortality = 0.61% &10.00%, respectively,	Similar rates of ICH= (0.93% forTNKase&0.94% for t-PA), but ▼ non-cerebral bleeding complications (26.43 vs. 28.95%, p=0.0003) & ▼blood transfusion (4.25 vs. 5.49%, p=0.0002) with TNKase. Death or non-fatal stroke rate at 30 days = 7.11% withTNKase&7.04% with t-PARR; 1.01 [95% CI 0.91-1.13]).

Trial	Patients	Treatment	Outcome	Results
ASSENT-3 (2001) [57,58]	6,095 AMI In Efficacy & safety trail	TNKase + Enoxvs. abciximabvs. UFHa	Significantly ▼ efficacy & safety endpoints in the Enox. & abciximab groups than in the UFH group	Significantly ▼ efficacy & safety endpoint: 280/2037 (13.7%) vs. 347/2036 (17.0%); 0.81 [0.70-0.93], p=0.0037] for Enox.&287/2016 (14.2%) vs. 347/2036 (17.0%; 0.84 [0.72-0.96], p=0.01416) for abciximab.
ENTIRE-TIMI 23 (2002) [59]	483STEMI patient	TNKase + Enoxvs. abciximabvs. UFHa	-TIMI 3 flow at 60 minutes: *52% &48% to 51% with Enox. *48% with UFH & 47% to 58% with Enox. The rate of TIMI 3 flow among all UFH patients * 50% &51% in Enox. pts. ---30 days, death/recurrent MI in the full-dose TNK grp= 15.9% of patients with UFH &4.4% with Enox. (P=0.005). In the combination therapy grp., the rates = 6.5% with UFH &5.5% with Enox.	The rate of major hemorrhage with full-dose TNK = 2.4% with UFH &1.9% with Enox. With combination therapy= 5.2% using UFH & 8.5% with Enox.
ASSENT-3-PLUS 2003 [62]	1,639 STEMI patient	TNKase + Enoxvs. UFHa, pre-hospital delivery	▼ the composite of 30-day mortality or in-hospital re-infarction, or in-hospital refractory ischemia to 14.2% vs. 17.4% for UFH(P=0.080)	No difference for composite end point of death, in-hospital ICH or major bleeding (18.3% vs. 20.3%, P=0.30). ▼ in-hospital re-infarction (3.5% vs. 5.8%, P=0.028) & refractory ischemia (4.4% vs. 6.5%, P=0.067) ▲ in total stroke (2.9% vs. 1.3%, P=0.026) &ICH (2.20% vs. 0.97%, P=0.047). The ▲ in ICH seen in patients >75 years

▼ = Decrease/less, ▲ = Increase/higher, ▶ = Equal, PPCI = primary percutaneous coronary intervention, UFH = unfractionated heparin, F = facilitated. ICH = intracranial hemorrhage, Enox = enoxaparin

5. ANGIOGRAPHIC TRIALS

5.1 Streptokinase

Many trials were conducted to evaluate the angiographic findings after treatment with SK in STEMI patients (Table 5), these trials accomplished as soon as possible after SK administration looking for coronary artery patency (defined as TIMI grade 2 or 3 flow) [9,11,15,18,19,22,24,26,27,73,80-94]. Overall, the angiographic data suggested patency rates with SK of ≈ 44%, 48% at 60 and 90 min respectively and 72% at 2 to 3 h after beginning therapy, and a rate of 75-85% at 24 h to 21 days after therapy from a pooled meta-analysis. These rates are substantially higher than those of control patients [27] while the bleeding and other complications rates in these studies are summarized in Table 5.

5.2 Alteplase (t-PA) (Table 6)

The first comparative trial between t-PA and SK was the *TIMI-1 trial*; 290 patients had angiography after receiving either SK or t-PA, in addition to IV heparin. The primary end point; 90 min reperfusion of an initially IRA was achieved in 62% of t-PA group vs. 31% of SK group (p <0.001). The patency rate at 90 min was 70% for the t-PA vs. 43% for the SK group (p<0.001) achieved (Table 5). There was comparable bleeding events, transfusions requirements and re-occlusion rates of the IRA between the two groups [11]. Subsequently t-PA was tested in numerous other angiographic trials [17,20,21,23,25,83,92-110] (table 6), reporting that the 3-h dosing regimen of t-PA resulted in higher patency and TIMI grade 3 flow at 60 min and 90 min. Neuhaus and colleagues [102] developed an "accelerated" 90-min dosing regimen for t-PA, which achieved higher rates of early reperfusion compared to the 3-h regimen of t-PA, anistreplase treatment or SK treatment [34,35,98,102,107-110]. The *GUSTO-1 angiographic sub study* (2,400 patients) randomized patients to angiography at 90 min, 180 min, 24 h, or 5 days. At the important, 90-min time point, t-PA-treated patients had a significantly higher patency rate and a much higher rate of TIMI grade 3 flow [33,34] and this was associated with improved survival at 24 h and at 30 days, thus stressing the benefits of rapid reperfusion [39].

5.3 Reteplase (r-PA) (Table 7)

Two angiographic trials compared t-PA with r-PA. The first, the Reteplase Angiographic Phase II International Dose-finding, *RAPID trial*, compared 3 dosing strategies for r-PAwith an infusion of alteplase (Table 7). The TIMI grade 3 flow rates at 90 min were 63% vs. 49% (p < 0.05) respectively. The 30-day mortality rate in the 10+10-MU group was 1.9% vs. 3.9% in the t-PA group. Similar re-infarction rates and congestive heart failure rates, 1 stroke in the r-PA groups (1/452) compared with 6 in the t-PA group (6/154). The incidence of stroke in the 10+10-MU r-PA group was less than that observed in the t-PA group (P=0.03) (Table 7) [111].

A second, larger trial (*RAPID-2*) compared the best regimen from RAPID with accelerated t-PA. The r-PA was superior to accelerated t-PA. When these two trials were combined, TIMI grade 3 flow rates at 90 min were 61% vs. 45% (p<0.01) respectively. The 16% absolute increase in TIMI grade 3 rates with r-PA over accelerated t-PA was less than the 24% increase seen with t-PA over SK in the GUSTO-1 angiographic sub-study, but this smaller difference translated into a much larger difference in mortality in the RAPID trials (3.1% for r-PA vs. 8.4% for t-PA). 35-day mortality was 4.1% for r-PA and 8.4% for t-PA (P = NS). No significant differences in bleedings requiring transfusion or hemorrhagic stroke (between the 2 groups (Table 7) [112].

5.4 Tenecteplase (TNKase) (Table 8)

Many angiographic trails evaluated TNKase [113-116]. In *CAPITAL AMI*; (170 high-risk STEMI patients) which compared TNKase alone vs. facilitated PCI. The primary end-points were: composite of death, re-infarction, recurrent unstable ischemia or stroke at 6 months. The median symptoms to needle time: 120 minutes and symptoms to balloon inflation: 204 minutes. The primary end-point was reduced by immediate PCI from 24.4% to 11.6% (p = 0.04). No significant differences in the rates of death or stroke between the 2 groups. Major bleeding risk was comparable; 7.1% vs. 8.1% of the TNK-alone vs. TNK-facilitated angioplasty group respectively (p = 1.00) (Table 8) [113].

The *WEST study*, an open-label, randomized feasibility study (304 STEMI patients) randomized to either TNKase, or to TNKase followed by PCI within 24 hours and primary angioplasty, all patient received aspirin and enoxaparin, symptoms to randomization time: 113, 130 and 176 minutes respectively. No differences between the 3 groups in the primary composite of death or re-infarction, refractory ischemia, CHF, cardiogenic shock or major ventricular arrhythmia. Higher rate of the death/re-infarction combination in TNKase group, but not of death (Table 8). The WEST trial confirms the data from CAPTIM 9 in regards to pre-hospital thrombolysis, TNKase is very competitive with primary PCI [114].

The larger *ASSENT-4 PCI trial*; an open-label trial (1667 patients); investigated TNKase facilitation on the prognosis of patients expected to have time-delay of 1 to 3 hours before primary PCI. The primary end-point was the composite of death or CHF or shock within 90 days. The trial was interrupted by the data and safety monitoring board for an excess of in-hospital mortality in the group where primary PCI was facilitated by TNKase. A TIMI-3 flow of 43% in primary PCI/TNKase-treated patients vs. 15% in the control group (p = 0.0001). The primary end-point at 90 days was increased in the facilitated group (19% vs. 13%, p = 0.0045), along with the stroke rates (1.8% vs. 0%, p = 0.0001) (Table 8) [115].

The *GRACIA-2* study (212 patients) a non-inferiority trial compared pharmaco-invasive" approach (TNKase followed by early routine PCI within 3–12 hours) with primary PCI with primary end-points of epicardial and myocardial reperfusion and the extent of left ventricular damage evaluated by infarct size and LVEF. Electrocardiographic ST-segment resolution spotted more frequently in the TNKase group (61% vs. 43%, p = 0.01). ICH occurred in 1.0%, 0.6%, and 1.7% of patients treated with any combination, eptifibatide 180/2/180 and half-dose TNK, and TNK monotherapy, respectively. Infarct size and LVEF were similar in the two groups [116]. ASSENT-4 PCI found that TIMI grade 3 flow in the IRA before PCI, occurring either spontaneously or obtained by fibrinolysis, is associated with a higher TIMI patency after PCI, better ST resolution and a trend towards a favorable 90 days clinical outcome [117]. GRACIA-2 confirmed the WEST study results, suggesting the analogous efficacy of TNKase (with rescue/routine PCI) and primary PCI. Utmost pertinent to pathophysiology and clinical practice, is the finding of GRACIA-2 (in combination with ASSENT-4 PCI) that routine

PCI after TNKase should be deferred at least 3 to 12 hours to achieve the benefit [118].

6. FIBRINOLYSIS AND ADJUNCTIVE THERAPIES

6.1 Fibrinolytics and Antiplatelet Agents

Persuasive evidence of the effectiveness of aspirin was demonstrated by the ISIS-2 trial, [29] in which the benefits of aspirin and SK were additive. The benefit of initial aspirin therapy was sustained long-term in the ISIS-2 trial. Treatment with aspirin (75-162 mg) should be continued indefinitely. The *Antiplatelet Trialists Collaboration* reported 40 further deaths, re-infarctions, or strokes prevented/1,000 patients in the first few years of sustained treatment [119,120].

Clopidogrel, a potent platelet inhibitor of thienopyridine derivative. In the *CLARITY* trial, patient's ≤75 years were treated with a standard fibrinolytic regimen and randomized to 300 mg clopidogrel loading dose followed by 75 mg/day or placebo on top of aspirin up to and including the day of angiography with a maximum of 8 days (mean=3 days). By 30 days, clopidogrel reduced the odds of the composite end-point of death from cardiovascular causes, recurrent MI/ischemia, with 20% reduction for urgent revascularization. No differences inmajor bleeding and ICH in the two groups [121] (Table 9).

In the *COMMIT study*, 45 852 Chinese patients (<1000 patients aged >75 years) with MI (93% with STEMI) randomized to clopidogrel 75 mg (without loading dose) or placebo in addition to aspirin. Significant 9% (95% CI 3-14) reduction in death, re-infarction, or stroke (9.2% vs. 10.1%; p = 0.002) in favor of clopidogrel, with significant 7% proportional reduction in any death (7.5% vs. 8.1%; p = 0.03). Such benefits appeared consistent across a wide range of patients and independent of other treatments. *In terms of risk;* no significant excess risk noted with clopidogrel, either overall (0.58% vs. 0.55%; p=0.59), or in patients aged older than 70 years or in those given fibrinolytic therapy [122].

Table 5. Angiographic studies with streptokinase

Author	Time to patency	Patient no.	Strep dose MU	Door needle time	Benefits:Patency rate %	risk
Cribier et al. [15]		21	1.5	115 min	52%	-------
PRIMI study group [73]	60 min	203	1.5	140 min	48%	Less bleeding complications with rscu-PA vs.SK
Spann et al. [80]		43	1.5	60 min	49% recanalization rate	No serious bleeding
Rogers et al. [81]		16	1.0	45 min	44% recanalization rate	Bleeding requiring transfusion1/51
de Marneffe et al. [82]		10	1.5	30min	80% recanalization rate	Few bleeding events1/10
ECSG-2 ; Verstraete et al. [83]	90 min	65	1.0	156 min	55%	Bleeding & other complications; less common in the rt-PA vs. SK
Chesebro et al. [11]		159	1.5	286 min	43%	No ICH, minor bleeding only
Stack et al. [84]		216	1.5	180 min	44%	GI bleeding in 14% of patients. All over bleeding : 72%
Lopez-Sendon et al. [85]		25	1.5	<6 h	60%	-------
PRIMI study group [73]		203	1.5	140 min	64%	See above
Charbonnier et al. [86]		58	1.5	168 min	51%	Hemorrhages ; 9/58pts with APSAC (15.5 p. 100) & 13/58 treated with SK (22.4 p. 100);
Hogg et al. [87]		63	1.5	209 min	53%	-------
Hillis et al. [88]		34	1.5	60 min	32% recanalization rate	-------
Chesebro et al. (TIMI-1) [11]	2 - 3 h	119	1.5	60min	31% recanalization rate	See above
Monnier et al. [89]		11	1.5	135 min	64%	No life threating complication
Golf et al. [90]		135	1.5	138 min	70	-------
Six et al. [9]		56	1.5	150 min	60%	Blood transfusion 2%, Major bleeding; 1 patient
PRIMI study grp [73]	24hr	203	1.5	140	88%	Less bleeding in urokise compared to steptokinase
Durand et al. [19]		35	1.5	149 min	82%	-------
Lopez-Sendon et al. [85]		25	1.5	<6h	75%	-------
Hogg et al. [87]		63	1.5	209	88%	-------
Ribeiro et al. [91]		50	1.2	180 min	80%	no major bleeding events,
White et al. [24]		107	1.5	180 min	75%	Deaths with SK vs. placebo; 2.5 % vs. 12.9 %, P = 0.012).
Bassand et al. [26]		52	1.5	210 min	68%	7/55 deaths in heparin grp&4/52 deaths in SKgp.
Kennedy et al. [22]		191	1.5	210 min	69%	Bleeding, in SK group (13.1% vs. 0.6%), allergic reactions (2.1% vs.0%).
Lopez-Sendon et al. [85]		25	1.5	<6h	90%	-------
Magnani (PAIMS) [92]		85	1.5	127min	77%	ICH occurred 1/85 patient
White et al. [93]		135	1.5	150 min	75%	No ICH in the SK group
Cherng et al. 1992 [94]		63	1.5	294 min	57%	In hospital bleeding 11.1% in SK vs. t-PA 13.6%

MU=million unit. APSAC= anisoylated plasminogen streptokinase activator complex, ICH =intracranial hemorrhage, SK =streptokinase

Table 6. Alteplase (t-PA) angiographic trials

Author/year	Time-patency	Patient no.	Alteplase dose	Symptoms-needle time	Benefits; patency rate %	Risk
Topol et al. [95]	60 min	75	1.25 mg/kg/3 h	216 min	57 %	Moderate or severe bleeding: 39% of t-PAvs. 32% of placebo/intracoronary SK (p = NS).
Smalling et al. [96]		91	1.25 mg/kg/3 h	228 min	45 %	Bleeding rate were comparable in both dose protocol
de Bono [97]		183	100 mg/3 h	156 min	60 %	Non-significant ▲ in bleeding in heparin group(include (ICH)
Carney et al. [98]		138	00 mg/3 h	168 min	63 %	Similar rates of recurrent ischemia, re-infarction, angiographic re-occlusion, stroke& death) & bleeding complications
Verstraete et al. [83]	90 min	64	0.75 mg/kg/1.5h	180 min	70 %	Less common in the bleeding episodes and other complications t-PA patients than in the SK group. Hospital mortality was identical in the 2 treatment groups.
Chesebro et al. [11]		157	80 mg/3 h	287 min	70 %	No ICH, minor bleeding only
Topol et al. [95]		75	1.25 mg/kg/3 h	216 min	69 %	See above
Topol et al. [95]		142	1 mg/kg/h	190 min	72 %	See above
Johns et al. [100]		68	1 mg/kg/1.5 h	180 min	76 %	Bleeding complication occur more frequently in T PA (P =NS)
TIMI-IIA [101]		133	100 mg/6 h	168 min	75 %	
Neuhaus et al. [102]		124	70 mg/1.5 h	,<4 h	69 %	Five cardiac deaths in each group, 1 fatal ICH in the t-PA group. In-hospital re-infarction rate =8.9% vs. 13.2% for patients treated with t-PA & urokinase, respectively.
Topol et al. [103]		134	1.5 mg/kg/4 h	168 min	79 %	Bleeding complications=13% in t-PA & heparin group vs. 18% in patients treated with t-PA only (p = 0.53). The only ICH occurred in a patient initially treated without heparin.
Topol et al. [104]		50	100 mg/3 h	243 min	52 %	———————
Smalling et al. [96]		91	1.25 mg/kg/3 h	228 min	70 %	See above
Califf et al. [105]		95	100 mg/3 h	200 min	71 %	No difference in bleeding complication rates was observed with any thrombolytic regimen.
Whitlow & Bashore [106]		206	100 mg/3 h	<6 h	63 %	In-hospital mortality (6% vs. 4%) &serious bleeding similar between the two groups(12% vs. 11%)
Grines et al. [99]		107	100 mg/3 h	180 min	64 %	
Carney et al. [98]	2 to 3 h	138	100 mg/3 h	168 min	77 %	See above
Topol et al. [95]		75	1.25 mg/kg/3 h	216 min	79 %	See above
Guerci et al. [17]		72	80–100 mg/3 h	192 min	66 %	No fatal or ICH occurred, and episodes of bleeding requiring transfusion were observed in 7.6 %t of the placebo group and 9.8%of the t-PA group
Neuhaus et al. [102]	24hr	124	70 mg/1.5 h	<4 h	78 %	See above
TIMI-IIA [101]		128	100–150 mg/6 h	174 min	82 %	
TIMI-II [107]		1,366	100 mg	156 min	85 %	ICH%=1.9 %with 150 mg of rt-PA &0.5 %with 100 mg of t-PA
Anderson et al. [108]		164	100 mg	168 min	86 %	Mortality (APSAC 6.2%, rt-PA 7.9%) stroke, ventricular

Study	Duration	Patients, no.	Fibrinolytic agent	Time	Patency %	Risk
TEAM III						tachycardia, ventricular fibrillation, heart failure within 1 month, recurrent ischemia &re-infarction were comparable in the 2 groups
de Bono [23]	3 to 21 d	367	100 mg/3 h	156 min	87 %	increased mortality in the intervention group
O'Rourke et al. [25]	-----	74	100 mg/3 h	120 min	81 %	More bleeding in the rt-PAgrp Most minor in nature
NHFA [21]		73	100 mg/3 h	195 min	70 %	
TIMI-IIA [101]		389	100–150 mg/6h	174 min	79 %	See above
Neuhaus et al. [102]		124	70 mg/3 h	<4 h	73 %	
Bassand et al. [20]		93	100 mg/3 h	172 min	76 %	ICH occurred 1/85 patient
Magnani [92]		86	100 mg/3 h	124 min	81 %	No ICH in the SK group
White et al. [93]		135	100 mg/3 h	150 min	76 %	-----
Rapold et al. [109]		34	100 mg/3 h	186 min	81 %	No difference in bleeding complications
Thompson et al. [110]		241	100 mg/3 h	155 min	80 %	See above
de Bono et al. [97]		652	100 mg/3 h	170 min	79 %	
Cherng et al. [94]		59	100 mg/3 h	312 min	77 %	In hospital bleeding 11.1% in SK vs. r-TPA 13.6%

ICH = intracranial hemorrhage, SK =streptokinase

Table 7. Reteplase (r-PA) angiographic trials

Study	Patients, no.	Fibrinolytic agent	Benefits: patency % vs. TIMI grade 3 flow at 90 min, %	Risk
RAPID [111]	146	r-PA 15 U	63 % vs. 41%	-Bleeding complications were similar between the gps -The incidence of re-occlusion was not different between the groups
	152	r-PA 10 U plus 5 U	67% vs. 46%	
	154	r-PA 10 U plus 10 U	85% vs. 63%	
RAPID II [112]	154	Alteplase 100 mg/3 h	77% vs. 49%	-35-day mortality = 4.1% for-PA & 8.4% for t-PA (P = NS. -No significant differences between r-PA & t-PA in bleedings requiring a transfusion (12.4% vs. 9.7%) or hemorrhagic stroke (1.2% vs. 1.9%).
	169	r-PA 10 U plus 10 U	83% vs. 60%	
	155	Alteplase (accelerated)	73% vs. 45%	

Table 8. Angiographic tenecteplase (TNKase) trials in AMI

Trial (year)	Patients no.	Comparison	Benefits	risk
INTEGRITI trial [60]	438	eptifibatide + ½ dosage TNK asevs. TNK asemonotherapy	TIMI-3 flow, overall patency& ST-segment resolution is similar	-More major hemorrhage (7.6% vs. 2.5%, p=0.14) &transfusions (13.4% vs. 4.2%, p=0.02). ICH=1.0%, 0.6%, & 1.7% of patients treated with any combination, eptifibatide 180/2/180 &1/2dose TNK, and TNK monotherapy, respectively.
CAPITAL-AMI [113]	170	F-PCIvs. TNKase	▼ residual ischemia with F-PCI	-No significant differences in the rates of death or stroke. -Major bleeding; 7.1% of the TNK-alone group vs. 8.1% of the TNK-facilitated angioplasty group (p = 1.00).
WEST [114]	304	TNKasevs. F-PCIcvs. PPCI	TNKase & F-PCI comparable to P-PCI	-No differences in 3 groups in the primary composite of death or reinfarction, refractory ischemia, CHF, cardiogenic shock or major ventricular arrhythmia (25% vs. 24% vs. 23%, p=NS). -In the plain TNKasegp. ▲ rate of the death/re-infarction combination (13.0% vs. 6.7% vs. 4.0%, p=0.021), but not of death (4.0% vs. 1.0% vs. 1.0%, p=NS).
ASSENT-4 [115]	1,667	F-PCIvs.PPCI	----------------	-Trial prematurely interrupted by the data &safety monitoring board for an excess of in-hospital mortality in the group where primary PCI facilitated by TNKase (6% vs. 3%, p=0.0105).
GRACIA-2 [116]	212	TNKase vs. PPCI	Similar infarct size (area under the curve of CK-MB: 4613 +/- 3373 vs. 4649 +/- 3632 microg/L/h, P=0.94); 6-week LVF(EF: 59.0 +/- 11.6 vs. 56.2 +/- 13.2%, P=0.11; ESVI: 27.2 +/- 12.8 vs. 29.7 +/- 13.6, P=0.21);in both groups	-Major bleeding (1.9 vs. 2.8%, P=0.99) & 6-month cumulative incidence of the clinical endpoint (10 vs. 12%, P=0.57; relative risk: 0.80; 95% confidence interval: 0.37-1.74).

▼ ---- Decrease; ▼ = Increase; ▲ = Equal, PPCI = primary percutaneous coronary intervention, UFH = unfractionated heparin, F = facilitated. LVF = left ventricular function, EF = ejection fraction. ESVI = endsystolic volume index

Ticagrelor an oral, reversible, direct-acting inhibitor of the adenosine diphosphate receptor P2Y12 with more rapid onset and pronounced platelet inhibition has not adequately studied in STEMI treated with fibrinolytics. The *PLATO trail* a multicenter, double-blind, randomized trial, compared ticagrelor (180-mg loading dose, 90 mg twice daily thereafter) to clopidogrel (300-to-600-mg loading dose, 75 mg daily subsequently) for the prevention of cardiovascular events in 18,624 ACS patients with or without STEMI. Ticagrelor as compared with clopidogrel significantly reduced the rate of death from vascular causes, MI, or stroke without an increase in the rate of overall major bleeding but with an increase in the rate of non-procedure-related bleeding [123].

Fibrinolytics and gp IIb/IIIa inhibitors were studied in many trials. Initial trials were performed with full doses of both agents (Table 9) [124,125]. *In terms of risk and benefits;* these trials consistently showed improvement in the angiographic and ECG measures of reperfusion, but with concerns of bleeding risks with this combination therapy that guided the evaluation of partial-dose fibrinolytic therapy with GP IIb/IIIa inhibition combination [126,127].

The dose-finding phase of the *TIMI-14* (677 patients). Subjects studied received partial-dose t-PA (20 mg, 35mg, 50 mg, or 65 mg) with abciximab (ABX) (0.25 mg/kg bolus/0.125 microg/kg/min infusion) or ABX with SK, 0.5, 0.75, 1.25, or 1.5 million units. Heparin 60 U/kg bolus/7 U/kg infusions. *In terms of risk and benefits:* ABX accelerates thrombolysis, with marked increases in TIMI 3 flow when combined with half dose alteplase without an increase in the risk of major bleeding. Substantial reductions in heparin dosing may reduce the risk of bleeding. Modest improvements in TIMI 3 flow can be achieved when combination of ABX and SK is used, but with increased risk of bleeding [127].

Similarly, the Strategies for Patency Enhancement in the Emergency Department study (*SPEED study*) (Table 9) randomized 304 patients to full-dose Abciximab (ABX) alone or ABX + r-PA. The preferred combination of r-PA (5 U + 5 U) with ABX compared to standard dosage (10 U + 10 U) of r-PA in 224 additional patients. In this angiographic trial, TIMI-3 flow rates at 60 to 90 min with half-dose r-PA and ABX, standard r-PA, and ABX alone were 62%, 47%, and 27%, respectively. Major bleeding

rates in phase A were 3.3% for ABX alone, 5.3% for abciximab + r-PA; rates in phase B were 9.8% for ABX + r-PA 5+5 U and 3.7% for r-PA alone. The increased patency rates observed with combination therapy may further decrease mortality [126].

GUSTO-V enrolled 16,588 patients within 6 h of STEMI. Patients were randomized in a 1:1 ratio to receive standard-dose r-PA (10U + 10U,30-min apart) andheparin (5,000-U bolus followed by 1,000 U/h) or a combination of ABX (0.25 mg/kg bolus, 0.125 microg/kg/min infusion—maximum 10 microg/min) for 12 h with half-dose r-PA (5 U + 5 U, 30 min apart) with 60 U/kg (5,000 U maximum) followed by 7 U/kg/h. The primary end point of 30-day mortality is similar in both r-PA - and combination treated patients (5.9% vs. 5.6%; OR, 0.95; 95% CI, 0.83 to 1.08; p = 0.43). *In term of risks:* Similar incidence of nonfatal disabling stroke or any stroke between the two groups with double risk of ICH in patient >75 years (1.1% vs. 2.1%; p =0.069).*In terms of benefits;* Re-infarction rates (3.5% vs. 2.3%, p<0.0001) and recurrent ischemia (12.8% vs. 11.3%, p<0.0001) were significantly reduced with combination therapy. Similar 1-year all-cause mortality in the r-PA -alone and combination therapy was found (Table 9) [61,128].

The ASSENT-3 described above; showed similar rates of all stroke (1.49% vs. 1.52%) and ICH (0.94% vs. 0.93%) for combination therapy as compared to standard treatment. Total, major, and minor bleeding rates were all significantly higher with combination treatment. Major bleeding with combination therapy in the elderly was noticeably higher than with TNKase therapy alone (13.3% vs. 4.1%) [118]. Consequently GUSTO-V and ASSENT-3 findings call attention to abciximab combination with half-dose fibrinolytic has a beneficial effect on the end point of re-infarction, with no impact on short or long-term mortality.

INTRO AMI trial randomized patients to receive double-bolus eptifibatide, with 50-mg t-PA; eptifibatide, with standard, full-dose, weight-adjusted t-PA. TIMI-3 flow rates at 60 min for the 3 groups were: 42%, 56%, and 40%, respectively. The median TIMI frame count was significantly lower with combination therapy, with similar rates of major bleeding and ICH [129].

The *INTEGRITI* trial, the Integrilin and TNKase in Acute Myocardial Infarction phase II angiographic trial [60] (Table 8) enrolled 438 patients within 6 h of STEMI. The combination of eptifibatide with half-dosage TNKase and UFH selected after the dose-finding phase. TIMI-3 flow was similar (59% vs. 49%, P = 0.15), as well as overall patency (85% vs.77%, p = 0.17), and ST-segment resolution (71% vs. 61%, p = 0.08) as standard TNKase monotherapy (0.53 mg/kg). ICH risk was 0.6% with combination therapy vs. 1.7% with standard therapy. Other trial (130) on other potent antiplatelet is summarized in Table 9.

6.2 Fibrinolytics with Unfractionated (UFH) vs. Low Molecular Weight Heparin (LMWH)

Fibrinolytic in combination with anticoagulants had been tested in many trials (Table 10) [57,59,62, 131-139]. Patient receiving SK, anistreplase, or t-PA in the ISIS-3 and GISSI-2 trials [36,37] received adjunctive SC heparin or no heparin. Treatment with SC heparin 12,500 IU initiated 12 hrs. in GISSI-2 and 4 hrs. in ISIS-3. In ISIS-3, an initial mortality reduction was observed but not at one month. There was an increase in hemorrhagic stroke (0.1- 0.2%) and excess bleeding (0.3-0.5%) with heparin. A combined analysis of the two trials showed *in terms of benefits*: early mortality reduction (0.5%) with heparin during the treatment period (6% vs. 7.3%) but not at 35 days or 6 months. *In term of risk;* heparin increases the absolute major bleeding of 3.2±0.7%. Heparin (IV and SC with SK) in the GUSTO-I trial bore similar clinical outcomes of death and re-infarction (with a propensity to increased rates of bleeding and hemorrhagic stroke with IV UFH).

The evidence for use of heparin with t-PA is sounder with higher patency rate. The superiority of front-loaded t-PA with UFH over SK in the GUSTO-I trial led to widespread clinical use of the t-PA/UFH. In large trials with t-PA GUSTO-I, GUSTO-IIb, TIMI 9B, COBALT, and GUSTO-III—all utilized heparin (5,000-U bolus + 1,000 U/h). Newer t-PA derivatives have all been tested in combination with UFH; therefore, information regarding its contributory beneficial effects is not available [29,131,132].The rate if ICH in GUSTO-I trial was 0.72% [133]. Higher heparin infusion rate (higher PTT) in the GUSTO-IIA and TIMI 9-A studies resulted in a prohibitive increase in ICH that was more evident with SK (3%). Heparin dosages decreased afterwards in the TIMI-9B and GUSTO-II B trials. It is preferable to use weight-adjusted bolus heparin (aPTT: 50 –70 s) irrespective of the reaction of the thromboplastin

[57]. The use of an early 3-h aPTT in TIME-II trial resulted in an observed ICH rate of 0.62%. These Data suggest 60 U/kg bolus with maintenance of 12U/kg/h is adequate with fibrin-specific agents [61], though no differences in patency rate in the combination of heparin (IV or SC) with SK vs. t-PA [127]. Patency appeared to be better with IV heparin with t- PA [128,97]. Close dose weight adjustment of IV heparin may decrease the risk of non-cerebral bleeding [57,110].

The largest trial comparing LMWH to UFH after fibrinolytic therapy completed to date was the ASSE*NT-3 trial* (standard dose of enoxaparin + TNKase for 7 days), enoxaparin reduced in-hospital re-infarction/refractory ischemia in contrast to heparin (Tables 10 and 4) [57]. Though, in the *ASSENT-3 PLUS* (n=1639) trial, pre-hospital administration of the same dose of enoxaparin showed significant increase in ICH rate in elderly patients [62]. In the large *ExTRACT trial* (Table 10) (n = 20,506), a lower dose of enoxaparin was given to patients >75 years and impaired renal function patients (estimated GFR: 30 mL/min).Significant reduction in the risk of death and re-infarction at 30 days vs. weight adjusted heparin dose on the cost of a significant increase in non-cerebral bleeding complications was observed (Tables 10 and 4) [134,135].

Second Trial of Heparin and Aspirin Reperfusion Therapy (HART II) (400 patients); non-inferiority of enoxaparin versus UFH for 3 days with an accelerated t-PA and aspirin in regard to IRA patency (Table 10). The 90 minutes patency rates (TIMI flow grade II/III) of 80.1% and 75.1% respectively. Re-occlusion at 5-7 days from TIMI grade 2/3 - TIMI 0 or 1 flow and TIMI grade 3 - TIMI 0/1 flow, respectively, occurred in 5.9% and 3.1% of the enoxaparin group vs. 9.8% and 9.1% in the UFH group with similar adverse events [136].It is worthy to mention that GP IIb/IIIa antagonists were not used in this trial. Guidelines issued by the ACC and AHA for the treatment AMI at the time of this trial recommend the adjunctive use of intravenous UFH in patients undergoing reperfusion therapy with thrombolytic agents. The guidelines advocate starting UFH at the initiation of thrombolytic therapy and continuing for 48 hours, or longer for patients at high risk of systemic or venous thromboembolism [136].

In the large *OASIS-6 trial*, a low dose of fondaparinux (synthetic indirect anti-Xa agent)

was superior to placebo or heparin in preventing death and re-infarction in 5436 patients who received fibrinolytic therapy. In the subgroup of 1021 patients in whom concomitant heparin was felt to be indicated fondaparinux was not superior to heparin in preventing death, re-infarction, or major bleeding complications (Table 10). However, this trial has limitation; it is not proposed to have sufficient power to independently examine the impact of fondaparinux in various subgroups, it is planned to have adequate power to detect clinically outcomes founded on the overall study population. The separate analysis of the main types of reperfusion therapy (primary PCI, thrombolytic and no reperfusion) was pre-specified in statistical analysis plan [137].

In *FRAMI study,* a multicenter, randomized, double blind; placebo-controlled trial investigated the efficacy and safety of dalteparin in the prevention of arterial thromboembolism after anterior AMI of subcutaneous dalteparin. Thrombolytic therapy and aspirin were administered in 91.5% and 97.6% of patients, respectively; dalteparin significantly reduced LV thrombus formation in anterior AMI but on the expense of increased hemorrhagic risk. (Table 10) [138], one more trial (139) described in Table 10.

6.3 Fibrinolytics and Direct Thrombin Inhibitors

Direct thrombin inhibitors (DTIs) have endured broad evaluation in conjunction with fibrinolytic therapy. DTI should be utilized as an alternative to heparin in the setting of STEMI when heparin induced thrombocytopenia (HIT) is an issue. Individual trials have not shown a dramatic improvement in clinical outcomes with DTIs as adjuncts to fibrinolytic therapy in AMI. The effects of hirudin with thrombolysis were tested in the TIMI-5, TIMI-6, and TIMI-9, *GUSTO-IIb,* Hirudin for the Improvement of Thrombolysis-3 *(HIT-III)* and Hirudin for the Improvement of Thrombolysis-4 trials *(HIT-III).*

In *TIMI-5,* a randomized, dose-ranging of hirudin vs. heparin as adjunctive with rt-PA administered to patients with AMI. Lower rate of re-infarction was observed with hirudin vs. heparin (4.3% vs. 11.9%, p = 0.03) and less re-occlusion (1.6% vs. 6.7%, p = 0.07) [140]. In the pilot trial *TIMI-6,* (193patients)*:* high dose hirudin achieved lower death and nonfatal re-infarction after 6 weeks vs. lowest dose (5.7% vs. 17.6%) with similar

incidence of major hemorrhage in heparin and hirudin dose groups At hospital discharge the occurrence of death, nonfatal re-infarction, CHF, or cardiogenic shock was greater with lowest dose of hirudin (21.6%) than in those receiving the higher doses of hirudin (dose 2 = 9.7%, dose 3 = 11.4%) [141].

In *HIT-III study*; 7000 AMI patients within 6 hours of chest pain were randomized to IV heparin or hirudin. Thetrial was stopped after increased rate of ICH observed in the hirudin group than heparin group (3.4% vs. 0 %) with stroke rate of 3.4% vs. 1.3% respectively. The safety findings from HIT-III were not strictly conclusive; the high rates of life-threatening bleeding in 3 independent trials (TIMI-9 and GUSTO-II and HIT III) with two hirudins and two different fibrinolytics gave important concern. In addition to patient selection (age, comorbidity), the combination of hirudin with fibrinolytics per se might increase the risk of bleeding by potentiating effects on lytic agent and/or hemostasis mechanisms. It may be simply an unrecognized dosing issue in phase II studies. The similar observed bleeding rates with significantly lower doses of hirudin in the HIT-III trial than in the GUSTO II and TIMI 9 trials point to a finer therapeutic range when combined with thrombolytics [142]. In HIT-4 trial: Lepirudin as adjunct to thrombolysis with SK did not significantly improve restoration of blood flow in the IRA as assessed by angiography with no increase in the risk of major bleedings with lepirudin [143].

GUSTO-IIb trial, hirudin tested in >12,000 ACS patients. Re-infarction rates were less with hirudin (5.4% vs. 6.3% for heparin, p = 0.04), with a trend toward reduction in death or MI at 30 days. In patients with STEMI, the incidence of death or MI was slightly lower with hirudin (9.9% vs. 11.3%, p = 0.13). A captivating trend toward a greater advantage of hirudin in patients treated with SK vs. t-PA, which is not observed in TIMI-9B. In the phase III, *TIMI-9B trial,* less re-infarction was noted during hospitalization (2.3% vs. 3.4%, p = 0.07), however there was no differences in the primary end point of death, MI, CHF, or shock at 30 days for hirudin vs. heparin (12.9% vs. 11.9% p = NS) [144,145].

A meta-analysis of 9,947 subjects (from 5 trails) reported a significant reduction in the end point of recurrent MI with DTI, compared to heparin therapy (2.5% vs. 3.4%), with overall mortality 4.1% vs. 3.9% respectively. No significant reduction in the combined end point of death and recurrent MI (6.3% vs. 6.9%) [145].

In a pilot study; *Hirulog Early Reperfusion/Occlusion (HERO) trial*, double-blind, randomized angiographic trial randomized patients to Hirulog 0.5 mg/kg/hour for 12 hours followed by 0.1 mg/kg per hour (low dose), Hirulog 1.0 mg/kg per hour for 12 hours followed by placebo (high dose), or to heparin 5000 U bolus followed by 1000 U/h titrated to aPTT of 2-2.5 times control after 12 hours. Hirulog achieved higher patency rates in the culprit artery with Hirulog combined with SK and aspirin in the early phase of AMI. Serious bleeding complications were observed in 22% of patients treated with the low dose of Hirulog, 18% with the high dose of Hirulog, and 31% with heparin. Blood transfusion needed in 5% of the Hirulog-treated patients and 31% of the heparin (P<0.02). No ICH or stroke was reported [146]. The superior TIMI grade 3 flow achieved with the combination of SK and bivalirudin in the *HERO-1* study had hearten to conduct of the *HERO-2 trial*, (17,073 patients with STEMI) randomized to adjunctive therapy with heparin vs. bivalirudin following initial SK treatment. In this trial; *in terms of benefits:* No reduction in the primary 30-day mortality end point with bivalirudin (10.8% vs. 10.9%; p = 0.85). *In terms of risk:*Severe bleeding occurred in 0.7% of bivalirudin group vs. 0.5% of the heparin group (p = 0.07), and ICH occurred in 0.6% vs. 0.4%, respectively (p=0.09). Moderate and mild bleeding was significantly higher in the bivalirudin group. Transfusions needed in 1.4% in the bivalirudin group vs. 1.1% in the heparin group (p = 0.11) [147].

7. FIBRINOLYSIS AND PRIMARY PERCUTANEOUS CORONARY REVASCULARIZATION, WHICH IS BETTER? (TABLE 11)

Several trials compared primary coronary revascularization with thrombolysis and subsequently several investigators performed meta-analysis of these trials in an attempt to determine if one strategy is superior to the other. (Table 11)

In an overview of 7 trials comprising 1,145 patients with STEMI treated with either primary angioplasty or thrombolysis (streptokinase or t-PA). Those undergoing PPCI had a considerable reduction in short term mortality up to 6 weeks with no long-term follow up data for mortality comparisons [148].

A review of 10 trials [149] totaling 2,606 patients included the in PAMI study [150] and GUSTO IIB cohorts was done [151]. PPCI was compared to thrombolytic therapy in which 4 trials utilized strepokinase, 3 used accelerated t-PA and 3 used standard dose t-PA. At 30-days, PPCI resulted in lower mortality (4.4% vs. 6.5%), lower death or re-infarction (7.2% vs. 11.9%) but similar hemorrhagic stroke (0.1% vs. 1.1%), such results were similar among the various thrombolytic agents used. Again there was insufficient long-term data available for evocative comparisons but GUSTO IIB 6 month follow-up showed significant decrease in the short term benefits ascribed to primary angioplasty [151].

The Cochrane database reviewed 10 trials (2,573 patients), PPCI was associated with significant relative risk reduction in short-term mortality (RRR 32%, 95% CI 5-50%), death or re-infarction (RRR 46%, 95% CI 30-58%) and stroke (RRR 66%, 95% CI 28-84%) [152]. A subgroup analysis comparing results from the largest study, GUSTO IIB, to the pooled analysis was done. The results from GUSTO IIB were less imposing than the pooled data, suggesting that the mortality benefit of primary angioplasty is less impressive when performed in community hospitals, as in GUSTO IIB. Another possible explanation is the use of non-optimal thrombolytic therapy (streptokinase or standard dose t-PA) in the other pooled trials vs. accelerated t-PA that was used in GUSTO IIB. Every et al. analyzed at data from the *Myocardial Infarction Triage and Intervention (MITI)* registry comparing 1,050 patients underwent primary angioplasty with 2,095 patients had thrombolytic therapy (2/3 t-PA, 1/3 streptokinase), established no difference in 4 years mortality [153]. Data from the second National Registry of Myocardial Infarction (NRMI-2) Comparing 4,939 patients undergoing primary angioplasty with 24,705 patients undergoing thrombolytic therapy (92% accelerated t-PA). For patients not in cardiogenic shock, in hospital mortality was similar for groups (5.2% vs. 5.4%) and death/non-fatal stroke (5.6% vs. 6.2%). Cardiogenic shock patients had significantly lower in hospital mortality in the primary angioplasty group (32.4% vs. 52.3%, p<0.0001) [154].

Many other studies [155-176] that compare primary angioplasty with thrombolysis are summarized in (Table 11).

Table 9. Clinical trials of full-dose fibrinolytic therapy with anti-platelet; agents clopedogril, GP IIb/IIIa inhibition

Trial/year	Patients no.	Primary treatment	Benefits:TIMI 3 Flow at 90 Min, %	Risk
CLARITY-TIMI 28 [120]	3491	Clopidogrel (300-mg loading dose, followed by 75 mg once daily) or placebo+ fibrinolytic + Wt. adjusted heparin	improves the patency rate of the infarct-related artery, ▼ ischemic complications	-Similar rates of major bleeding and ICH in the two groups
COMMIT [121]	45,852	Clopedogril 75 mg+aspirin 162 mg + slandered fibrinolysis	▼ mortality and major vascular events in hospital	-No significant excess risk was noted with clopidogrel, in regards fatal, transfused, or cerebral bleeds together,
PLATO trail [122]	18,624 ACSpts. with /without ST elevation.	Ticagrelcr (180-mg loading dose, 90 mg twice daily thereafter) vs. clopidogrel (300-to-600-mg loading dose, 75 mg daily thereafter)	Ticagrelorvs. clopidogrel significantly ▼ the rate of death from vascular causes, MI, or stroke 9.8% vs. 11.7%	No ▲ in the rate of overall major bleeding but with ▲ in the rate of non-procedure-related bleeding.
INTEGRITI [60]	438	-Eptifibatide + TNK +heparin 60 U/kg bolus; 7 U/kg/h infusion -TNK alore 60 U/kg bolus; 12 U/kg/h infusion	TIMI 3 Flow/ 90 Min =62%, TIMI 3 Flow/ 90 Min =49%	▲ Major hemorrhage (7.6% vs. 2.5%, p = 0.14) and transfusions (13.4% vs. 4.2%, p = 0.02). ICH = 1.0%, 0.6%, & 1.7% of patients treated with any combination, eptifibatide 180/2/180 & 1/2dose TNK, &TNK monotherapy, respectively.
TAMI-8 [123]	68	m7E3 +t-PA	▲ angiographic patency. Less recurrent ischemia m7E3 Fab-treated patients vs. control subjects (13%vs 20%)	- 25% m7E3 Fab-treated patients vs. 50%)control patients had major bleeding
IMPACT-AMI [124]	132	Eptifibatide +t-PA	▲ acute TIMI grade 3 flow &faster ECG resolution vs. t-PA	-Similar rates of the composite end point (43% versus 42% for placebo-treated patients) & severe bleeding (4% vs. 5%, respectively).
GUSTO-V [61,127]	16,588	-r-PA +heparin vs. r-PA ½ dose +abciximab	Rates of re-infarction (p <0.0001) &recurrent ischemia no difference in the incidence of nonfatal disabling stroke or any stroke in two groups but not above 75 yr	-No difference in the incidence of nonfatal disabling stroke or any stroke between 2 groups. Patient aged > 75 years receiving combination therapy, had a double ICH risk (1.1% vs. 2.1%; p =0.069
SPEED [125]	528	-Abciximab + r-PA + heparin 60 U/kg boluses -Abciximab + r-PA + heparin 40 U/kg boluses -r-PA + heparin 70 U/kg boluses	TIMI 3 Flow/ 90 Min 61% TIMI 3 Flow/ 90 Min =51% TIMI 3 Flow/ 90 Min =47%	-Major bleeding rates in phase A were 3.3% for abciximab alone & 5.3% for abciximab + r-PA 5+5 U; rates in phase B were 9.8% for abciximab + r-PA 5+5 U and 3.7% for r-PA alone. - Major bleeding was similar with standard- or low-dose heparin (6.3% vs. 10.5%, P=0.30).
TIMI-14 [126]	888	-t-PA+ abciximab + heparin60 U/kg bolus; 7 U/kg/h infusion-t-PA + abciximab +heparin 30 U/kg bolus; 4 U/kg/h infusion-t-PA alone +heparin70 U/kg bolus; 15 U/kg/h infusion	TIMI 3 Flow/ 90 Min =78% TIMI 3 Flow/ 90 Min =69% TIMI 3 Flow/ 90 Min =62%	-The SK study arm was abandoned due to unacceptable bleeding risk. -With standard t-PA treatment with no difference in the overall major bleeding rate (7%)
INTRO AMI [128]	649	-Eptifibatide + t-PA + heparin 60 U/kg bolus; 7 U/kg/h infusion -t-PA alone + heparin60 U/kg bolus; 7 U/kg/h infusion	TIMI 3 Flow/ 90 Min= 56% TIMI 3 Flow/ 90 Min= 40%	-Similar rates of major bleeding & ICH.in both groups
PARADIGM [129]	345	Lamifiban + t-PA or SK	▲ST-segment resolution vs. fibrinolytic alone	-More bleeding associated with lamifiban (transfusions in 16.1% lamifiban-treated vs. 10.3% placebo-treated patients)

▼ = Decrease, ▲ = Increase, = Equal,r-PA= reteplase, t-PA = Alteplase, SK = streptokinase

Table 10. Trials of fibrinolytics with unfractionated heparin (UFH) versus low-molecular weight heparin (LMWH)

Trial/year	Patients no.	Fibrinolytic agent	LMWH group vs. control group	Primary efficacy outcome	Benefits & risks
OASIS-6 trial [135]	5436	Predominantly SK	Fundapurinoxvs UFH	30-d death, in-hospital re-infarction,	-Significant ▼the risk of death, re-MI &severe bleeds
ExTRACT trial [133,134]	20506	SK or fibrin specific fibrinolysis	Enox. throughout hospitalization or UFH for at least 48 h	30-d death, in-hospital re MI, in-hospital refractory ischemia	-Significant ▼in the risk of death &re-infarction at 30 vs. weight adjusted heparin dose, but with a significant ▲ in non-cerebral bleeding complications.
ASSENT-3 PLUS [62]	1,639	Tenecteplase	Enox 30 mg IV bolus pre-hospital + 1 mg/kg sc. bid (up to 7 days) vs. UFH	30-d death, in-hospital re-infarction, in-hospital refractory ischemia	-53% of pts.to receive pre-hospital fibrinolysis within 2 hrs. of symptom onset. combination of tenecteplase + Enox ▼early ischemic events,
ENTIRE-TIMI 23 [59]	483	full or half-dose tenecteplase + abciximab	Enox30 mg IV bolus+ 1 mg/kg SC bid (up to 8 d) vs. UFH	TIMI 3 flow (60 min)	-Enox associated with similar TIMI 3 flow rates as UFH at an early time point
Baird et al. [138]	300	SK, anistreplase,or t-PA	Enox40 mg IV bolus+ 40 mg SC tid (96 h) vs. UFH	Death, reinfarction, or unstable angina readmission (30 d)	-Fewer recurrent cardiac events at 90 days. -Independent of other important clinical and therapeutic factors.
AMI-SK [131]	496	SK	Enox 30 mg IV bolus+1 mg/kg bid (3–8 d) vs. placebo	TIMI 3 flow (5–10 d)	-Triple clinical end-point of death, re-infarction & recurrent angina at 30 days ▼ with Enox 13% vs. placebo21%,P=0.03
ASSENT-3 [57]	4,075	Tenecteplase	Enox 30 mg IV bolus+ 1 mg/kg SC bid (upto 7 d) vs. UFH	30-d death, in hospital re infarction, refractory ischemia	- ▼ The risk of in-hospital re-infarction or in-hospital refractory ischemia compared to heparin.
HART II [135]	400‡	t-PA	Enox 30 mg IV bolus + 1 mg/kg SC bid (3 d) vs. UFH	IRA patency (90 min)	-▲ recanalization rates & ▼ re-occlusion at 5 to 7 days -Similar frequency of adverse events in both treatment groups
BIOMACS II [130]	101	SK	Dalteparin 100 IU/kg pre SK + 120 IU/kg at 12 h vs. placebo	TIMI 3 flow (20–28 h)	-▲ rate of TIMI grade 3 flow in infarct-related artery compared to placebo, 68% vs.51% (p = 0.10). -Dalteparin had no effects on noninvasive signs of early reperfusion
FRAMI [137]	776	SK	Dalteparin 150 IU/kg bid (in hospital) vs. Placebo	LV thrombus + Arterial thromboembolism (9 d)	-Significantly ▼ LV thrombus formation in anterior AMI , ▲ hemorrhagic risk

IRA = infarct related artery, Enox = Enoxaparin, UFH; unfractionated heparin, LV ; left ventricular , ▼ = Decrease, ▲ = Increase , SK = streptokinase

Table 11. Studies comparing fibrinolysis and primary angioplasty

Author	Registry	Patient no	Mean age	Result
Yan AT et al. Canada [155]	TRANSFER-AMI trial	1200 pts. high-risk STEMI presenting to non-PCI centers.	---------	-Early routine PCI associated with ▼ rate of death/re-MI at 30 days in the low-intermediate risk stratum (8.1 vs. 2.9%, P<0.001), but an ▲ rate of death/re-MI in the high-risk group (13.8 vs. 27.8%, P=0.025)
Pipilis et al. (156) Greece	HELIOS Registry(a cohort)	PCI n=84, 9.7% & FL n=497,57.1%	61 ± 12 vs62 ± 13	In hospital mortality 3.6% In PCI group & 4.6% in FL group. MR 30 days& at 6 months = 7.2% &11.3% in PCI group &5.8% & 7.1% in FL group, respectively.
Gao RL et al. China [157]	multicenter randomized clinical trial	PCI group n=101; (r-Sk) group (n=104); & (rt-PA) group (n=106)	57.33±9.18	FL with rescue PCI associated with ▼ rates of coronary patency & TIMI flow grade 3, ▼MR, death/MI & hemorrhagic complications at 30 days vs. PPCI in this group of STEMI pts with late presentation & delayed treatments. life-threatening hemorrhage =2.9%
Itoh T et al. Japan [158]	IMPORTANT study multicenter, prospective, randomized study	101 pts. have prior-t-PA group (n=50) & PPCI group (n=51).	55.8±10.6	Patency rate & LVEF in the prior-t-PA group▲than in the P-PCI group (69% vs. 17%, P<0.001; 61.6±9.5% vs. 55.0±11.6%, P=0.01). The MACE-free rate in the prior-t-PA group ▼ than PPCI group (58.7% vs. 80.9%; P=0.03). The MACE-free rate in the F-PCI group = to PPCI group (73.7% vs. 80.9%; P=0.39), MACE-free rate in the prior-t-PA-alone group ▼ in the PPCI group (48.1% vs. 80.9%; P=0.01)
StoltSteiger V et al. Switzerland [159]	Swiss prospective national registry data ACS in (AMIS Plus).	12 026 STEMI pts In 68 hospitals.	64 ± 13 years ,73% male	In-hospital MR & re-infarction rate ▼ significantly in Swiss STEMI pts in the last 7 years, parallel to a significant ▲ in the number of PCI + medical therapy. Outcome is not related to the site of admission but to PCI access.
Soares et al. Brazil [160]	cohort, observational, prospective	158 pts. with STEMI	60.8 years (22-89)	TT used in only 33% of cases. Death rate 21.2% vs. 2.1 in angioplasty treated pt. major bleeding =2.2%
Busk M et al. Denmark [161]	DANAMI-2 trial	1572 pts. with STEMI	63 (54–73) years	angioplasty vs. FL.; the composite endpoint occurred in 20.1 vs. 26.7% (P =0.007), death in 13.6 vs. 16.4% (P = 0.18), I re-infarction in 8.9 vs. 12.3% (P = 0.05). stroke in 3.2 vs. 4.7% (P = 0.23)
Prieto et al. Chile [162]	GEMI network, from 2001 to 2005	3,255 pts.	FL= 60 ± 11 in PCI =60 ± 13	MR in TT group= 10.2% (7.6% in men &18.7% in women, p <0.01). for pts treated with PPCI, was 4.7% (2.5% in men & 13% in women, p <0.01).
Di Mario et al. [163] France, Italy,& Poland	CARESS-in-AMI trial	600 pts. ▶ PPCI vs. rescue PCI 1/2-dose after FL	75 years or younger	Death, re-infarction, refractory ischemia at 30 days occurred in 4.4%.in the immediate PCI group compared 10.7% in the standard care/rescue PCI group (HR 0.40; 95% CI 0.21-0.76, log rank p=0.004). Major bleeding ▶ (3.4%vs 2.3%, p=0.47). Strokes ▲ (0.7%vs 1.3%, p=0.50).
Grajek et al. Poland [164]	Wielkopolska regional 2002 Registry (WIRE Registry)	3780 pts. with STEMI	59.1±11.6 yr. - PCI. 56.1±10,4 yr. in r-TPA gp. 65.6±11.8 l yr. SK gp.	t-PA in pts.under 70 years of age &up to 4 hours from pain onset may be an alternative to an invasive strategy. 25% pts. require urgent PCI. In long-term mortality benefit can be clearly seen only in early PCI Patient.
Greig et al. Chile [165]	Chilean National Registry of Acute MI	1,634 STEMI pts. 72% ▶ FL	967 pts, 60±12 yrs, 77% Males.	Hospital MR among pts. treated with FL =10.9% & PCI= 5.6% (p =0.01),
Nallamothu B et al. [166]	GRACE a prospective, observational cohort study 106 hospitals	1786 (45.1%) pts. have FL	63 (53 to 73)	Treatment delays associated with ◀6-month mortality in both FL & PPCI pts (p<0.001) with FL, 6-month MR ▲ by 0.30% per 10-min delay in door-to-needle time= 30 & 60 min compared with 0.18% per 10-min delay in door-to-balloon time between 90 & 150 min for PPCI pts.

	in 14 countries			
Widimsky et al. Czech Rep [167]	The PRAGUE-2 trial	850 STEMI pts. in non cath lab hospitals in 12 h	64 (31–86)years	At 5 years follow up TT compared to transfer PCI 53% vs. 40%.cumulative all-cause mortality 23 vs.19% recurrent infarction 19 vs. 12%, stroke 8 vs. 8%, revascularization 51 vs. 34%
Kalla et al. Austria.[168]	Vienna STEMI Registry	1053 pts with acute STEMI	60.8±13.0	PPCI usage ▲ from 16% to almost 60%, the use of FL ▼ from 50.5% to 26.7% in the participating centers. In-hospital MR ▼from 16% to 9.5%, including pts not receiving RT. PPCI & FL have comparable in-hospital MR when initiated within 2 to 3 hrs. from onset of symptoms, PPCI more effective in acute STEMI of >3 but <12 hours' duration.
Boersma E et al. [169]	25 randomized trials analysis testing the efficacy of PPCI vs. FL	7743 pt. / 3383 receive FL	62 (53–71)	In FL ; over all Death 7.9%, re-infarction 6.7%, Death or re-infarction 13.5%, Stroke =2.2% PPCI associated 37% ▼ in 30-day mortality [adj. OR; 0.63; 95% CI (0.420.84)].
McNamara RL et al. USA [170]	Retrospective observational study from the National Registry of MI 3 & 4	FL; n=68,439 pts. PCI n=33,647 pts.	61.7 (13.0) in FL 61.8 (13.2) in PCI	46% of the pts.in the FL cohort treated within the recommended 30-minute door-to-needle time; 35% of the pts. in the PCI cohort treated within 90-minute door-to-balloon time
Rathore et al. [171]	a randomized controlled trial	47882 AMI pts.	76 (70-82)yr	30-day MR ▲ in pts.with ▲TIMI scores (TIMI score 2: 4.4% vs. TIMI score >8:35.6%, P <0.0001 for trend).
Magid DJ et al. USA [172]	Cohort study 1999 2002.	68 439 pts. with STEMI,FL & 33 647 treated with PCI)	Age, mean (SD), y 63 ±(13)	Overall, after adjusting for all pts. covariates. pts. presenting during off-hours had significantly ▲ in-hospital mortality than pts. presenting during regular hours (OR, 1.07; 95% CI, 1.01-1.14; P=0.02).
Fassa AA et al. Switzerland [173]	AMIS Plus project : prospective ACS registry	PPCI, n = 1419 FL ;n = 2833	60.2 (12.5) vs. 62.7 (12.4)	In-hospital MR ▼over the study period (p , 0.001). in-hospital mortality predictors by multivariate analysis ;PPCI (OR) 0.52, 95% (CI) 0.33 to 0.81, TT (OR 0.63, 95% CI 0.47 to 0.83), and Killip class III (OR 3.61, 95% CI 2.49 to 5.24) & class IV (OR 5.97, 95% CI 3.51 to 10.17) at admission
Danchin et al. [174]	French Nationwide USIC 2000 Registry /FAST MI	1922 AMI pts.	median age, 67 yrs.; 73% men)	In-hospital death = 3.3% for pre-hospital FL, 8.0% for in-hospital FL 6.7% for PPCI, 1-year survival = 94%, 89%, 89%,respectively
Dalby et al. [175]	meta-analysis 6 clinical trials	3750 pts.	-----	Re-infarction ▼by 68% (95% CI, 34% to 84%; P=0.001) & stroke by 56% (95% CI, _15% to 77%; P_0.015). ▼ In all-cause mortality of 19% (95% CI,=3% to 36%; P=0.08) with transfer PCI.
Sakurai k et al. [176] Japan	Registry of Miyagi Study Group for AMI (MsAMI)	3,258 AMI pts.	66.5 years	30-day in-hospital MR = 12.7% for IV-T, 3.7% for IC-T, 4.8% for rescue PCI, covariate-adjusted OR (95% CI) =0.38 (0.28–0.52) for PPCI, 0.30 (0.15–0.60) for IC-T, 1.04 (0.51–2.10) for IV-FL & 0.77 (0.46–1.30) in rescue PCI.
Keeley et al. [179] USA	Meta- analysis of 23 trials	7739thrombolytic-eligible patients with STEMI-to PPCI (n=3872) or TT (n=3867).	short-term : 4-6 weeks long-term; 6–18 months	-PPCI was better than TT at:1)- ▼ overall short-term death (7% vs. 9%,p=0-0002), death excluding the SHOCK trial data (5%vs 7% , p=0-0003), non-fatal re-infarction (3% vs. 7%; p<0-0001), stroke (1% vs. 2% ;p=0-0004), & the combined endpoint of death, non-fatal re-infarction, &stroke (8% [253] vs. 14% [442]; p<0-0001). -PPCI was better than TT on long-term follow-up independent of both the type of thrombolytic agent used, and whether or not the patient was transferred for primary PTCA.

PCI = percutaneous coronary intervention, AMI = acute myocardial infarction, PPCI = primary percutaneous coronary intervention, FL = fibrinolysis, ACS= acute coronary syndrome, STEMI = ST elevation myocardial infarction, LVEF = left ventricular ejection fraction, RT = reperfusion therapy, TT =thrombolytic therapy, IC- T = intracoronary thrombolysis, F-PCI = facilitated percutaneous coronary intervention, MR = mortality rate, ▼ = Decrease, ▲ = Increase , ▶ = Equal, pts.= patients, hrs.= hours, yr.= year, yrs.= years

8. ROLE OF PRE-HOSPITAL THROMBOLYTIC THERAPY

Acute myocardial infarction (AMI) is the prototype of a real emergency that requires efficacy and speed for effective management. Reperfusion therapy should be initiated as early as possible. It is clear that in the early management of acute ischemic syndromes, saving time hoards lives, and several large studies have demonstrated that pre-hospital initiation of thrombolysis is feasible and safe with respect to contraindications. Pre-hospital thrombolytic therapy has been shown to reduce both short-term relative in hospital mortality by 11% to 51% and long-term mortality at 10 years [32,177]. The mortality gain is dependent on the delay time of early reperfusion, such relationship is best described as exponential: in the first 1 to 2 hours after the onset of chest pain, the benefit of thrombolysis is greater. In the last 15 years, a large number of strategies to reduce the time to reperfusion have been evaluated, including initiation of thrombolytic therapy prior to arrival to hospital. For example, in France, pre-hospital emergency medicine is a fundamental part of the medical care system, a hospital department whose function is to centralize emergency medical calls and organize an appropriate response with the intention of ensuring the shortest delay between the initial call and the appropriate treatment. Pre-hospital thrombolysis is currently the best treatment strategy. Such experience has proven that pre-hospital thrombolysis is both safe and effective. During the last 10-15 years the field of reperfusion during AMI was a real struggle zone between the proponents of thrombolysis and those of PPCI. Many physicians considered that the best way is not to oppose these two effective methods but to find the most appropriate role for each or even better to combine them to accomplish reperfusion. In this concept, the idea of facilitated percutaneous intervention is a very attractive one with promising results. A large number of studies demonstrated its efficacy and to help us choosing the ideal combination of anti-thrombotic agents to be used. That is one of the main interests of the *CAPTIM* study. French trial studied whether pre-hospital thrombolysis could counterbalance the efficacy of primary angioplasty in AMI, found no significant differences between the treatment strategies in the combined primary endpoint of 30-day death, re-infarction or stroke (8.2% in the pre-hospital thrombolysis group, 6.2% in the angioplasty group). The mortality rate, however, was lower in the pre-hospital thrombolysis group, with 33% of patients requiring rescue angioplasty [178]. In an ideal situation, thrombolysis should be started within the 2 first hours of injury (Golden Hour). But, most of the time, the patient calls for an ambulance later than these 2 first hours after onset of symptoms. That could be determinant in the real life for AMI. We have to deem in this study the fact than 33% of the patients had a pre hospital thrombolysis followed by a fast angioplasty. The results are impressing: the 30-day mortality in the pre-hospital thrombolysis arm is only 3.8%. But if the delay between pain to pre hospital thrombolysis is under 2 hours this 30 day mortality fall down to 2.2%. Such outcome: superior in allrecent trials published comparing on site thrombolysis to primary angioplasty (DANAM II, PRAGUE II) [161,167] and other trials [179] (Table 10). These good results in the CAPTIM study when the delay pain to treatment is less than 2 hours include also the occurrence of cardiogenic shock in favor of pre hospital thrombolysis (1.3%).

The good strategy in a next future could be the association of pre hospital thrombolysis and angioplasty. In a recent French registry (USIC 2000) [174] including all the patients arriving in coronary intensive care unit during a month and regardingone-month mortality (3.6%), this strategy seemed to be the best. TNK-t-PA is now changing the general management of pre-hospital AMI by reducing the time to treatment. This is clearly now the new standard of pre-hospital treatment. The reduction of UFH dose is recommended and the LMWH is considered as the next step as recently demonstrated in the ASSENT 3 and ASSENT 3 Plus trials. Several recent registries have shown than reperfusion offered to only half of the patients and may not offered which is unjustified in nearly half of the cases resulting in a very poor prognosis. The other major problem is that patients are treated too late mainly because the call for the emergency system too late. There are several ways to improve the time to treatment: information of the patients, shortening of the intra-hospital delays by better organization and finally and perhaps more importantly, pre hospital triage and treatment. The efficacy and safety of the pre hospital strategy is now recognized worldwide. The best strategy for AMI should involve emergency physicians and cardiologist in a real local task-force to join and coordinate their efforts.

9. FUTURE PERSPECTIVES

Thrombolytic therapy has been a foremost encroachment in the treatment of AMI, that is easy to administer compared to angioplasty. The therapeutic goal is early restoration of complete flow of IRA after the acute coronary occlusion that had great impact on the immediate and long-term morbidity and mortality. Several ways in which reperfusion rates and clinical outcomes can be improved: 1) Different dosing regimens of established agents. 2) Combinations of different agents. 3) Improved adjunctive therapy such as direct anti-thrombin agents, LMWH, or GP IIb/IIIa receptor antagonists. 4) Development of novel thrombolytic agents with enhanced fibrin specificity, resistance to native inhibitors, or prolonged half-lives allowing bolus administration. 5) Pre-hospital administration of fibrinolysis. Till the date of writing this article, the extensive developed researches include both clinical and angiographic trials with considerable patients population from different parts of the world. Most of these major trials included the early generations of non-fibrin selective fibrinolytic agent. To best of our knowledge, this is the first article, which summarizes all the clinical and angiographic trial in term of risks and benefits in detailed description.

In spite of the extensive researches, still there is missing information about the stratification of risk vs. benefit of fibrinolytics, regarding the time of administration (pre hospital administration). This target has been poorly studied. The combination of fibrinolytic therapy with newer antiplatelet agents with or without the use of newer antithrombotics may have great impact; it may increase the risk or improve the outcome of such mode of therapy.

As mentioned above the principal goal of benefits of thrombolytic (fibrinolytic) therapy is to achieve earliest reperfusion after the proper clinical diagnosis of STEMI, such aim may be compromised by many factors including: 1) when and where to administer the fibrinolytic agent. 2) The proper antiplatelet agent. 3) The target aim that the patency of the culprit vessel may be condensed by ensuing re-occlusion of the IRA which can result in loss of ventricular function that doubles the mortality rate. In addition to the risk of ICH and major bleed requiring emergency transfusion, such risk augmented with new advent of anti-platelets, anti-thrombin, patient age and associated morbidities. Physician using thrombolytic in AMI should be very meticulous in judging the risk benefit ratio and more careful patient's selection for thrombolysis, keeping in mind the absolute and relative contraindication for acute fibrinolysis. It is very sensitive decision making, giving the fact the ceiling of the time interval with aim to reduce the door - needle time as per guidelines recommendations.

Fibrinolytics are the most broadly studied drug in the history of medicine (200 000 patients) in both clinical (mortality and safety trials) and angiographic trials. It is still safe medicine in spite of the low risk of bleeding with relatively good re-canalization (up to 80%) rate specifically with the new adjuvant of platelets inhibitors. Further clinical trial needed in particular with the newer antiplatelet like third generation thienopyridine, Prasugrel and Ticagrelor which had not been tested adequately in combination with the fibrinolytics. To achieve this aim, researches are needed to administer these treatment as soon as the patient presented which is measured now as door to needle time, in fact we need to achieve shorter symptoms to needle time, to reach this aim, we need to establish proper system for diagnosis of STEMI; this can be accomplished starting from patients, family and public education. Pre-hospital administration of thrombolytics requires highly skilled staff, trained in ECG diagnosis of STMI with proper communication with cardiologist which may be possible with new electronics, keeping in mind the contraindication to use of thrombolytics. This in our opinion is the biggest challenge to optimize the potential and undiscovered benefits of thrombolytic.

Unfortunately the clinical trials are shifting to the angioplasty side probably due to the influence of industry. In spite of the emergence of the newer antiplatelet, no trial tested these with the newer fibrinolytics, though the fibrinolytics continue to be the most suitable and the mostly used way of recanalization of STEMI. It looks that fibrinolytics became part of the past from the research point of view though it is the most expanded in this field of thrombo-cardiology.

Again we think that research should directed to pre-hospital administration of thrombolytic that carries potential for higher recanalization rate in the setting of acute occlusion of coronary arteries though this carried a lot of legal and ethical challenges.

10. CONCLUSION

The management of AMI has been revolted in the last few decades with innovations in both the pharmacological and interventional field of clinical cardiology. Fibrinolytic agent considered the best easily accessible and administered pharmacologic agent keeping in mind the good patency and relative safety profile when used accurately and meticulously. Many improvements in pharmacological reperfusion appear possible. Not only a higher initial patency rates can be achieved and maintained, but the net clinical benefit resulting from successful reperfusion can probably also be increased. The "ideal" thrombolytic agent has not yet been developed. Judiciously accomplished dose-ranging studies to select the best dose for attainment of TIMI grade 3 flow with satisfactory safety profile are needed to improve the results with t-PA, together with large clinical trials to assess clinical end points and safety.

CONSENT

Not applicable.

ETHICAL APPROVAL

Not applicable.

COMPETING INTERESTS

Authors have declared that no competing interests exist.

REFERENCES

1. White HD, Van de Werf FJ. Thrombolysis for Acute Myocardial Infarction. Circulation. 1998;97:1632-1646.
2. Reimer KA, Lowe JE, Rasmussen MM, Jennings RB. The wave front phenomenon of ischaemic cell death. 1. Myocardial infarct size vs duration of coronary occlusion in dogs. Circulation. 1977;56:786-794.
3. Bishop SP, White FC, Bloor CM. Regional myocardial blood flow during acute myocardial infarction in the conscious dog. Circ Res. 1976;38:429-438.
4. Rivas F, Cobb FR, Bache RJ, Greenfield JC Jr. Relationship between blood flow to ischaemic regions and extent of myocardial infarction. Serial measurement of blood flow to ischaemic regions in dogs. Circ Res. 1976;38:439-447.
5. Fletcher AP, Alkjaersig N, Smyrniotis FE, Sherry S. The treatment of patients suffering from early myocardial infarction with massive and prolonged streptokinase therapy. Trans Assoc Am Physicians. 1958;71:287-296.
6. Yusuf S, Collins R, Peto R, et al. Intravenous and intracoronary fibrinolytic therapy in acute myocardial infarction: overview of results on mortality, reinfarction and side-effects from 33 randomized controlled trials. Eur Heart J. 1985;6:556-585.
7. Chazov EI, Matveeva LS, Mazaev AV, et al. Intracoronary administration of fibrinolysin in acute myocardial infarct. Ter Arkh. 1976;48:8-19.
8. Rentrop KP, Blanke H, Karsch KR, Wiegand V, et al. Acute myocardial infarction: intracoronary application of nitroglycerin and streptokinase. Clin Cardiol. 1979;2:354-363.
9. Six AJ, Louwerenburg HW, Braams R, et al. A double-blind randomized multicenter dose-ranging trial of intravenous streptokinase in acute myocardial infarction. Am J Cardiol. 1990;65:119-123
10. Anderson JL, Marshall HW, Askins JC, et al. A randomized trial of intravenous and intracoronary streptokinase in patients with acute myocardial infarction. Circulation. 1984;70:606-618
11. Chesebro JH, Knatterud G, Roberts R, et al. Thrombolysis in Myocardial Infarction (TIMI) Trial: Phase I. A comparison between intravenous tissue plasminogen activator and intravenous streptokinase. Circulation. 1987;76:142-154.
12. Timmis AD, Griffin B, Crick JC, Sowton E. Anisoylated plasminogen streptokinase activator complex in acute myocardial infarction: a placebo-controlled arteriographic coronary recanalization study. J Am Coll Cardiol. 1987;10:205-210.
13. Collen D, Topol EJ, Tiefenbrunn AJ, et al. Coronary thrombolysis with recombinant human tissue-type plasminogen activator: a prospective, randomized, placebo-controlled trial. Circulation. 1984;70:1012-1017.
14. Topol EJ, O'Neill WW, Langburd AB, et al. A randomized, placebo-controlled trial of intravenous recombinant tissue type plasminogen activator and emergency

coronary angioplasty in patients with acute myocardial infarction. Circulation. 1987;75:420–428.

15. Cribier A, Berland J, Saoudi N, et al. Intracoronary streptokinase, OK! . . . intravenous streptokinase first? Heparin or intravenous streptokinase in acute infarction: preliminary results of a prospective randomized trial with angiographic evaluation in 44 patients. Haemostasis. 1986;16:122–129.

16. Verstraete M, Bleifeld W, Brower RW, et al. Double-blind randomized trial of intravenous tissue-type plasminogen activator versus placebo in acute myocardial infarction (ECSG-1). Lancet. 1985;2:965–969.

17. Guerci AD, Gerstenblith G, Brinker JA, et al. A randomized trial of intravenous tissue plasminogen activator for acute myocardial infarction with subsequent randomization to elective coronary angioplasty. N Engl J Med. 1987;317:1613–1618.

18. Armstrong PW, Baigrie RS, Daly PA, et al. Tissue plasminogen activator: Toronto (TPAT) placebo-controlled randomized trial in acute myocardial infarction. J Am Coll Cardiol. 1989;13:1469–1476.

19. Durand P, Asseman P, Pruvost P, et al. Effectiveness of intravenous streptokinase on infarct size and left ventricular function in acute myocardial infarction. Clin Cardiol. 1987;10:383–392.

20. Bassand JP, Machecourt J, Cassagnes J, et al. Multicenter trial of intravenous anisoylated plasminogen streptokinase activator complex (APSAC) in acute myocardial infarction: effects on infarct size and left ventricular function. J Am Coll Cardiol. 1989;13:988–997.

21. National Heart Foundation of Australia Coronary Thrombolysis Group. Coronary thrombolysis and myocardial salvage by tissue plasminogen activator given up to 4 hours after onset of myocardial infarction. Lancet. 1988;1:203–208.

22. Kennedy JW, Martin GV, Davis KB, et al. The Western Washington Intravenous Streptokinase in Acute Myocardial Infarction Randomized Trial. Circulation 1988; 77:345–352.

23. de Bono DP. The European Cooperative Study Group trial of intravenous recombinant tissue-type plasminogen activator (rt-PA) and conservative therapy versus rt-PA and immediate coronary angioplasty. J Am Coll Cardiol. 1988;12:20A–23A.

24. White HD, Norris RM, Brown MA, et al. Effect of intravenous streptokinase on left ventricular function and early survival after acute myocardial infarction. N Engl J Med. 1987;317:850–855.

25. O'Rourke M, Baron D, Keogh A, et al. Limitation of myocardial infarction by early infusion of recombinant tissue- type plasminogen activator. Circulation. 1988;77:1311–1315.

26. Bassand JP, Faivre R, Becque O, et al. Effects of early high-dose streptokinase intravenously on left ventricular function in acute myocardial infarction. Am J Cardiol. 1987;60:435–439.

27. Granger CB, White HD, Bates ER, et al. A pooled analysis of coronary arterial patency and left ventricular function after intravenous thrombolysis for acute myocardial infarction. Am J Cardiol. 1994;74:1220–1228.

28. ISIS-2 (Second International Study of Infarct Survival) Collaborative Group. Randomised trial of intravenous streptokinase, oral aspirin, both, or neither among 17,187 cases of suspected acute myocardial infarction: ISIS-2. Lancet. 1988;2:349–360.

29. Gruppo Italiano per lo Studio della Streptochinasi nell' Infarto Miocardico (GISSI). Effectiveness of intravenous thrombolytic treatment in acute myocardial infarction. Lancet. 1986;1:397–402.

30. The ISAM Study Group. A prospective trial of intravenous streptokinase in acute myocardial infarction (ISAM): mortality, morbidity, and infarct size at 21 days. N Engl J Med. 1986;314:1465–1471.

31. EMERAS (Estudio Multicentrico Estreptoquinasa Republicas de America del Sur) Collaborative Group. Randomised trial of late thrombolysis in patients with suspected acute myocardial infarction. Lancet. 1993; 342:767–772.

32. Fibrinolytic Therapy Trialists' (FTT) Collaborative Group. Indications for fibrinolytic therapy in suspected acute myocardial infarction: collaborative overview of early mortality and major morbidity results from all randomised trials of more than 1000 patients. Lancet. 1994;343:311–322.

33. The GUSTO Investigators. An international randomized trial comparing four thrombolytic strategies for acute

myocardial infarction. N Engl J Med. 1993;329:673–682.

34. The GUSTO Angiographic Investigators. The effects of tissue plasminogen activator, streptokinase, or both on coronary- artery patency, ventricular function, and survival after acute myocardial infarction. N Engl J Med. 1993;329:1615–1622.

35. Cannon CP, McCabe CH, Diver DJ, et al. Comparison of front-loaded recombinant tissue-type plasminogen activator, anistreplase and combination thrombolytic therapy for acute myocardial infarction: results of the Thrombolysis in Myocardial Infarction (TIMI) 4 trial. J Am Coll Cardiol. 1994;24:1602–1610.

36. GISSI-2: A factorial randomised trial of alteplase versus streptokinase and heparin versus no heparin among 12,490 patients with acute myocardial infarction. Gruppo Italiano per lo Studio della Sopravvivenza nell'Infarto Miocardico. Lancet. 1990;336(8707):65-71.

37. ISIS-3: a randomised comparison of streptokinase vs tissue plasminogen activator vs anistreplase and of aspirin plus heparin vs aspirin alone among 41,299 cases of suspected acute myocardial infarction. ISIS-3 (Third International Study of Infarct Survival) Collaborative Group. Lancet. 1992;339(8796):753-70.

38. Ohman EM, Califf RM, Topol EJ, et al. Consequences of reocclusion after successful reperfusion therapy in acute myocardial infarction. Circulation. 1990;82:781–791.

39. Simes RJ, Topol EJ, Holmes DR Jr, et al. Link between the angiographic substudy and mortality outcomes in a large randomized trial of myocardial reperfusion: importance of early and complete infarct artery reperfusion. Circulation. 1995;91:1923–1928.

40. Purvis JA, McNeill AJ, Siddiqui RA, et al. Efficacy of 100 mg of double-bolus alteplase in achieving complete perfusion in the treatment of acute myocardial infarction. Am J Cardiol. 1994;23(1):6-10.

41. The COBALT Investigators. A comparison of continuous infusion of alteplase with double-bolus administration for acute myocardial infarction. N Engl J Med 1997; 337:1124– 1130.

42. Bleich SD, Adgey AA, McMechan SR Love TW.. An angiographic assessment of alteplase: double-bolus and front-loaded infusion regimens in myocardial infarction. Am Heart J 1998; 136:741–748.

43. Bode C, Nordt TK, Peter K, et al. Patency trials with reteplase (r-PA): what do they tell us? Am J Cardiol. 1996;78:16–19.

44. International Joint Efficacy Comparison of Thrombolytics. Randomised, double-blind comparison of reteplase doublebolus administration with streptokinase in acute myocardial infarction (INJECT): trial to investigate equivalence. Lancet. 1995;346:329–336.

45. The Global Use of Strategies to Open Occluded Coronary Arteries (GUSTO III) Investigators. A comparison of reteplase with alteplase for acute myocardial infarction. N Engl J Med. 1997;337:1118–1123.

46. Tsikouris JP, Tsikouris AP. A review of available fi brin-specific thrombolytic agents used in acute myocardial infarction. Pharmacotherapy. 2001;21:207–217.

47. Modi NB, Eppler S, Breed J, et al. Love TW. Pharmacokinetics of a slower clearing tissue plasminogen activator variant, TNK-tPA, in patients with acute myocardial infarction. Thromb Haemost. 1998;79:134–139.

48. Serebruany V, Malinin A, Callahan K, et al. Effect of tenecteplase versus alteplase on platelets during the first 3 hours of treatment for acute myocardial infarction: The Assessment of the Safety and Efficacy of a New Thrombolytic Agent (ASSENT-2) platelet substudy. Am Heart J. 2003;145:636–642.

49. Collen D, Stassen JM, Yasuda T, et al. Comparative thrombolytic properties of tissue-type plasminogen activator and of a plasminogen activator inhibitor-1-resistant glycosylation variant, in a combined arterial and venous thrombosis model in the dog. Thromb Haemost. 1994;72:98–104.

50. Cannon CP, McCabe CH, Gibson CM, et al. TNK-tissue plasminogen activator in acute myocardial infarction. Results of the Thrombolysis in Myocardial Infarction (TIMI) 10A dose-ranging trial. Circulation. 1997;95:351–356.

51. Cannon CP, Gibson CM, McCabe CH, et al. TNK-tissue plasminogen activator compared with front-loaded alteplase in acute myocardial infarction: results of the TIMI 10B trial. Circulation 1998;98:2805–2814

52. Van de Werf F, Cannon CP, Luyten A, et al. Safety assessment of single-bolus

administration of TNK tissue-plasminogen activator in acute myocardial infarction: the ASSENT- 1 trial. The ASSENT-1 Investigators. Am Heart J. 1999;137:786–91.

53. Giugliano RP, McCabe CH, Antman EM, et al. Lower-dose heparin with fibrinolysis is associated with lower rates of intracranial hemorrhage. Am Heart J. 2001;141:742–750.

54. Single-bolus tenecteplase compared with front-loaded alteplase in acute myocardial infarction: the ASSENT-2 double-blind randomised trial. Assessment of the Safety and Efficacy of a New Thrombolytic Investigators. Lancet. 1999;354:716–722.

55. Van de Werf F, Barron HV, Armstrong PW, et al. Incidence and predictors of bleeding events after fibrinolytic therapy with fi brin specific agents: a comparison of TNK-tPA and rt-PA. Eur Heart J. 2001;22:2253–2261.

56. Sinnaeve PA, Alexander JB, Belmans AC, et al. One-year follow-up of the ASSENT-2 trial: A double-blind, randomized comparison of single bolus tenecteplase and front-loaded alteplase in 16,949 patients with ST elevation acute myocardial infarction. Am Heart J. 2003;146:27–32.

57. Assessment of the Safety and Efficacy of a New Thrombolytic Regimen (ASSENT)-3 Investigators. Efficacy and safety of tenecteplase in combination with enoxaparin, abciximab, or unfractionated heparin: the ASSENT-3 randomised trial in acute myocardial infarction. Lancet. 2001;358:605–613.

58. Kaul P, Armstrong PW, Cowper PA, et al. Economic analysis of the Assessment of the Safety and Effi cacy of a New Thrombolytic Regimen (ASSENT-3) study: costs of reperfusion strategies in acute myocardial infarction. Am Heart J. 2005;149:637–644.

59. Antman EM, Louwerenburg HW, Baars HF, et al. The ENTIRE-TIMI 23 Investigators. Enoxaparin as Adjunctive Antithrombin Therapy for ST-Elevation Myocardial Infarction: Results of the ENTIRE Thrombolysis in Myocardial Infarction (TIMI) 23 Trial. Circulation. 2002;105:1642–1649.

60. Giugliano RP, Roe MT, Harrington RA, et al. Combination reperfusion therapy with eptifibatide and reduced-dose tenecteplase for ST-elevation myocardial infarction:

Results of the integrilin and tenecteplase in acute myocardial infarction (INTEGRITI) Phase II Angiographic urial. J Am Coll Cardiol. 2003;41:1251–1260.

61. Topol EJ. Reperfusion therapy for acute myocardial infarction with fibrinolytic therapy or combination reduced fibrinolytic therapy and platelet glycoprotein IIb/IIIa inhibition: the GUSTO V randomised trial. Lancet. 2001;357:1905–1914.

62. Wallentin L, Goldstein P, Armstrong PW, et al. Efficacy and safety of tenecteplase in combination with the low-molecular-weight heparin enoxaparin or unfractionated heparin in the prehospital setting: The Assessment of the Safety and Efficacy of a New Thrombolytic Regimen (ASSENT)-3 PLUS randomized trial in acute myocardial infarction. Circulation. 2003;108:135–142.

63. Armstrong PW, Chang WC, Wallentin L, et al. Efficacy and safety of unfractionated heparin versus enoxaparin: a pooled analysis of ASSENT-3 and -3 PLUS data. CMAJ. 2006;174:1421–1426.

64. Antman EM, Morrow DA, McCabe CH, et al. The ExTRACT-TIMI 25 Investigators. Enoxaparin versus Unfractionated Heparin with Fibrinolysis for ST-Elevation Myocardial Infarction. N Engl J Med. 2006;354:1477–1488.

65. Collen D, Van de Werf F. Coronary thrombolysis with recombinant staphylokinase in patients with evolving myocardial infarction. Circulation. 1993;87:1850–1853.

66. Vanderschueren S, Barrios L, Kerdsinchai P, et al. A randomized trial of recombinant staphylokinase versus alteplase for coronary artery patency in acute myocardial infarction. Circulation. 1995;92:2044–2049.

67. Armstrong PW, Burton JR, Palisaitis D, et al. Collaborative angiographic patency trial of recombinant staphylokinase (CAPTORS). Am Heart J. 2000;139:820–823.

68. Califf RM, Topol EJ, Stack RS, et al. Evaluation of combination thrombolytic therapy and timing of cardiac catheterization in acute myocardial infarction: results of thrombolysis and angioplasty in myocardial infarction phase 5 randomized trial. Circulation. 1991;83:1543–1556.

69. Neuhaus KL, Tebbe U, Gottwik M, et al. Intravenous recombinant tissue plasminogen activator (rt-PA) and

urokinase in acute myocardial infarction: results of the German activator urokinase study (GAUS). J Am Coll Cardiol 1988; 12:581– 587

70. Mathey DG, Schofer J, Sheehan FH, et al. Intravenous urokinase in acute myocardial infarction. Am J Cardiol. 1985;55:878–882.

71. Wall TC, Phillips HRI, Stack RS, et al. Results of high dose intravenous urokinase for acute myocardial infarction. Am J Cardiol 1990;65:124–131.

72. Rossi P, Bolognese L. Comparison of intravenous urokinase plus heparin versus heparin alone in acute myocardial infarction. Am J Cardiol. 1991;68:585–592.

73. PRIMI Trial Study Group. Randomised double-blind trial of recombinant pro-urokinase against streptokinase in acute myocardial infarction. Lancet. 1989;1:863–868.

74. Bar FW, Meyer J, Vermeer F, et al. Comparison of saruplase and alteplase in acute myocardial infarction: SESAM Study Group; the Study in Europe with Saruplase and Alteplase in Myocardial Infarction. Am J Cardiol. 1997;79:727–732.

75. Tebbe U, Michels R, Adgey J, et al. Randomized, double blind study comparing saruplase with streptokinase therapy in acute myocardial infarction: the COMPASS equivalence trial. J Am Coll Cardiol. 1998;31:487–493.

76. White HD. Thrombolytic therapy and equivalence trials [editorial]. J Am Coll Cardiol. 1998;31:494–496.

77. den Heijer P, Vermeer F, Ambrosioni E, et al. Evaluation of a weight-adjusted single-bolus plasminogen activator in patients with myocardial infarction: a double-blind, randomized angiographic trial of lanoteplase versus alteplase. Circulation. 1998;98:2117–2125.

78. The In TIME-II Investigators. Intravenous NPA for the treatment of single-bolus lanoteplase vs accelerated alteplase for the treatment of patients with acute myocardial infarction. Eur Heart J. 2000;2005–2013.

79. Rawles J. Halving of mortality at 1 year by domiciliary thrombolysis in the Grampian Region Early Anistreplase Trial (GREAT). J Am Coll Cardiol. 1994;23:1–5.

80. Spann JF, Sherry S, Carabello BA, et al. High-dose, brief intravenous streptokinase early in acute myocardial infarction. Am Heart J. 1982;104:939–945.

81. Rogers WJ, Mantle JA, Hood WP Jr, et al. Prospective randomized trial of intravenous and intracoronary streptokinase in acute myocardial infarction. Circulation. 1983;68:1051–1061.

82. de Marneffe M, Van Thiel E, Ewalenko M, et al. High-dose intravenous thrombolytic therapy in acute myocardial infarction: efficiency, tolerance, complications and influence on left ventricular performance. Acta Cardiol. 1985;40:183–198.

83. Verstraete M, Bernard R, Bory M, et al. Randomised trial of intravenous recombinant tissue-type plasminogen activator versus intravenous streptokinase in acute myocardial infarction (ECSG-2). Lancet. 1985;1:842.

84. Stack RS, O'Connor CM, Mark DB, et al. Coronary reperfusion during acute myocardial infarction with a combined therapy of coronary angioplasty and high-dose intravenous streptokinase. Circulation. 1988;77:151–161.

85. Lopez-Sendon J, Seabra-Gomes R, Macaya C, et al. Intravenous anisoylated plasminogen streptokinase activator complex versus intravenous streptokinase in myocardial infarction: a randomized multicenter study. Circulation. 1988;78:II-277.

86. Charbonnier B, Cribier A, Monassier JP, et al. Etude europeenne multicentrique et randomisee de l'APSAC versus streptokinase dans l'infarctus du myocarde. Arch Mal Coeur Vaiss. 1989;82:1565–1571.

87. Hogg KJ, Gemmill JD, Burns JM, et al. Angiographic patency study of anistreplase versus streptokinase in acute myocardial infarction. Lancet. 1990;335:254–258.

88. Hillis LD, Borer J, Braunwald E, et al. High dose intravenous streptokinase for acute myocardial infarction: preliminary results of a multicenter trial. J Am Coll Cardiol. 1985;6:957–962.

89. Monnier P, Sigwart U, Vincent A, et al. Anisoylated plasminogen streptokinase activator complex versus streptokinase in acute myocardial infarction. Drugs. 1987; 33(suppl 3):175–178.

90. Golf S, Vogt P, Kaufmann U, et al. Intravenous thrombolytic treatment for acute myocardial infarction: effects of early intervention and early examination. Acta Med Scand. 1988; 224:523–529.

91. Ribeiro EE, Silva LA, Carneiro R, et al. A randomized trial of direct PTCA vs

intravenous streptokinase in acute myocardial infarction. J Am Coll Cardiol. 1991;17:152A.

92. Magnani B. Plasminogen Activator Italian Multicenter Study (PAIMS): comparison of intravenous recombinant singlechain human tissue- type plasminogen activator (rt-PA) with intravenous streptokinase in acute myocardial infarction. J Am Coll Cardiol. 1989;13:19–26.

93. White HD, Rivers JT, Maslowski AH, et al. Effect of intravenous streptokinase as compared with that of tissue plasminogen activator on left ventricular function after first myocardial infarction. N Engl J Med. 1989;320:817–821.

94. Cherng WJ, Chiang CW, Kuo CT, et al. A comparison between intravenous streptokinase and tissue plasminogen activator with early intravenous heparin in acute myocardial infarction. Am Heart J. 1992;123:841–846.

95. Topol EJ, Morris DC, Smalling RW, Schumacher RR, Taylor CR, Nishikawa A, et al. A multicenter, randomized, placebo-controlled trial of a new form of intravenous recombinant tissue-type plasminogen activator (activase) in acute myocardial infarction. J Am Coll Cardiol. 1987;9:1205–1213.

96. Smalling RW, Schumacher R, Morris D, et al. Improved infarct-related arterial patency after high dose, weightadjusted, rapid infusion of tissue-type plasminogen activator in myocardial infarction: results of a multicenter randomized trial of two dosage regimens. J Am Coll Cardiol. 1990;15:915–921.

97. de Bono DP, Simoons ML, Tijssen J, et al. Effect of early intravenous heparin on coronary patency, infarct size, and bleeding complications after alteplase thrombolysis: results of a randomised double blind European Cooperative Study Group trial. Br Heart J. 1992;67:122–128.

98. Carney RJ, Murphy GA, Brandt TR, et al. Randomized angiographic trial of recombinant tissue-type plasminogen activator (alteplase) in myocardial infarction. J Am Coll Cardiol. 1992;20:17–23.

99. Grines CL, Nissen SE, Booth DC, et al. A prospective, randomized trial comparing combination half-dose tissue type plasminogen activator and streptokinase with full-dose tissue-type plasminogen activator. Circulation. 1991;84:540–549.

100. Johns JA, Gold HK, Leinbach RC, et al. Prevention of coronary artery reocclusion and reduction in late coronary artery stenosis after thrombolytic therapy in patients with acute myocardial infarction: a randomized study of maintenance infusion of recombinant human tissue-type plasminogen activator. Circulation. 1988;78:546–556.

101. TIMI Study Group. Immediate versus delayed catheterization and angioplasty after thrombolytic therapy for acute myocardial infarction. N Engl J Med. 1988;260:2849–2858.

102. Neuhaus KL, Tebbe U, Gottwik M, et al. Intravenous recombinant tissue plasminogen activator (rt-PA) and urokinase in acute myocardial infarction: results of the German activator urokinase study (GAUS). J Am Coll Cardiol 1988; 12:581– 587.

103. Topol EJ, George BS, Kereiakes DJ, et al. A randomized controlled trial of intravenous tissue plasminogen activator and early intravenous heparin in acute myocardial infarction. Circulation 1989; 79:281–286

104. Topol EJ, Ellis SG, Califf RM, et al. Combined tissue- type plasminogen activator and prostacyclin therapy for acute myocardial infarction. J Am Coll Cardiol. 1989;14:877–884.

105. Califf RM, Topol EJ, Stack RS, Ellis SG, George BS, Kereiakes DJ, et al. Evaluation of combination thrombolytic therapy and timing of cardiac catheterization in acute myocardial infarction: results of thrombolysis and angioplasty in myocardial infarction phase 5 randomized trial. Circulation. 1991;83:1543–1556.

106. Whitlow PL, Bashore TM. Catheterization/Rescue Angioplasty after Thrombolysis (CRAFT) study: acute myocardial infarction treated with recombinant tissue plasminogen activator versus urokinase. J Am Coll Cardiol. 1991;17:276A.

107. TIMI Study Group. Comparison of invasive and conservative strategies after treatment with intravenous tissue plasminogen activator in acute myocardial infarction: Results of the Thrombolysis In Myocardial Infarction (TIMI) phase II trial. N Engl J Med. 1989;320:618–627.

108. Anderson JL, Becker LC, Sorensen SG, et al. Anistreplase versus alteplase in acute myocardial infarction: Comparative effects

on left ventricular function, morbidity and 1-day coronary artery patency. J Am Coll Cardiol. 1992;20:753–766.

109. Rapold HJ, Kuemmerli H, Weiss M, Baur H, Haeberli A. Monitoring of fibrin generation during thrombolytic therapy of acute myocardial infarction with recombinant tissue-type plasminogen activator. Circulation. 1989;79:980–989.

110. Thompson PL, Aylward PE, Federman J, et al. A randomized comparison of intravenous heparin with oral aspirin and dipyridamole 24 hours after recombinant tissue-type plasminogen activator for acute myocardial infarction. Circulation. 1991;83:1534–1542.

111. Smalling RW, Bode C, Kalbfleisch J, et al. More rapid, complete, and stable coronary thrombolysis with bolus administration of reteplase compared with alteplase infusion in acute myocardial infarction. Circulation. 1995;91:2725–2732.

112. Bode C, Smalling RW, Berg G, et al. Randomized comparison of coronary thrombolysis achieved with double-bolus reteplase (recombinant plasminogen activator) and front-loaded, accelerated alteplase (recombinant tissue plasminogen activator) in patients with acute myocardial infarction. The RAPID II Investigators. Circulation. 1996;94(5):891-8.

113. Le May MR, Wells GA, Labinaz M, et al. Combined angioplasty and pharmacological intervention versus thrombolysis alone in acute myocardial infarction (CAPITAL AMI study). J Am Coll Cardiol. 2005;46:417–424.

114. Armstrong PW, WEST Steering Committee. A comparison of pharmacologic therapy with/without timely coronary intervention vs primary percutaneous intervention early after ST-elevation myocardial infarction: the WEST (Which Early ST-elevation myocardial infarction Therapy) study. Eur Heart J. 2006;27:1530–1538.

115. Assessment of the Safety and Efficacy of a New Treatment Strategy with Percutaneous Coronary Intervention (ASSENT-4 PCI) investigators. Primary versus tenecteplase-facilitated percutaneous coronary intervention in patients with ST-segment elevation acute myocardial infarction (ASSENT-4 PCI): randomised trial. Lancet. 2006;367:569–578.

116. Fernandez-Aviles F, Alonso JJ, Pena G. et al. Primary angioplasty vs early routine post-fibrinolysis angioplasty for acute myocardial infarction with ST-segment elevation: the GRACIA-2 non-inferiority, randomized, controlled trial. Eur Heart J. 2007;28:949–960.

117. Zeymer U1, Huber K, Fu Y, et al. (for the ASSENT-4 PCI Investigators). Impact of TIMI 3 patency before primary percutaneous coronary intervention for ST-elevation myocardial infarction on clinical outcome: results from the ASSENT-4 PCI study. Eur Heart J Acute Cardiovasc Care. 2012;1(2):136-42.

118. Gibson CM, Karha J, Giugliano RP, Roe MT, Murphy SA, Harrington RA, et al. Association of the timing of ST-segment resolution with TIMI myocardial perfusion grade in acute myocardial infarction. Am Heart J. 2004;147:847–852.

119. Antiplatelet Trialists' Collaboration. Collaborative meta analysis of randomized trials of antiplatelet therapy for prevention of death, myocardial infarction, and stroke in high-risk patients. BMJ. 2002;324:71–86.

120. Collins R, Peto R, Baigent C, Sleight P. Aspirin, heparin, and fibrinolytic therapy in suspected acute myocardial infarction. N Engl J Med. 1997;336:847–860.

121. Sabatine MS, Cannon CP, Gibson CM, et al. Addition of clopidogrel to aspirin and fibrinolytic therapy for myocardial infarction with ST-segment elevation. N Engl J Med. 2005;352:1179–1189.

122. COMMIT (ClOpidogrel and Metoprolol in Myocardial Infarction Trial) collaborative group. Addition of clopidogrel to aspirin in 45 852 patients with acute myocardial infarction: randomized placebo-controlled trial, Lancet. 2005;366:1607–1621.

123. Wallentin L, Becker RC, Budaj A et al. Ticagrelor versus clopidogrel in patients with acute coronary syndromes. N Engl J Med. 2009;361(11):1045-57.

124. Kleiman NS, Ohman EM, Califf RM, et al. Profound inhibition of platelet aggregation with monoclonal antibody 7E3 Fab after thrombolytic therapy: results of the Thrombolysis and Angioplasty in Myocardial Infarction (TAMI) 8 pilot study. J Am Coll Cardiol. 1993;22:381–389.

125. Ohman EM, Kleiman NS, Gacioch G, et al. Combined accelerated tissue-plasminogen activator and platelet glycoprotein IIb/IIIa integrin receptor blockade with integrilin in

acute myocardial infarction: results of a randomized, placebo-controlled, dose-ranging trial. IMPACT-AMI Investigators. Circulation. 1997;95:846–854.

126. Trial of abciximab with and without low-dose reteplase for acute myocardial infarction: Strategies for Patency Enhancement in the Emergency Department (SPEED) Group. Circulation. 2000;101:2788–2794.

127. Antman EM, Giugliano RP, Gibson CM, et al. Abciximab facilitates the rate and extent of thrombolysis: results of the thrombolysis in myocardial infarction (TIMI) 14 trial. Circulation. 1999;99:2720–2732.

128. Lincoff AM, Califf RM, Van de Werf F, et al. Mortality at 1 year with combination platelet glycoprotein IIb/IIIa inhibition and reduced-dose fibrinolytic therapy vs conventional fibrinolytic therapy for acute myocardial infarction: GUSTO V randomized trial. JAMA. 2002;288:2130–2135.

129. Brener SJ, Zeymer U, Adgey AA, et al. Eptifibatide and low-dose tissue plasminogen activator in acute myocardial infarction: the Integrilin and Low-Dose Thrombolysis in Acute Myocardial Infarction (INTRO AMI) trial. J Am Coll Cardiol. 2002;39:377–386.

130. Combining thrombolysis with the platelet glycoprotein IIb/ IIIa inhibitor lamifiban: results of the Platelet Aggregation Receptor Antagonist Dose Investigation and Reperfusion Gain in Myocardial Infarction (PARADIGM) trial. J Am Coll Cardiol. 1998;32:2003–2010.

131. Frostfeldt G, Ahlberg G, Gustafsson G, et al. Low molecular weight heparin (dalteparin) as adjuvant treatment of thrombolysis in acute myocardial infarction: a pilot study; biochemical markers in acute coronary syndromes (BIOMACS II). J Am Coll Cardiol. 1999;33:627–633.

132. Simoons M, Krzeminska-Pakula M, Alonso A, et al. Improved reperfusion and clinical outcome with enoxaparin as an adjunct to streptokinase thrombolysis in acute myocardial infarction: the AMI-SK study. Eur Heart J. 2002;23:1282–1290.

133. The effects of tissue plasminogen activator, streptokinase, or both on coronary-artery patency, ventricular function, and survival after acute myocardial infarction. The GUSTO Angiographic Investigators. N Engl J Med. 1993;329:1615–1622.

134. Giraldez RR, Nicolau JC, Corbalan R, et al. Enoxaparin is superior to unfractionated heparin in patients with ST elevation myocardial infarction undergoing fibrinolysis regardless of the choice of lytic: An ExTRACT-TIMI 25 analysis. Eur Heart J. 2007;28:1566–1573.

135. White HD, Braunwald E, Murphy SA, et al. Enoxaparin vs. unfractionated heparin with fibrinolysis for ST-elevation myocardial infarction in elderly and younger patients: results from ExTRACT-TIMI 25. Eur Heart J. 2007;28:1066–1071.

136. Ross AM, Molhoek P, Lundergan C, et al. HART II Investigators. Randomized comparison of enoxaparin, a low-molecular-weight heparin, with unfractionated heparin adjunctive to recombinant tissue plasminogen activator thrombolysis and aspirin: Second trial of Heparin and Aspirin Reperfusion Therapy (HART II). Circulation. 2001;104(6):648-52.

137. Peters RJ, Joyner C, Bassand JP, et al. For the OASIS-6 Investigators. The role of fondaparinux as an adjunct to thrombolytic therapy in acute myocardial infarction: a subgroup analysis of the OASIS-6 trial. Eur Heart J. 2008;29:324–331.

138. Kontny F, Dale J, Abildgaard U, Pedersen TR. Randomized trial of low molecular weight heparin (dalteparin) in prevention of left ventricular thrombus formation and arterial embolism after acute anterior myocardial infarction: The Fragmin in Acute Myocardial Infarction (FRAMI) Study. J Am Coll Cardiol. 1997;30(4):962-9.

139. Baird SH, Menown IB, McBride SJ, Trouton TG, Wilson C. Randomized comparison of enoxaparin with unfractionated heparin following fibrinolytic therapy for acute myocardial infarction. Eur Heart J. 2002;23:627–632.

140. Scharfstein JS1, Abendschein DR, Eisenberg PR, et al. Usefulness of fibrinogenolytic and procoagulant markers during thrombolytic therapy in predicting clinical outcomes in acute myocardial infarction.TIMI-5 Investigators. Thrombolysis in Myocardial Infarction. Am J Cardiol. 1996;78(5):503-10.

141. Lee LV. Initial experience with hirudin and streptokinase in acute myocardial infarction: Results of the Thrombolysis in Myocardial Infarction (TIMI) 6 trial. Am J Cardiol. 1995;75:7–13.

142. Neuhaus KL, von Essen R, Tebbe U, et al. Safety observations from the pilot phase of the randomized r-Hirudin for Improvement of Thrombolysis (HIT-III) study: a study of the Arbeitsgemeinschaft Leitender Kardiologischer Krankenhausarzte (ALKK). Circulation. 1994;90:1638–1642.

143. Neuhaus KL, Molhoek GP, Zeymer U, et al. Recombinant hirudin (lepirudin) for the improvement of thrombolysis with streptokinase in patients with acute myocardial infarction: results of the HIT-III) study. J Am Coll Cardiol. 1999;34:966–973.

144. Metz BK, White HD, Granger CB, et al. Randomized comparison of direct thrombin inhibition versus heparin in conjunction with fibrinolytic therapy for acute myocardial infarction: results from the GUSTO-IIb Trial. Global Use of Strategies to Open Occluded Coronary Arteries in Acute Coronary Syndromes (GUSTO-IIb) Investigators. J Am Coll Cardiol. 1998;31:1493–1498.

145. Direct thrombin inhibitors in acute coronary syndromes: principal results of a meta-analysis based on individual patients' data. Lancet. 2002;359:294–302.

146. Theroux P, Perez-Villa F, Waters D, et al. Randomized double-blind comparison of two doses of Hirulog with heparin as adjunctive therapy to streptokinase to promote early patency of the infarct-related artery in acute myocardial infarction. Circulation. 1995;91:2132–2139.

147. White H. Thrombin-specific anticoagulation with bivalirudin versus heparin in patients receiving fibrinolytic therapy for acute myocardial infarction: the HERO-2 randomised trial. Lancet. 2001;358:1855–1863.

148. Michels KB, Yusuf S. Does PTCA in acute myocardial infarction affect mortality and reinfarction rates? A quantative overview (meta-analysis) of the randomized clinical trials. Circulation. 1995;91:476-485.

149. Weaver WD, Simes J, Betrui A, Grines CL, Zijlstra F, Garcia E, et al. Comparison of primary coronary angioplasty and intravenous thrombolytic therapy for acute myocardial infarction. A quantative review. JAMA. 1997;278:2093-98.

150. Grines CL, Browne KF, Marco J, Rothbaum D, Stone GW, O'Keefe J, et al. A comparison of immediate angioplasty with thrombolytic therapy for acute myocardial infarction: The Primary Angioplasty in Myocardial Infarction Study Group. N Engl J Med. 1993;328:673-679.

151. Gusto Investigators. A clinical trial comparing primary coronary angioplasty with tissue plasminogen activator for acute myocardial infarction: The Global Use of Strategies to Open Occluded Coronary Arteries in Acute Coronary Syndromes (Gusto IIB) Angioplasty Substudy Investigators. N Engl J Med. 1997;336:1621-1628.

152. Cucherat M, Bonnefoy E, Tremray G. Primary angioplasty versus intravenous thrombolysis for acute myocardial infarction. Cochrane Database Syst Rev. 2000;2:CD001560.

153. Every N, Parsons LS, Hlatky M, Martin JS, Weaver WD. A comparison of thrombolytic therapy with primary coronary angioplasty for acute myocardial infarction: Myocardial Infarction Triage and Intervention Investigators. N Engl J Med. 1996;335:1253-1260.

154. Tiefenbrunn AJ, Chandra NC, French WJ, Gore JM, Rogers WJ. Clinical experience with primary PTCA compared to altepase in patients with acute myocardial infarction. J Am Coll Cardiol. 1998;31:1240-1245.

155. Yan AT, Yan RT, Cantor WJ, Borgundvaag B, Cohen EA, Fitchett DH, et al. TRANSFER-AMI Investigators. Relationship between risk stratification at admission and treatment effects of early invasive management following fibrinolysis: Insights from the Trial of Routine ANgioplasty and Stenting After Fibrinolysis to Enhance Reperfusion in Acute Myocardial Infarction (TRANSFER-AMI). Eur Heart J. 2011;32(16):1994-2002.

156. Pipilis A, Andrikopoulos G, Lekakis J, Gotsis A, Oikonomou K, Toli K, Kyrpizidis C, et al. Do we reperfuse those in most need? Clinical characteristics of ST-elevation myocardial infarction patients receiving reperfusion therapy in the countrywide registry HELIOS. Hellenic J Cardiol. 2010;51(6):486-91.

157. Gao RL, Han YL, Yang XC, Mao JM, Fang WY, Wang L, et al. Collaborative Research Group of Reperfusion Therapy in Acute Myocardial Infarction (RESTART). Thorombolytic therapy with rescue percutaneous coronary intervention versus primary percutaneous coronary intervention in patients with acute myocardial infarction: a multicenter

randomized clinical trial. Chin Med J (Engl). 2010;123(11):1365-72.

158. Itoh T, Fukami K, Suzuki T, Kimura T, Kanaya Y, Orii M, et al. Important investigators. Comparison of long-term prognostic evaluation between pre-intervention thrombolysis and primary coronary intervention: A prospective randomized trial: five-year results of the important study. Circ J. 2010;74(8):1625-34.

159. Stolt Steiger V, Goy JJ, Stauffer JC, Radovanovic D, Duvoisin N, Urban P, et al. AMIS Plus Investigators. Significant decrease in in-hospital mortality and major adverse cardiac events in Swiss STEMI patients between 2000 and December 2007. Swiss Med Wkly. 2009;139(31-32):453-7.

160. Soares Jda S, Souza NR, Nogueira Filho J, Cunha CC, Ribeiro GS, Peixoto RS. Treatment of a cohort of patients with acute myocardial infarction and ST-segment elevation. Arq Bras Cardiol. 2009;92(6):430-6,448-55,464-71.

161. Busk M, Maeng M, Rasmussen K, Kelbaek H, Thayssen P, Abildgaard U, et al. DANAMI-2 Investigators. The Danish multicentre randomized study of fibrinolytic therapy vs. primary angioplasty in acute myocardial infarction (the DANAMI-2 trial): outcome after 3 years follow-up. Eur Heart J. 2008;29(10):1259-66.

162. Prieto JC, Sanhueza C, Martínez N, Nazzal C, Corbalán R, Cavada G, et al. Grupo de Estudio Multicéntro del Infarto. In-hospital mortality after ST-segment elevation myocardial infarction according to reperfusion therapy. Rev Med Chil. 2008;136(2):143-50.

163. Di Mario C, Dudek D, Piscione F, Mielecki W, Savonitto S, Murena E, CARESS-in-AMI (Combined Abciximab RE-teplase Stent Study in Acute Myocardial Infarction) Investigators.Immediate angioplasty versus standard therapy with rescue angioplasty after thrombolysis in the Combined Abciximab REteplase Stent Study in Acute Myocardial Infarction (CARESS-in-AMI): an open, prospective, randomised, multicentre trial. Lancet. 2008;371(9612):559-68.

164. Grajek S, Lesiak M, Araszkiewicz A, Pyda M, Skorupski W, Grygier M, et al. Short- and long-term mortality in patients with ST-elevation myocardial infarction treated with

different therapeutic strategies. Results from Wlelkopolska REgional 2002 Registry (WIRE Registry). Kardiol Pol. 2008;66(2):154-63;

165. Greig D, Corbalán R, Castro P, Campos P, Lamich R, Yovaniniz P. Mortality of patients with ST-elevation acute myocardial infarction treated with primary angioplasty or thrombolysis. Rev Med Chil. 2008;136(9):1098-106.

166. Nallamothu B, Fox KA, Kennelly BM, Van de Werf F, Gore JM, Steg PG, et al. GRACE Investigators.Relationship of treatment delays and mortality in patients undergoing fibrinolysis and primary percutaneous coronary intervention. The Global Registry of Acute Coronary Events. Heart. 2007;93(12):1552-5.

167. Widimsky P, Bilkova D, Penicka M, Novak M, Lanikova M, Porizka V, et al ; PRAGUE Study Group Investigators. Long-term outcomes of patients with acute myocardial infarction presenting to hospitals without catheterization laboratory and randomized to immediate thrombolysis or interhospital transport for primary percutaneous coronary intervention. Five years' follow-up of the PRAGUE-2 Trial. Eur Heart J. 2007;28(6):679-84.

168. Kalla K, Christ G, Karnik R, Malzer R, Norman G, Prachar H, et al. Vienna STEMI Registry Group. Implementation of guidelines improves the standard of care: the Viennese registry on reperfusion strategies in ST-elevation myocardial infarction (Vienna STEMI registry). Circulation. 2006;113(20):2398-405.

169. Boersma E; Primary Coronary Angioplasty vs. Thrombolysis Group. Does time matter? A pooled analysis of randomized clinical trials comparing primary percutaneous coronary intervention and in-hospital fibrinolysis in acute myocardial infarction patients. Eur Heart J. 2006;27(7):779-88.

170. McNamara RL, Herrin J, Bradley EH, Portnay EL, Curtis JP, Wang Y, Magid DJ, et al. NRMI Investigators. Hospital improvement in time to reperfusion in patients with acute myocardial infarction, 1999 to 2002. J Am Coll Cardiol. 2006;47(1):45-51.

171. Rathore SS, Weinfurt KP, Foody JM, Krumholz HM. Performance of the Thrombolysis in Myocardial Infarction (TIMI) ST-elevation myocardial infarction

risk score in a national cohort of elderly patients. Am Heart J. 2005;150(3):402-10.

172. Magid DJ, Wang Y, Herrin J, McNamara RL, Bradley EH, Curtis JP, Pollack et al. Relationship between time of day, day of week, timeliness of reperfusion, and in-hospital mortality for patients with acute ST-segment elevation myocardial infarction. JAMA. 2005;294(7):803-12.

173. Fassa AA, Urban P, Radovanovic D, Duvoisin N, Gaspoz JM, Stauffer JC, et al. AMIS Plus Investigators. Trends in reperfusion therapy of ST segment elevation myocardial infarction in Switzerland: six year results from a nationwide registry. Heart. 2005;91(7):882-8.

174. Danchin N, Coste P, Ferrières J, Steg PG, Cottin Y, Blanchard D, et al. FAST-MI Investigators. Comparison of thrombolysis followed by broad use of percutaneous coronary intervention with primary percutaneous coronary intervention for ST-segment-elevation acute myocardial infarction: data from the french registry on acute ST-elevation myocardial infarction (FAST-MI). Circulation. 2008;118(3):268-76.

175. Dalby M, Bouzamondo A, Lechat P, Montalescot G. Transfer for primary angioplasty versus immediate thrombolysis in acute myocardial infarction: a meta-analysis. Circulation. 2003;108(15):1809-14.

176. Sakurai K, Watanabe J, Iwabuchi K, Koseki Y, Kon-no Y, Fukuchi M, et al. Comparison of the efficacy of reperfusion therapies for early mortality from acute myocardial infarction in Japan: registry of Miyagi Study Group for AMI (MsAMI). Circ J. 2003;67(3):209-14.

177. Franzosi MG, Santoro E, De Vita C. Ten-year follow-up of the first megatrial testing thrombolytic therapy in patients with acute myocardial infarction: results of the Gruppo Italiano per lo Studio della Soprav vivenzanell'Infarcto-I Study. Circulation. 1998;98:2659-65.

178. Bonnefoy E, Lapostolle F, Leizorovicz A. Primary angioplasty versus prehospital fibrinolysis in acute myocardial infarction. Lancet. 2002;360:825-9.

179. Keeley EC, Boura JA, Grines CL. Primary angioplasty versus intravenous thrombolytic therapy for acute myocardial infarction: a quantitative review of 23 randomised trials. Lancet. 2003;361(9351): 13-20.

Kindergarten Children with Congenital Heart Disease Show Good Physical Activity but Reduced Motor Skills in Comparison with Healthy Children

Andrea Engelhardt[1*], Pinar Bambul Heck[1], Renate Oberhoffer[1,2], Peter Ewert[1] and Alfred Hager[1]

[1]*Department of Paediatric Cardiology and Congenital Heart Disease, Deutsches Herzzentrum München, Technische Universität München, Germany.*
[2]*Institute of Preventive Pediatrics, Technische Universität München, Germany.*

Authors' contributions

Authors AE, PBH and AH were responsible for conception and design of the study. Author AE sampled the data in the clinic and the kindergartens. Authors AE and AH were responsible for data monitoring, integrity, analysis and drafted the manuscript. Authors RO and PE gave important input for revising the manuscript. All authors have read and approved the final version of the manuscript.

Editor(s):
(1) Francesco Pelliccia, Department of Heart and Great Vessels University La Sapienza, Rome, Italy.
Reviewers:
(1) Anonymous, Medical University, Poland.
(2) Pietro Scicchitano, Cardiology Department, "San Giacomo" Hospital, Monopoli, Italy.

ABSTRACT

Objective: For the interaction of individuals with their environment, motor competence is of major importance. It is known that school children with congenital heart disease (CHD) have motoric limitations even without hemodynamic residuals. Data from kindergarten children is lacking. This study was to compare the motor competence of kindergarten children with congenital heart disease (4-6 years) with healthy children of the same age group.
Patients and Methods: A motor test "MOT 4-6" with 18 tasks in different groups of motor skills was performed in 62 children (19 female, 43 male) with various forms of CHD and compared to 39 healthy children (22 female, 17 male). In addition to the motor test all subjects answered the Kiddy-KINDL® quality of life questionnaire, and wore an accelerometer to capture daily physical activity for seven consecutive days.
Results: The median (quartile 1; quartile 3) motor quotient in the CHD group (104 [96;113]) was

Corresponding author: E-mail: engelhardt@dhm.mhn.de

significantly lower than in the control group (111 [104;116]; Mann-Whitney-U test p=0.005). Quality of life did not differ significantly (p=0.774, parents' questionnaire p=0.066), nor the minutes in moderate and vigorous physical activity (p=0.093). No correlation between the motor quotient and the other variables could be shown.

Conclusion: Kindergarten children with CHD should be screened for a normal motor development. This delay seems to be independent from daily physical activity.

Keywords: Congenital heart disease; motor development; physical activity.

1. INTRODUCTION

Motor development is one of the essential aspects in young children [1]. The perceptual and motor experience of children influences not only physical and motor, but also emotional, psychosocial, and cognitive development [2]. Deficits in motor activities might affect the child's entire personal development [1,3]. Most children born with congenital heart disease (CHD), who were repaired successfully in infancy, are able to participate in all normal age-appropriate physical activities with their healthy peers [4]. However, in more detailed tests several children show neurodevelopmental deficits. The deficits in motor development are dependent of the severity of the cardiac lesion [5], and are also seen in children without hemodynamic residuals. These deficits might result from immobilisation periods after surgery or catheter intervention, but also because of an overprotective behaviour of the parents.

Few studies have focused on motor development of children with congenital heart disease [1-3, 5-7]. Most of them examined school children. Earlier data about the motor development of kindergarten children with CHD are rare. In a review about motor and cognitive outcomes after early surgery for CHD [8], only three studies focused on kindergarten children. Only one of these three studies investigated motor development in this age group. None of these studies have included physical activity data to investigate the deficits in relation to daily physical activity [8].

The aim of the present study was to examine kindergarten children with CHD, to compare their gross and fine motor skills with healthy peers of the same age and to relate these findings to daily physical activity.

2. PATIENTS AND METHODS

2.1 Study Design

From May to October 2010 and May to September 2011, we recruited all children at the age of 4-6 years, attending our outpatient department for routine follow-up of their CHD. We chose to recruit only in spring and summertime, when outdoor activity is performed regularly to avoid a bias in daily activity by seasonal effects. Children with syndromes, physical disabilities (severe neurodevelopmental retardation such as hydrocephalus, microcephaly or trisomy 21), who were expected to be unable to perform any task of the motoric test and children with cardiac intervention less than six month ago were excluded (Fig. 1). The sample of the tested children represented the complete spectrum of congenital cardiac disease. The detailed diagnoses corresponding to complex, moderate and mild lesions [9] are presented in Table 1. In parallel, healthy preschool children of three kindergartens were recruited. The age range of the included children was 4-6 years. All anthropometric data is depicted in Table 2.

All subjects performed the "motoric test for kindergarten children (MOT 4-6)", answered the "Kiddy-KINDL® questionnaire", and wore an accelerometer to capture daily activity for the next seven days after the test. In addition the parents were asked to rate their children's quality of life.

The study was designed as a prospective cross-sectional cohort study. The study protocol was in accordance with the declaration of Helsinki. It was approved by the local ethical board (project number 2782/10). All patients' parents gave written informed consent. All authors read the final version of the manuscript and agreed with its publication.

2.2 Motor Development Assessment

To assess the motor development, the "MOT 4-6" from R. Zimmer and M. Volkamer was used [10]. It was developed in 1984 to capture the motor development of 4-6 year old children. The test consists of 18 tasks in different groups of motor skills: gross motor skills of the whole body (5 tasks), fine motor skills (3 tasks), balance (5 tasks), reaction (2 tasks), bounce (2 tasks), speed (3 tasks), and control of motion (2 tasks). The first task for the children is to acclimatize and get comfortable with the test situation. The other tasks are scored with zero (not able to perform), one (intermediate performance) or two points (correct performance). Precise instructions are given for the 18 tasks, as well as the definition of "intermediate" and "correct" performance. At the end all task scores are summed up to a raw value and transformed into a motor quotient, according to the age-dependent reference values [10]. A higher motor quotient represents a better motor ability with a mean of 100 and a standard deviation of 15 in a reference population.

The motoric test for children with CHD was performed in our hospital in a physio therapy room. The healthy children were tested in their kindergarten in a gym. All examinations were performed by one of the authors (A.E.).

2.3 Daily Activity Assessment

Daily physical activity was measured by the tri-axial accelerometer "RT3" (Stayhealthy, Monrovia, California, USA) for seven days after the motoric tests. The accelerometer was allowed to be taken off only during showering, swimming or at bedtime. Data sets accounting for less than 5 days were discarded.

The "RT3" is designed as a complete activity recording and measurement device for clinical and research applications. Worn on the waist, it continuously tracks activities throughout the day with the use of piezo-electric accelerometer technology. It measures motion in three dimensions and provides tri-axial vector data in activity units.

In our study, vector magnitudes were used to calculate the three dimensions with a sampling epoch of one minute. The daily minutes in moderate (3-6 metabolic equivalents) and vigorous activity (>6 metabolic equivalents) were calculated, using the published cut-off-points for moderate (> 970 count/min) and vigorous (> 2333 counts/min) activity [11]. Data were averaged for the sampling days. For statistics, the data from moderate to vigorous activity representing all activity >3 metabolic equivalents were pooled.

2.4 Quality of Life Assessment

The KINDL® questionnaire was applied to assess the health-related quality of life for children. It is used both for clinical assessment as well as for healthy children. It was developed for three different age groups (4-7 years, 8-12 years and 13-16 years) and additionally for parents to classify their children. The questionnaire was tested and evaluated in several studies with 3000 healthy children and children with chronic disease [12]. It has proven to be a flexible, modular, and accepted psychological method to evaluate the quality of life for children.

In our study we used the Kiddy-KINDL® for children aged 4-7 years and the Kiddy-KINDL® questionnaire for parents of children from the same age group. The questionnaire for children consists of 12 items about body, feelings, self-estimation, family, friends, and kindergarten (two items each). For the parents' questionnaire, the same items as in the children's questionnaire are used but supplemented by 22 general questions about their relation to the child.

Table 1. primary cardiac diagnosis in the CHD group

15	Simple CHD
7	Atrial septal defect
2	Ventricular septal defect
2	Persistant foramen ovale
1	Persistent arterial duct
3	Primary arrhythmia (supraventricular tachycardia/premature ventricular contraction)
22	Moderate CHD
4	Tetralogy of Fallot
5	Aortic stenosois
5	Coarctation of the aorta
2	Pulmonary stenosis
2	Totally anomalous pulmonary venous connection
2	Ebstein's malformation
1	Aortic regurgitation
1	Shone complex
25	Complex CHD
6	Transposition of the great arteries
5	Pulmonary atresia
4	Congenital corrected transposition of the great arteries
4	Double outlet right ventricle
3	Complex lesions/functionally univentricular heart
3	Tricuspid atresia

Diagnosis corresponding to complex, moderate and mild lesions [9] CHD (congenital heart disease)

All questions were read to the children by the investigator and each child had to choose one of three given answers (1=never, 2=sometimes, 3=very often). None of the questions were explained to the child, if it was not able to answer a question, the question was ignored. From the answers a score was calculated from 0-100 with higher scores representing a better quality of life.

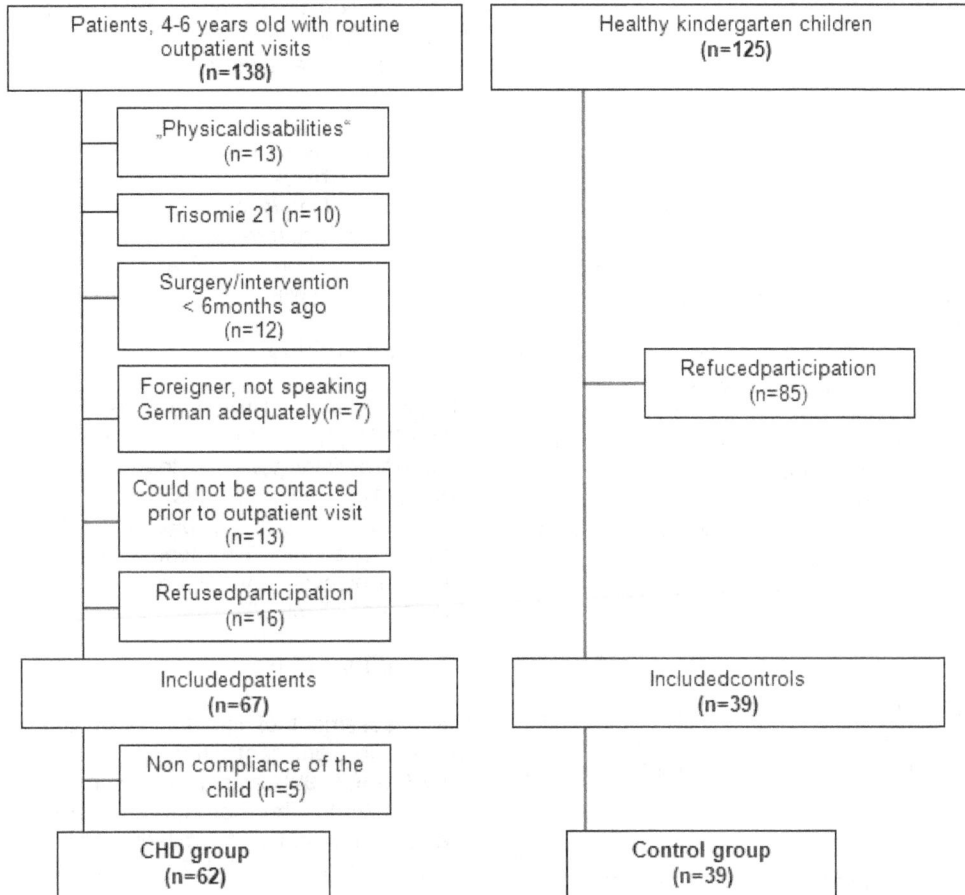

```
┌─────────────────────────────────┐        ┌─────────────────────────────────┐
│ Patients, 4-6 years old with     │        │ Healthy kindergarten children    │
│ routine outpatient visits        │        │            (n=125)               │
│            (n=138)               │        │                                  │
└─────────────────────────────────┘        └─────────────────────────────────┘
        │                                            │
        ├──┌──────────────────────────┐              │
        │  │ „Physicaldisabilities"    │              │
        │  │        (n=13)            │              │
        │  └──────────────────────────┘              │
        ├──┌──────────────────────────┐              │
        │  │ Trisomie 21 (n=10)        │              │
        │  └──────────────────────────┘              │
        ├──┌──────────────────────────┐              │
        │  │ Surgery/intervention      │              │
        │  │ < 6months ago             │              │
        │  │        (n=12)            │              │
        │  └──────────────────────────┘              │
        ├──┌──────────────────────────┐              ├──┌──────────────────────────┐
        │  │ Foreigner, not speaking   │              │  │ Refucedparticipation      │
        │  │ German adequately(n=7)    │              │  │        (n=85)            │
        │  └──────────────────────────┘              │  └──────────────────────────┘
        ├──┌──────────────────────────┐              │
        │  │ Could not be contacted    │              │
        │  │ prior to outpatient visit │              │
        │  │        (n=13)            │              │
        │  └──────────────────────────┘              │
        ├──┌──────────────────────────┐              │
        │  │ Refusedparticipation      │              │
        │  │        (n=16)            │              │
        │  └──────────────────────────┘              │
┌─────────────────────────────────┐        ┌─────────────────────────────────┐
│ Includedpatients (n=67)          │        │ Includedcontrols (n=39)          │
└─────────────────────────────────┘        └─────────────────────────────────┘
        │                                            │
        ├──┌──────────────────────────┐              │
        │  │ Non compliance of the     │              │
        │  │ child (n=5)               │              │
        │  └──────────────────────────┘              │
┌─────────────────────────────────┐        ┌─────────────────────────────────┐
│ CHD group (n=62)                 │        │ Control group (n=39)             │
└─────────────────────────────────┘        └─────────────────────────────────┘
```

Fig. 1. Recruitment and participation of the children from our outpatient department and from three local kindergartens

CHD, congenital heart disease

Table 2. Anthropometric data and results of the tested parameters

	CHD Median (Q1;Q3)	Control group Median (Q1;Q3)	P*
Sex (male/female)	43/19	17/22	0.059
Age (years)	5.1 (4.5;5.9)	5.5 (4.8;6.2)	0.099
Body mass (kg)	18.0 (17.0;22.0)	21.0 (17.5;22.5)	0.129
Body length (cm)	110 (104;116)	118 (110;122)	**0.003**
Body mass index (kg/m²)	15.2 (14.2;16.7)	14.8 (13.9;15.5)	0.173
Motor quotient"MOT4-6"	104 (96;113)	111 (104;116)	**0.005**
Daily moderate activity (minutes per day)	123 (106;163)	109 (91;124)	0.060
Daily vigorous activity (minutes per day)	25 (16;42)	22 (16;32)	0.534
Daily moderate and vigorous activity	155 (124;190)	136 (112;163)	0.093
"Kiddy-KINDL®" questionnaire	75 (67;91)	79 (70;87)	0.744
"KINDL parents®" questionnaire	75 (70;80)	78 (73;82)	0.066

children with congenital heart disease (CHD) compared with the control group
(* p values from a Wilcoxon rank sum test, except for sex: Chi² test was used)

The parents (either mother or father) had to complete the parents' questionnaire without any help.

2.5 Statistical Analysis

All statistic calculations were performed with SPSS 19.0.0 (SPSS Inc., an IBM Company, Chicago, Illinois, USA). All investigated variables were skewed and normal distribution was rejected by a Shapiro Wilk test. Therefore, all measurements were depicted as median (1st quartile; 3rd quartile) and non-parametric tests were used. For the primary question, to describe the difference of the motor quotient for children with CHD in comparison with healthy children, the Wilcoxon rank sum test was performed. To compare activity and Kiddy-KINDL® questionnaire as secondary questions also Wilcoxon rank sum test was performed. With the Spearman rank correlation the relation of the motor quotient with sex, age, body mass index (BMI), activity and life quality was tested. Two-sided p-values <0.05 were considered significant.

3. RESULTS

Our study group did not differ significantly from the control group in respect to age, sex, body weight, and body mass index. Healthy children had a slightly higher body length (p=0.003, Table 2).

The motoric test could be performed in all children except in five patients who were all four years old and too much afraid of the test situation. These five children were excluded from the analysis. In the CHD group 27 children and in the control group 6 children refused to wear the accelerometer or had incomplete data sets. Six children with CHD were not able to answer the Kiddy-KINDL® questionnaire because of poor German or they didn't want to answer it. Among the parents only one was not able to answer the questions due to language barrier.

3.1 Motor Development

The median motor quotient of the CHD group was 104 (96;113) and significantly lower than in the control group with 111 (104;116) (p=0.005, Table 2). Only 6% of the CHD children showed motor quotient values below 85, but none of the healthy children.

This result was confirmed in an additional post-hoc stepwise multiple regression analysis. CHD was the most prominent factor for an deminished motor quotient, responsible for a loss of MQ of 5.6 (p=0.020). This was followed by the body mass index, responsible for a loss of 1,4 per every additional 1 kg/m² of BMI (p=0.029). After including those two factors, sex, age, body length, body mass did not reach significance in the model.

A post-hoc power analysis revealed, that a sample size of 32 subjects in each of the two groups would have been enough to detect the measured MQ difference of 6 with the measured standard deviations of 8.8 and 11.9 and a given p-value of 0.05 with a power of 90%.

3.2 Daily activity

Children with CHD trended to be slightly more active (155 [124; 190]) minutes of moderate and vigorous activity per day) than healthy children (136 [112; 163] minutes of moderate and vigorous activity per day, p=0.093). This was the result of a slightly increased time at moderate activity. However, both differences did not reach significance (Table 2).

3.3 Quality of Life

The assessment of life quality by the children showed no significant difference in children with CHD (75 [67; 92]) and healthy children (79 [71; 87] p=0.744). The parents estimated the life quality of their children similarly, (CHD group 75 [67; 92], control group 78 [74; 83] p=0.066).

3.4 Correlation to Motor Development

No correlation of the motor quotient to age, sex, daily activity or quality of life was found, neither in the CHD group nor in the control group (Table 3).

4. DISCUSSION

This study showed that kindergarten children with CHD have a slightly reduced motor ability in comparison with healthy children. These limitations could not be related to physical activity or quality of life.

During the last fifteen years, several studies have investigated the motor development of children with various congenital heart defects. Some of them analysed a mixed group of CHD [1,3,5], others investigated specific groups of CHD [6,7, 13-15]. Only two studies compared their results with healthy children of the same age group [1,5].

Table 3. Spearman correlation of the motor quotient with other tested parameters

	CHD	Controls
	r (p)	r (p)
Activity (min/day)	0.009 (0.959)	0.186 (0.308)
Body mass index (kg/m²)	-0.176 (0.175)	-0.084 (0.643)
"Kiddy-Kindl®" questionnaire	0.260 (0.053)	0.117 (0.479)
"KINDL parents®" questionnaire	0.067 (0.605)	-0.091 (0.580)

Furthermore, two studies examined very large age ranges between 5-14 years, whereas only one focussed on kindergarten children [8].

All studies found deficits in the motor development of children with congenital heart disease. Our findings confirm these results that there is a reduced motor ability in children with congenital heart diseases compared to a current control group. Nevertheless, in our group most of the children with congenital heart diseases had normal values in their motor development, when they are compared to the established reference values. This was also shown in our study on motor training, where most of the children with CHD also showed values within the reference range in their motor ability [16]. It was our control group that showed supranormal values. This might be a regional phenomenon. However, it cannot be ruled out that a selection bias of the control group was responsible for the supranormal values. In the patient group, far less subjects denied participation and such a bias is less likely.

To test the motor ability of the children some of the studies used the body coordination test for children (KTK) [1,3,5]. The "KTK" has only four gross motor skill tests and is recommended for children from 5 to 15 years. With its four tasks it is rather limited in the estimation of the complete motor development. In contrast we used the "MOT 4-6". It is a special motoric test for kindergarten children (4-6 years). With its 18 tasks it analyses many areas of motor development. The results of the motoric test were summed up to a single score. So we could not differentiate whether children had deficits in one area of motor development. But most children enjoyed the motoric test, maybe because it is so much diversified. Only five patients, all of them were four years old, were so afraid about the test situation that they denied participation.

Bjarnason-Wehrens [1] speculated that over-protection of the parents could be the main reason for motor deficits. They investigated school children and found motor limitations that were independent from the severity of the defect. These limitations could even be shown in patients with simple defects that were repaired with no or only mild residuals, which are very unlikely to cause any hemodynamic limitations. However, they did not investigate daily activity or parental education style itself to affirm their speculation. Our findings do not support this speculation. Our children with congenital heart disease were at least as active as healthy children. Children with CHD even seem to be more active than the healthy control group. This was surprising. McCrindle [17] as well as our group [18] could show in school children with Fontan circulation that they indeed have a reduced daily activity. However, in most previous studies on children with simpler congenital heart defects no daily activity was measured.

Honestly, some of the enhanced activity might also be explained by the fact that the CHD group had slightly more boys than the control group and boys are known to be physically more active than girls [18].

To our opinion the best explanation for the normal activity of children with congenital heart disease is a change in the attitude towards sport activities in these children during the last decade. Nowadays, the recommendation of the medical societies concerning leisure and even competitive sport participation became much more liberal [19]. For the last decade, in our institution physical activity has been promoted in patients with CHD, if no clear medical contraindications are present.

5. LIMITATIONS

Our control group showed supranormal values in the motor test. This might be a regional phenomenon. However, it cannot be ruled out that a selection bias of the control group was responsible for the supranormal values. But the small number of the control group, in contrast to the CHD-group could be a limitation. Unfortunately a substantial number of parents, from the kindergarten children did not agree to the participation of their child. In the patient group, far less subjects denied participation and such a bias is less likely.

6. CONCLUSION

For the daily clinical work, it seems to be very important to focus more on the motor development during medical follow-up check-ups of the children. We agree with Hövels-Gürich [20] that at the age of 2 and 5 years a motoric test should be performed in all children with congenital heart disease. In addition, assessment of life quality should be implemented. At this age group such children showing limitations could be sent to a specialized motor training [16]. Once their condition improves, they can join regular sport classes at school. This avoids separation from their playmates, and helps to prevent consecutive social drawbacks. For those without deficits and no clear contraindications, physical activity of at least 60 minutes a day should be promoted, like for all children [19].

ETHICAL APPROVAL

The authors assert that all procedures contributing to this work comply with the ethical standards of the relevant national guidelines on human experimentation (Good clinical practice ISO 14155:2011) and with the Helsinki Declaration of 1975, as revised in 2013. The study has been approved by the institutional ethical board (ethical board of the medical faculty, Technische Universität München, project number 2782/10).

COMPETING INTERESTS

Authors have declared that no competing interests exist.

REFERENCES

1. Bjarnason-Wehrens B, Dordel S, Schickendantz S, Krumm C, Bott D, Sreeram N, et al. Motor development in children with congenital cardiac diseases compared to their healthy peers. Cardiol Young. 2007;17:487-98.

2. Bjarnason-Wehrens B, Schmitz S, Dordel S. Motor development in children with congenital cardiac diseases. Paediatric Cardiology. 2008;92-6.

3. Dordel S, Bjarnason-Wehrens B, Lawrenz W, Leurs S, Rost R, Schickendantz S, et al. Zur Wirksamkeit motorischer Förderung von Kindern mit (teil-)korrigierten angeborenen Herzfehlern. Deutsche Zeitschrift für Sportmedizin. 1999;50:41-6.

4. Reybrouck T, Mertens L. Physical performance and physical activity in grown-up congenital heart disease. Eur J Cardiovasc Prev Rehabil. 2005;12:498-502.

5. Stieh J, Kramer HH, Harding P, Fischer G. Gross and fine motor development is impaired in children with cyanotic congenital heart disease. Neuropediatrics. 1999;30:77-82.

6. Bellinger DC, Wypij D, du Plessis AJ, Rappaport LA, Jonas RA, Wernovsky G, et al. Neurodevelopmental status at eight years in children with dextro-transposition of the great arteries: The Boston Circulatory Arrest Trial. J Thorac Cardiovasc Surg. 2003;126:1385-96.

7. Bellinger DC, Wypij D, Kuban KC, Rappaport LA, Hickey PR, Wernovsky G, et al. Developmental and neurological status of children at 4 years of age after heart surgery with hypothermic circulatory arrest or low-flow cardiopulmonary bypass. Circulation. 1999;100:526-32.

8. Snookes SH, Gunn JK, Eldridge BJ, Donath SM, Hunt RW, Galea MP, et al. A systematic review of motor and cognitive outcomes after early surgery for congenital heart disease. Pediatrics. 2010;125:e818-27.

9. Warnes CA, Liberthson R, Danielson GK, Dore A, Harris L, Hoffman JI, et al. Task force 1: the changing profile of congenital heart disease in adult life. J Am Coll Cardiol. 2001;37:1170-5.

10. Zimmer R, Volkamer M. Manual MOT 4-6 Motoriktest für vier- bis sechsjährige Kinder. 2. überarbeitete und erweiterte Auflage ed. Weinheim: Belz; 1987.

11. Rowlands AV, Thomas PW, Eston RG, Topping R. Validation of the RT3 triaxial accelerometer for the assessment of physical activity. Med Sci Sports Exerc. 2004;36:518-24.

12. Ravens-Sieberer U, Bullinger M. LQ-Mesung bei Kindern-psychomotorische Ergebnisse zum KINDL. In: Bullinger M, Morfeld M, Ravens-Sieberer U, Koch U, editors. Medizinische Psychologie in einem sich wandelneen Gesundheitssystem:

Identität. Integration & Intedisziplinarität: Pabst Verlag; 1998.

13. Bellinger DC, Jonas RA, Rappaport LA, Wypij D, Wernovsky G, Kuban KC, et al. Developmental and neurologic status of children after heart surgery with hypothermic circulatory arrest or low-flow cardiopulmonary bypass. N Engl J Med. 1995;332:549-55.

14. Hovels-Gurich HH, Seghaye MC, Dabritz S, Messmer BJ, von Bernuth G. Cognitive and motor development in preschool and school-aged children after neonatal arterial switch operation. J Thorac Cardiovasc Surg. 1997;114:578-85.

15. Vahsen N, Kavsek M, Toussaint-Gotz N, Schneider K, Urban AE, Schneider M. Cognitive and motor abilities and behavioural outcome in children after neonatal operation with cardiopulmonary bypass. Klinische Padiatrie. 2009;221:19-24.

16. Muller J, Pringsheim M, Engelhardt A, Meixner J, Halle M, Oberhoffer R, et al. Motor training of sixty minutes once per week improves motor ability in children with congenital heart disease and retarded motor development: A pilot study. Cardiology in the Young; 2012.

17. Mc Crindle BW, Williams RV, Mital S, Clark BJ, Russell JL, Klein G, et al. Physical activity levels in children and adolescents are reduced after the Fontan procedure, independent of exercise capacity, and are associated with lower perceived general health. Arch Dis Child. 2007;92:509-14.

18. Muller J, Christov F, Schreiber C, Hess J, Hager A. Exercise capacity, quality of life, and daily activity in the long-term follow-up of patients with univentricular heart and total cavopulmonary connection. Eur Heart J. 2009;30:2915-20.

19. Takken T, Giardini A, Reybrouck T, Gewillig M, Hovels-Gurich HH, Longmuir PE, et al. Recommendations for physical activity, recreation sport, and exercise training in paediatric patients with congenital heart disease: A report from the Exercise, Basic & Translational Research Section of the European Association of Cardiovascular Prevention and Rehabilitation, the European Congenital Heart and Lung Exercise Group, and the Association for European Paediatric Cardiology. Eur J Cardiovasc Prev Rehabil; 2011.

20. Hövels-Gürich HH. Causes, prevalence and prevention of developmental disorders after cardiac surgery in childhood. Monatsschrift Kinderheilkunde. 2012;160: 118-28.

8

Signal Processing Tools for Heart Sounds Analysis Based on Time-Frequency Domain

Ali Moukadem[1], Christian Brandt[2], Emmanuel Andrès[3*], Samy Talha[4] and Alain Dieterlen[1]

[1]MIPS Laboratory, University of Haute Alsace, 68093 Mulhouse, France.
[2]Center of Clinical Investigations, University Hospital of Strasbourg, Inserm, BP 426, 67091 Strasbourg, France.
[3]Department of Internal Medicine, University Hospital of Strasbourg, BP 426, 67091 Strasbourg, France.
[4]Laboratory of Physiology and Functional Explorations, University Hospital of Strasbourg, BP 426, 67091 Strasbourg, France.

Authors' contributions

This work was carried out in collaboration between all authors. Author AM designed the study, wrote the protocol, and wrote the first draft of the manuscript. Authors AM, CB, AD managed the literature searches, analyses of the results of the study. All authors read and approved the final manuscript.

Editor(s):
(1) Francesco Pelliccia, Department of Heart and Great Vessels University La Sapienza, Rome, Italy.
(2) Fatih Yalcin, School of Medicine, Department of Cardiology, Johns Hopkins University, USA.
Reviewers:
(1) Prabakaran Kandasamy, Electronics And Instrumentation Engineering, Erode Sengunthar Engineering College & India.
(2) Rajkumar Palaniappan, School of Mechatronic Engineering, Universiti Malaysia Perlis, Malaysia.
(3) Anonymous, University Malaysia Pahang, Malaysia.
(4) Anonymous, University A.B. Belkaid-Tlemcen, Algeria.

ABSTRACT

This paper present several signal processing tools for the analysis of heart sounds. Cardiac auscultation is noninvasive, low-cost and accurate to diagnose some heart diseases. A new module for the segmentation of heart sounds based on S-Transform is presented. The heart sound segmentation process divides the Phono Cardio Gram (PCG) signal into four parts: S1 (first heart sound), systole, S2 (second heart sound) and diastole. The segmentation can be considered one of the most important phases in the auto-analysis of PCG signals. A segmentation method based on the Shannon energy of the local spectrum calculated by the S-transform is proposed. Then, the energy concentration of the S-transform is optimized to accurately detect the boundaries of the localized sounds. New features based on the energy concentration of the S-transform are

Corresponding author: E-mail: Emmanuel.ANDRES@chru-strasbourg.fr

proposed to classify S1 and S2 and other features based on the complexity measure via Time-Frequency (TF) domain are proposed to detect systolic murmurs.

Keywords: Heart sounds; segmentation; feature extraction; classification.

1. INTRODUCTION

The recent advances in signal processing lead to powerful applications in the real life conditions for Doctors and medical staff.

Simultaneous technological evolutions with the development of non connected devices allow new approaches for medical practice via telemedicine.

Combination of the two developments lead to an increase in clinical diagnostic power immediately if signal processing is available on an hosting device or after connection to a reference center.

Raw heart auscultation data have to be converted in a phonocardiogram.PCG can be associated or not to simultaneous registrations of blood pressure, SAO2 or ECG by example.

As well single heart auscultation treated as a PCG includes enough information to authorize segmentation of the heart cycle.

Therefore heart rate, duration of systole and diastole detection of pathologic events can be easily detected.

The focus of this paper is the PCG signal (Fig. 1) obtained from auscultation, first medical step in clinical examination, with an electronic stethoscope [1,2]. The PCG reveals the mechanical activity of the heart and it can be considered as non-stationary signal.

For an untrained human ear, it's not an evidence to localize heart sounds, recognize their internal components and classify the murmurs and their origins. For that, the signal processing tools allow better estimation and detection of these signals. In this respect, different approaches could be considered to improve the electronic stethoscope [3]:

- Tools providing embedded autonomous analysis, easy to use by the general public at home for auto-diagnosis, monitoring and warning if need be.
- Tools providing sophisticated analysis (coupled to a PC, Bluetooth link) for the use of professionals in order to make an in-depth medical diagnosis and to train medical students.

In the past twenty years, many studies have interested in the PCG signal processing field (see Fig. 2); for the de-noising of the PCG many advanced tools of signal processing are used as the Kalman filter [4], the wavelets, and more recently the Emperical Modal Decomposition (EMD). For the time-frequency representation of the PCG signal the famous STFT is used [5], the Continuous Wavelet Transform (CWT) [6], the S-transform [7] and the Wigner-Ville Distribution (WVD) [8,9] etc. For the segmentation process the methods can be classified depending on the domain on which they are applied: time domain (Shannon energy [10]), frequency domain (homomorphic filter [11], time-frequency domain (wavelet transform[12], S-transform [13]) and nonlinear domain (Radial basis function [14]). For the classification of heart sounds: Artificial Neural Networks (ANN) [15], K-Nearest Neighbors (KNN) [16] and Support Vector Machines (SVM) [17,18].

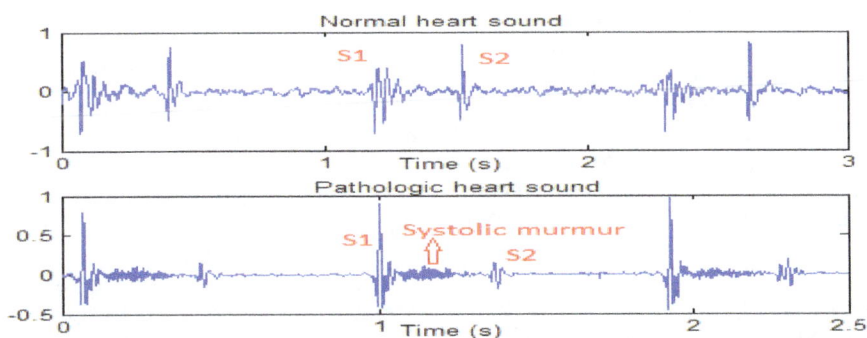

Fig. 1. Example of a normal (top) and pathologic (bottom) heart sounds with systolic murmur

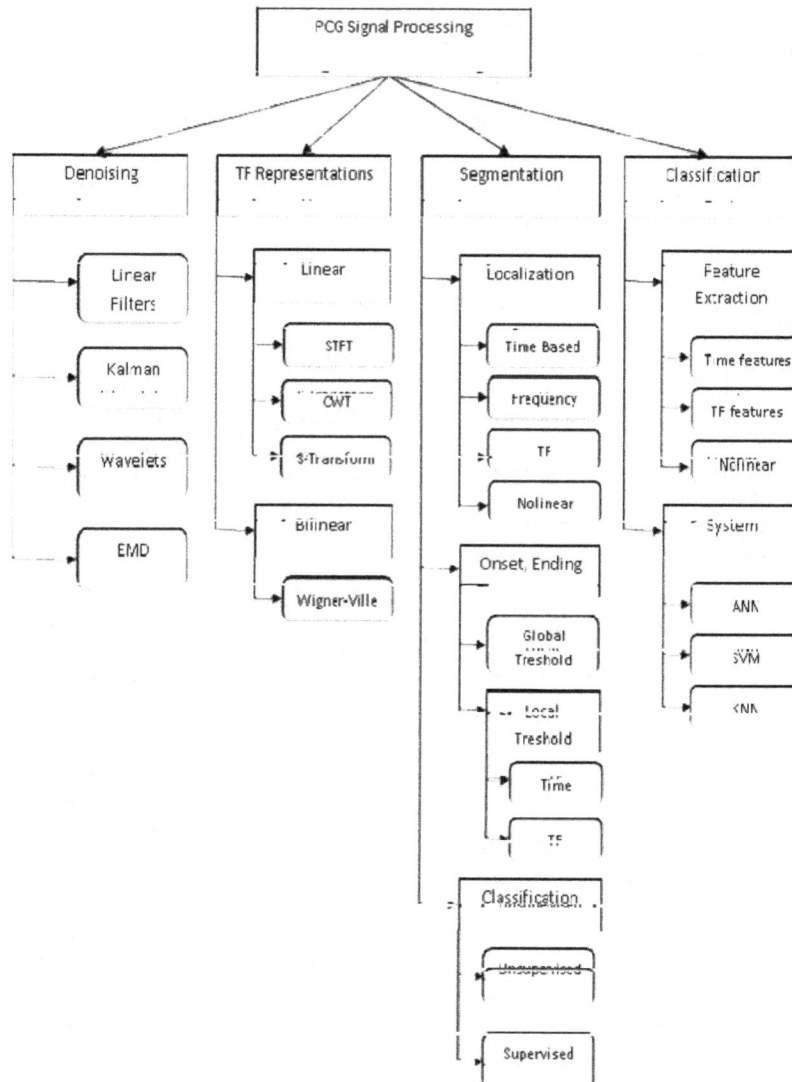

Fig. 2. An overview of the different contributions existing in the literature concerning the PCG signal processing algorithms and methods

The segmentation is one of the first phases of the heart sound analysis. Heart sound segmentation partitions the PCG signals into cardiac cycles and further into S1 (first heart sound), systole, S2 (second heart sound) and diastole [3]. Manypapers in the literature that tried to segment heart sounds without any help of ECG as Shannon energy [10], Hilbert Transform [19], high order statistics [20], a hidden Markov model [21], among others.

In this paper we present some signal processing tools based on time frequency domain to segment, classify and extract feature from heart sounds. The results are based on some real

examples used as preliminary validation of the proposed methods.

2. METHODS AND MATERIALS

2.1 Sounds Collection

The heart sounds have been collected in the Hospital of Strasbourg (France) where Different cardiologists equipped with a prototype electronic stethoscope. The sounds are recorded with 16 bits accuracy and 8000Hz sampling frequency in a wave format. Recruitment was made through clinical research project (HUS-PRI 4179) with the support of the clinical investigation center

(INSERM) All of the participants have given a written informed consent. The best auscultation focus has been registered. Duration of registration varied from 8 to 12 s while patients controlled their respiration. Just some examples are included in this paper to perform a preliminary validation of the proposed methods.

2.2 Localization and Segmentation of Heart Sounds

2.2.1 Preprocessing

At first the original signal is decimated by factor 4 from 8000 Hz to 2000 Hz and the a normalization process is applied as follows:

$$x_{norm}(t) = \frac{x(t)}{\left|\max(x(t))\right|} \tag{1}$$

2.2.2 Localization and segmentation of heart Sounds

The localization algorithms operating on PCG data try to emphasize heart sound occurrences with an initial transformation that can be classified into three main categories: frequency based transformation, morphological transformations and complexity based transformations [1].

Modified S-transform and Shannon Energy (MSSE) localization method: MSSE envelope(Fig. 3).

We have proposed a method named SSE in [13] to segment the heart sound. This method is based on the S-transform and the Shannon energy. The SSE method operates on the local spectrum calculated by the S-transform.

The proposed SSE method calculates the Shannon energy of each column of the extracted S-matrix as follows:

$$SSE(x_i) = -\int_{-\infty}^{+\infty} \left|S_x(\tau,f)\right|^n \log(\left|S_x(\tau,f)\right|^n) df \tag{2}$$

Where $S_x(\tau,f)$ is the S-transform of the signal $x(t)$ [22]:

$$S_x(\tau,f) = \int_{-\infty}^{+\infty} x(t)w(t-\tau,f)e^{-2\pi jft} dt \tag{3}$$

The parameter n in equation [23] is usually fixed to 2 which is the standard coefficient of the Shannon energy measure. The parameter n can be fixed to 1.5 for example to enhance the detection of low intensities sounds buried in noise. This occurs in heart sounds more often with S2 when the cardiac frequency is high. Fig. 4 shows the compromise of attenuation of low and high intensities, as a function of the value of n. we note here that for the SSE method, the intensities are the local spectrum coefficients of the S-transform and not the time sample intensities of the signal.

Figs. 5 and 6 shows the SSE envelope extract for normal noisy heart sounds and pathological heart sounds, respectively.
When the first and the second heart sounds are localized by the SSE method the OSSE [3,13] method is applied to segment these sounds.

The block diagram of the OSSE algorithm is shown below (Fig. 7).

First it consists to estimate the limit boundaries for each located sound by applying a window of 150 ms. Then the Stockwell transform of each segmented bound is optimized. The SSE envelope is recalculated based on the new (optimized) representation and finally a local threshold is applied to estimate the refined boundaries.

Figs. 8, 9 and 10 shows figures show the process to achieve the signal analysis and detection of S1 and S2.

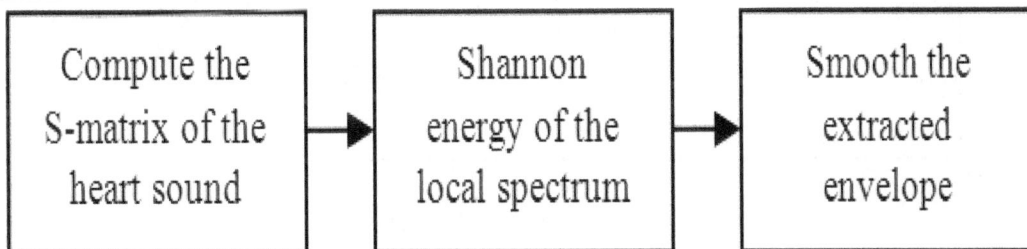

Compute the S-matrix of the heart sound	Shannon energy of the local spectrum	Smooth the extracted envelope

Fig. 3. Block diagram of SSE method

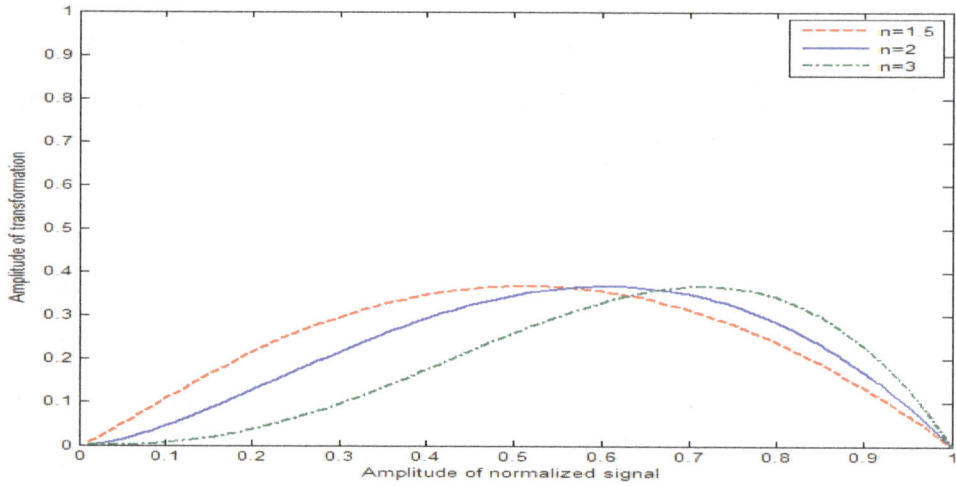

Fig. 4. The envelope of normalized signal for values of n=1.5, 2 and 3

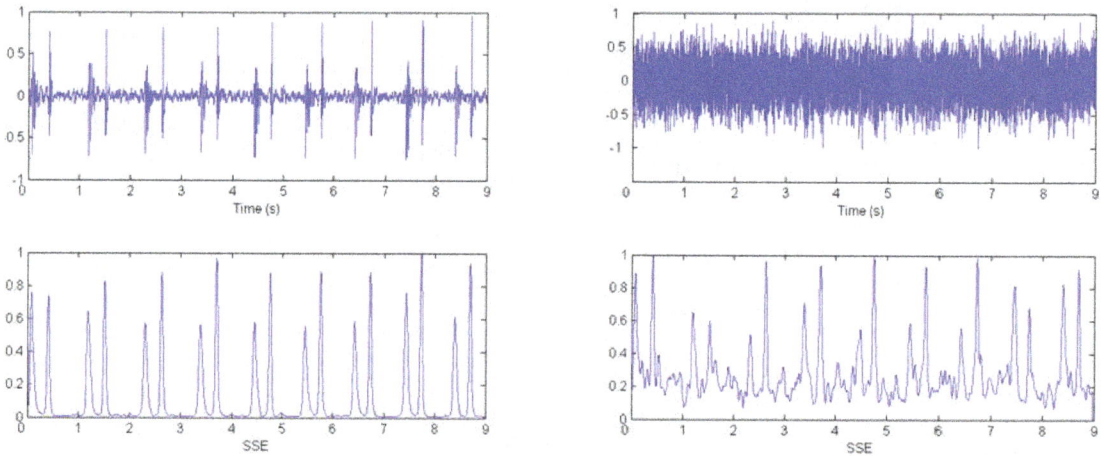

Fig. 5. (top) Envelope extraction for two normal PCG signal without and with additive Gaussian noise, (bottom) their SSE envelopes

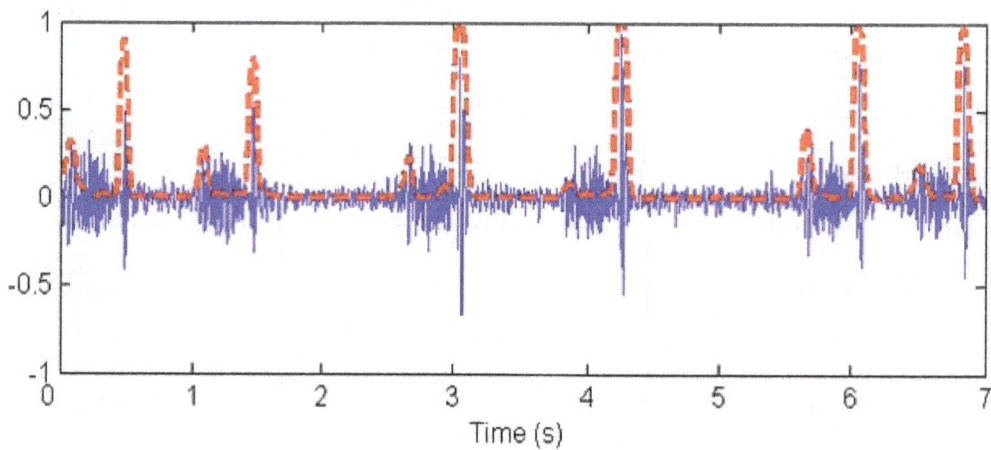

Fig. 6. The SSE Envelope (dashed lines) for a signal with systolic murmur

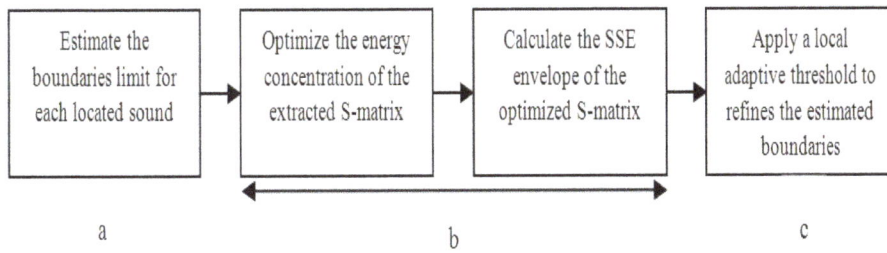

Fig. 7. The block diagram of the OSSE Method

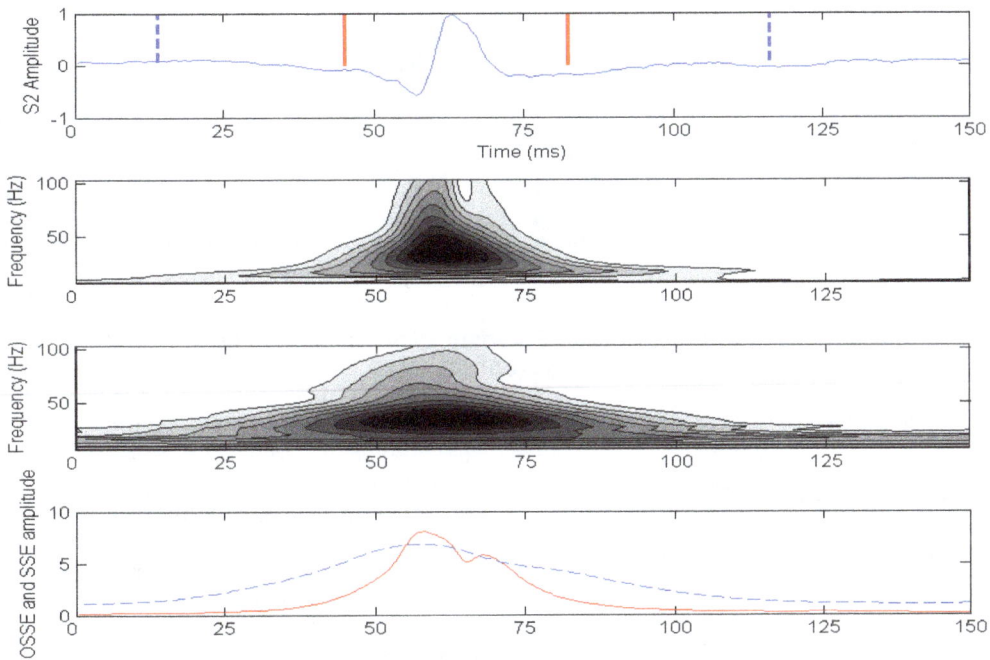

Fig. 8. (top) S2 signal with two detected boundaries calculated by the optimized S-transform and the standard S-transform (dashed line), S-transform with the optimum valueα=0.5, standard S-transform withα=1, (bottom) SSE envelope for the optimized S-transform and standard S-transform (dashed line)

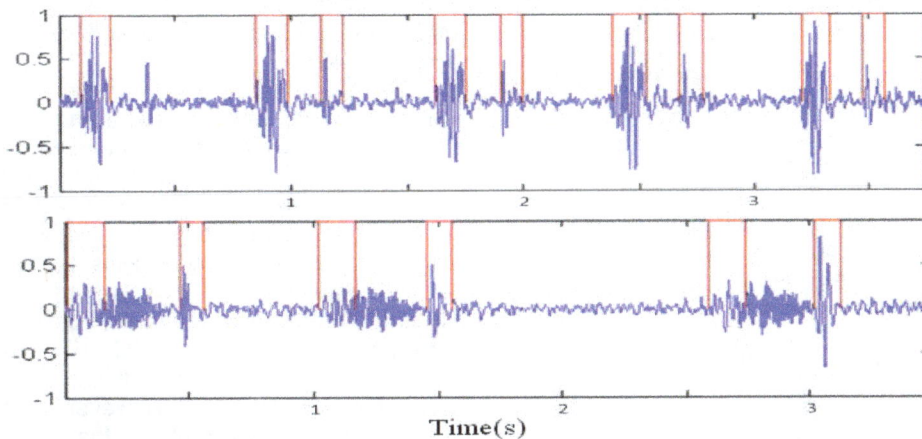

Fig. 9. OSSE method applied on a normal heart sound (top) and pathological heart sound (bottom)

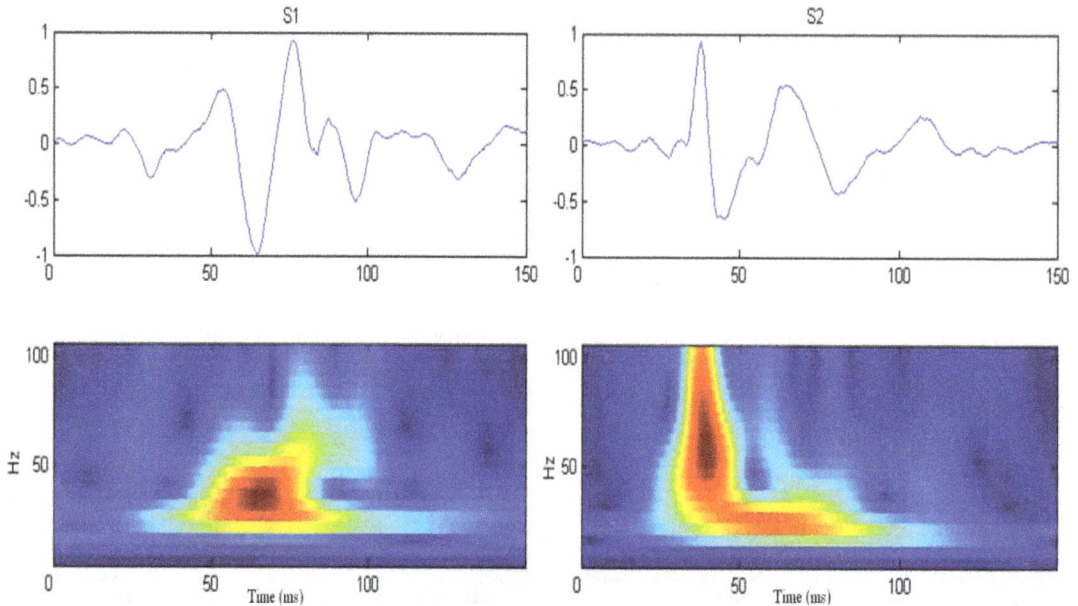

Fig. 10. S1 and S2 signals (top), optimized S-transform obtained with α=0.8 for S1 and α=0.5 for S2 (bottom)

2.3 Classification of Heart Sounds

2.3.1 S1 and S2 Classification

a. The Gaussian parameter α as discriminant feature

A new feature based on the energy concentration in time frequency domain is used to classify the first and the second heart sounds. This feature is used to optimize the energy concentration of the S-transform as follows:

$$\alpha_{opt} = \arg\max_{\alpha}(CM(\alpha)) \qquad (4)$$

Where CM is the energy concentration measure that we aim to optimize [13].

b. The SSE envelope feature: β

A second feature investigated in this study, named β, it aims to integrate the normalized SSE envelope over time, and it can be given as:

$$\beta = \int_{-\infty}^{+\infty}\left\{\int_{-\infty}^{+\infty}|S_x(t,f)|^2\log(|S_x(t,f)|^2)df\right\}dt \qquad (5)$$

The SSE envelope estimates the frequency energy at the local spectrum of the signal. It can be considered as a modified instantaneous frequency measure. The β feature aims to reveal the frequency contribution of each sound over time. Mathematically, it can be viewed as the integration over time of a modified instantaneous frequency measure. Physically, this feature reveals in some way the shape morphology of the signal. The measure is computed from the normalized SSE envelope to avoid the influence of the amplitude variations.

Fig. 11 shows an example of the β feature calculated on S1 and S2 sounds from their normalized SSE envelopes.

Murmurs detection: Normalized Shannon Entropy (NSE) [4]

Heart murmurs usually result from turbulence in blood flow or the vibration of heart tissues which can occur in a systolic or diastolic period. The presence of murmurs increases the heart sound complexity. Several recent studies use methods for nonlinear and chaotic signals to estimate the signal complexity and detect murmurs [20,23]. These methods are generally based on the reconstructed state space which explores the non-linear behavior and the non-Gaussian components of the signal. However, even though it seems reasonable to expect the nonlinear and chaotic characteristics of turbulence in blood flowthrough a vessel to be reflected in the murmurs, it is well accepted that recorded signals do not necessarily reflect the nonlinear and chaotic behavior of the underlying system [24,25]. Moreover, application of such methods suited for nonlinear or chaotic signals might be an unnecessary increase in algorithm complexity compared to linear methods based on autocorrelation and power spectrum [24,26]. Therefore, we apply the complexity measure on the TFR plane (ST-Spectrogram) instead of the reconstructed state space, to detect murmurs in heart sounds.

The Shannon Entropy is a natural candidate for measuring the complexity of a signal through TFR. It is applicable on the ST-Spectrogram coefficients (C_x) since the ST-spectrogram verifies the non-negativity condition. The Shannon Entropy is defined as follows:

$$H(C_x) = -\iint C_x(t,f) \log_2 C_x(t,f) dt df \quad (6)$$

To normalize the Shannon entropy, we normalize first the coefficients of the ST-spectrogram as follows:

$$C_x^{norm}(t,f) = \frac{C_x(t,f)}{\iint C_x(u,v) du dv} \quad (7)$$

The maximum of Shannon Entropy, which correspond to equiprobable events case, can be given as:

$$H_{\max}(C_x^{norm}) = \log_2(n \times m) \quad (8)$$

Where, n is the samples number of the signal $x(t)$, m is the number of frequency voices used to calculate the ST-spectrogram and $n \times m$ is the total number of coefficients in the $C_x^{norm}(t,f)$ distribution. Therefore, the normalized Shannon Entropy can be given as:

$$H_{norm}(C_x^{norm}) = \frac{H(C_x^{norm})}{\log_2(n \times m)} \quad (9)$$

The peaky TFRs of signals comprised of small numbers of elementary components would yield small entropy values, while the diffuse TFRs of more complicated signals would yield large entropy values. Fig. 12 shows an example of normal and pathologic systolic sounds and their NSEs based on ST-Spectrogram [27,28]. The number of component in pathologic sound with the presence of murmur is higher than the normal systole, which explains the higher NSE (0.88) [29].

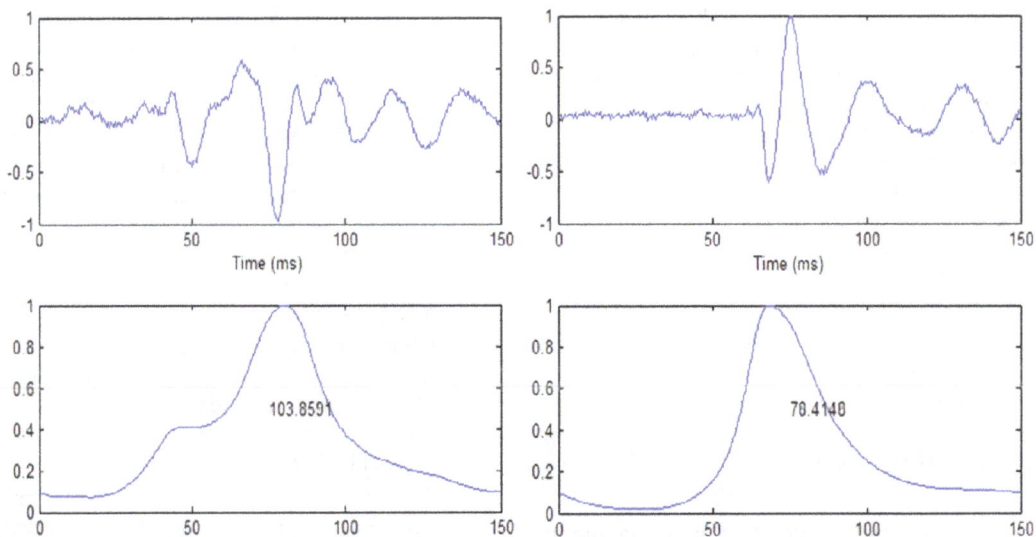

Fig. 11. S1 (left) and S2 signals (right) and their normalized SSE envelopes with the values of β (bottom)

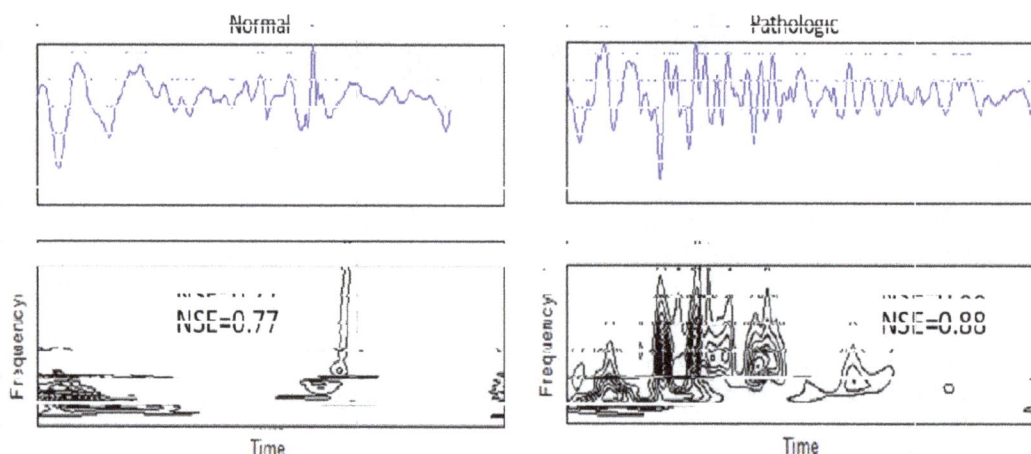

Fig. 12. NSEs applied on the ST-Spectrogram plane for normal and pathologic segmented

4. CONCLUSION

This paper presented several algorithms and methods to segment and classify the heart sounds (PCG signal) based on time-frequency domain. Heart sounds are accurate for diagnosing some heart diseases. They are non-stationary signals by nature (as most biosignals) which make the application of Time-Frequency based methods intuitive.

The paper focused on the application of the S-transform on heart sounds. Several theoretical methods are proposed and applied on real signals. Localization, segmentation, feature extraction and classification schemes of heart sounds are explored and discussed. A campaign of measurements is in motion in the Hospital University of Strasbourg to collect normal and pathological heart sounds which will allow us to test the proposed signal processing tools on large clinical datasets. The classification of murmurs from different origin and the assessing of their severity, the detection of additional sounds as S3 and S4 can be considered as future research perspectives to this work.

ETHICAL APPROVAL

All authors hereby declare that all experiments have been examined and approved by the ethics committee of the *University Hospital of Strasbourg* (Strasbourg, France, *PRI* Project) and have therefore been performed in accordance with the ethical standards laid down in the 1964 Declaration of Helsinki.

COMPETING INTERESTS

Authors have declared that no competing interests exist.

REFERENCES

1.   Palaniappan R, Kenneth Sundaraj, Nizam. Machine learning in lung sound analysis: A systematic review, Journal of Biocybernetics and Biomedical Engineering. 2013;33(3);129-135.

2.   Palaniappan R, Sundaraj K, Sundaraj S, Artificial intelligence techniques used in respiratory sound analysis - A systematic review, Biomedical Engineering/ Biomedizinische Technik. 2014;59(1):7-18.

3.   Moukadem A, Dieterlen A, Brandt C. Phonocardiogram signal processing module for auto-diagnosis and telemedicine applications, ehealth and Remote Monitoring INTECH. 2012;117–136 (Chapter 7).

4.   Charleston S, Azimi-Sadjadi MR. Reduced order Kalman filtering for the enhancement of respiratory sounds, IEEE Transactions on Biomedical Engineering. 1997;44;1006–1019.

5.   Djebarri A, Bereksi RF. Short-time fourier transform analysis of the phonocardiogram signal, in: The 7th IEEE International Conference on Electronics, Circuits and Systems (ICECS). 2000;844–847.

6.   Debbal SM, Bereksi-Reguig F. Computerized heart sounds analysis,

Computers in Biology and Medicine. 2008;38:263-280.

7. Sejdic E, Jiang J. Comparative study of three time-frequency representations with applications to a novel correlation method, in Proceedings of the IEEE International Conference on Acoustics, Speech and Signal Processing (ICASSP). 2004;2:633–636.

8. Boutana D, Benidir M, Barakat B. Segmentation and identification of some pathological phonocardiogram signals using time-frequency analysis, IET Signal Process. 2011;5(6):527-537. DOI:10.1049/iet-spr.2010.0013.

9. Djebbari, Bereksi – Reguig. Detection of the valvular split within thesecond heart sound using the reassigned smoothed pseudo Wigner–Ville distribution. Bio Medical Engineering OnLine. 2013;12:37.

10. Liang H, Lukkarinen S, & Hartimo I. Heart sound segmentation algorithm based on heart sound envelogram. Helsinki University of Technology, Espoo, Finland; 1997.

11. Gupta CN, Palaniappan R, Swaminathan S, Krishnan SM. Neural network classification of homomorphic segmented heart sounds, Applied Soft Computing. 2007;7:286–297.

12. Moussavi Z, Flores D, Thomas G. Heart sound cancellation based on multiscale products and linear prediction, proceedings of the 26th annual international conference of the IEEE EMBS san francisco, CA, USA. 2004;1-5.

13. Moukadem A, Dieterlen A, Brandt C. A robust heart sound segmentation module based on s-transform. Biomedical Signal Processing and Control. 2013;8:273–281

14. Moukadem, A.; Dieterlen, A.; Hueber, N. & Brandt C. Comparative study of heart sounds localization. Bioelectronics, Biomedical and Bio-inspired Systems SPIE, Prague. (2011);8068A-27.

15. Moukadem A, Dieterlen A, Hueber N, Brandt C. Localization of heart sounds based on s-transform and radial basis functions, 15TH Nordic-Baltic conference on Biomedical engineering and medical physics (NBC) IFMBE Proceedings. 2011;34:68-171. DOI: 10.1007/978-3-642-21683-1_42.

16. Sinha RK, Aggarwal Y, Das BN. Backpropagation artificial neural network classifier to detect changes in heart sound due to mitral valve regurgitation. J Med Syst. 2007;31(3):205–209.

17. Vepa J. Classification of heart murmurs using cepstral features and support vector machine, engineering in medicine and biology society. Annual international conference of the IEEE, EMBC; 2009.

18. Maglogiannis I, Loukis E, Zafiropoulos E, Stasis A. Support vectors machine-based identification of heart valve diseases using heart sounds. Comput Methods Programs Biomed. 2009;95(1):47-61. DOI: 10.1016/j.cmpb.2009.01.003.

19. Liang H, Lukkarinen S, Hartimo I. A boundary modification method for heart sound segmentation algorithm. Computers in Cardiology. 1998;593-595.

20. Choi S. & Jiang Z. Compariason of envelope extraction algorithms for cardiac sound signal segmentation. Micro-Mechatronics Laboratory, Yamaguchi University, Japan; 2006.

21. Ahlstrom C. Nonlinear phonocardiographic signal processing thesis. Linkoping University, Linkoping, Sweden. 2008;SE-581-85.

22. Moukadem A, Dieterlen A, & Brandt C. Automatic heart sound analysis module based on stockwell transform applied on auto-diagnosis and telemedicine applications. In eTELEMED, The Fifth International Conference on eHealth, Telemedicine, and Social Medicine. 2013;259-264.

23. Schmidt SE, Holst-Hansen C, Graff C, Toft E, Struijk JJ. Segmentation of heart sound recordings by a duration-dependent hidden Markov mode, Physiological Measurement. 2010;31(4):513-529.

24. Stockwell RG, Mansinha L, & Lowe RP. Localization of the complex spectrum: The s-transform, IEEE Trans. Sig. Proc. 1996;44(4):998–1001.

25. Ahlstrom C, Hult P, Rask P, Karlsson J-E, Nylander E, Dahlstrom U, Ask P. Feature extraction for systolic heart murmur classification. Annals of Biomedical Engineering. 2006;34(11):1666-1677.

26. Samit A, Kumar P, Goutam S. On an algorithm for boundary estimation of commonly occurring heart valve diseases in time domain. India Conference, Annual IEEE; 2006.

10.1109/INDCON.2006.302758.

27. Schlant RC, wayne R, Alexander (Eds.). The heart arteries and veins. McGraw Hill Inc; 1994.

28. Sejdic E, Djurovic I, Jiang J. A window width optimized s-transform. EURASIP Journal on Advances in Signal Processing. 2008;13. Article ID: 672941.

   DOI:10.1155/2008/672941.

29. Stankovic LJ, Measure of some time-frequency distributions concentration, signal processing. 2001;81(3):621–631.

9

Clinical Factors Associated with Atrial Fibrillation in Congestive Heart Failure Patients Admitted to the University Teaching Hospital, Lusaka, Zambia

Methuselah Jere[1*], Fastone M. Goma[1], Ben Andrews[2], Longa Kaluba[1] and Charity Kapenda[1]

[1]Department of Physiological Sciences, School of Medicine, University of Zambia, Lusaka, Zambia.
[2]Department of Internal Medicine, School of Medicine, University of Zambia, Lusaka, Zambia.

Authors' contributions

This work was carried out in collaboration between all authors. Author FMG born the idea, author MJ designed the study, wrote the proposal and authors MJ, LK and CK corrected the data. Author MJ did the analysis, wrote the report and prepared the manuscript. Authors FMG and BA supervised the whole process. All authors read and approved the final manuscript.

Editor(s):
(1) Wilbert S. Aronow, University of California, College of Medicine, Irvine, USA.
(2) Eirin Massat Alfonso, College of Medicine, Mayo Clinic, USA And Renovascular Research Laboratory, Mayo Clinic, Rochester, Minnesota, USA.
Reviewers:
(1) Cliff Richard Kikawa, Tshwane University of Technology, South Africa.
(2) Hugo Ramos, National University of Cordoba, Cordoba, Argentina.
(3) Romeu R. De Souza, Sao Judas Tadeu University, Sao Paulo, Brazil.

ABSTRACT

Introduction: Atrial fibrillation (AF) and Congestive Heart failure (CHF) have emerged as major global epidemics. Each of these conditions predisposes to the other, and their concomitant presence has additive adverse effects. This study examined the clinical factors associated with AF in CHF patients admitted to the University Teaching Hospital (UTH), Lusaka, Zambia.

Methods: This was a hospital-based cross-sectional study done in the admission wards of the UTH involving adult patients with the primary diagnosis of congestive heart failure. The data was collected from July 2014 to September 2014. A structured interview schedule was used to capture the socio-demographic and related historical data. Then all patients had a standard 12-lead ECG done on them to check for AF. Those participants with no AF on a standard 12-lead ECG had 24-hours ECG DR180+ Digital Recorder applied to try to pick-up paroxysmal AF. Finally all

Corresponding author: E-mail: jeremethuselah@gmail.com

participants with AF were assessed for clinical factors (i.e. sex, age, BMI, smoking, excessive alcohol intake, hypertension, coronary artery disease, dilated cardiomyopathy, diabetes mellitus, and chronic lung disease). Pearson chi-square of independence of the data was used to analyze the data in SPSS® 20.0 to determine clinical factors of AF in CHF patients.

Results: A total of 49 patients were included in the study and 13 (26.5%) of them had AF, 7 diagnosed by standard ECG and 6 diagnosed by holter ambulatory ECG monitoring. The prevalence of AF in CHF was found to be strongly associated with age 65 years and above, obesity, smoking, excessive alcohol intake, hypertension, dilated cardiomyopathy, diabetes mellitus and chronic lung disease. These findings suggest the need for clinicians to consider full scale use of ambulatory ECG monitors in all CHF patients with the above conditions.

Keywords: ECG DR180+ digital recorder; smoking; cardiomyopathy; diabetes; lung disease.

1. INTRODUCTION

1.1 Background

Atrial fibrillation (AF) and Congestive Heart failure (CHF) have emerged as major global epidemics [1]. These two conditions share similar risk factors, frequently coexist, and have additive adverse effects when occurring in conjunction [2]. The risk factors include hypertension (HTN), coronary artery disease (CAD), structural heart disease (non-ischaemic, valvular), diabetes mellitus (DM), obesity and obstructive sleep apnoea [3]. The co-prevalence also increases with advancing age and each predicts/ compounds the course of the other [1,4].

There has been increasing evidence regarding the adverse role of AF in patients with CHF both in terms of morbidity as well as prognosis [1]. Most of the studies done have revealed that AF through the loss of organized atrial activity and absence of coordinated atrial mechanical function, is associated with clinical and hemodynamic deterioration which may predispose the patient to systemic thromboembolism and poorer prognosis [1]. Impaired contraction of the atria may cause blood stasis and the potential for thrombus formation, particularly in the left atrial appendage, especially in CHF as there is already presumed stagnation of blood [5].

The pathoaetiological interplay between CHF and AF is complex. CHF predicts the development of AF and conversely AF predisposes to CHF [1]. The mechanisms, through which CHF provides arrhythmogenic atrial substrate include: elevated left-sided filling pressures, mitral regurgitation, atrial enlargement, interstitial fibrosis and electromechanical remodelling [4]; activation of

autonomic and renin-angiotensin axis; as well as changes in the intracellular calcium [5].

Conversely, AF can lead to CHF through multiple adverse effects including loss of atrial systole, functional mitral/tricuspid regurgitation, tachycardiomyopathy, and reduced ventricular diastolic filling time [1]. Irregularity in the RR interval can also have a potentially deteriorating influence on cardiac output irrespective of the heart rate [6]. Moreover, deterioration of sinus rhythm in AF patients with CHF can lead to acute decompensation.

1.2 Clinical Factors Known to be Associated with AF in CHF

Body Mass Index [7] is said to be associated with AF and may impact on outcomes. This is probably due to its association with cardiovascular conditions like hypertension. The severity of heart failure as determined by the New York Heart Association (NYHA) classification has also been reported to be a factor in AF whose prevalence is said to increase with increased severity of the NYHA class [8].

Hypertension is implicated in the initiation and maintenance of AF through structural changes, neurohormonal activation, fibrosis, atherosclerosis seen in this condition [9]. Coronary artery disease is implicated in atrial fibrillation in that a partially blocked artery might cause an imbalance of nutrient flow to an area of downstream heart muscle causing ischemia [10]. Ischemia can cause electrical irritability in the ventricle leading to the initiation and perpetuation of atrial fibrillation [10].

Dilated Cardiomyopathy has been associated with occurrence of AF as well. Electrophysiological features associated with left atrial dilation in dilated cardiomyopathy include shortening of the refractory period and prolongation of conduction time [11]. These alterations may both lead to development of multiple reentrant wave fronts starting and possibly perpetuating AF in dilated cardiomyopathy [11].

In diabetes mellitus both glucose and insulin disturbance may directly affect the myocardium in atrium and ventricle, leading to AF. Left ventricular (LV) hypertrophy has been associated with DM and abnormal glucose tolerance in several epidemiology studies and LV hypertrophy has been said to be a significant risk factor for AF. Analysis of the Framingham study subjects showed that LV mass increased with the worsening of glucose tolerance and the trend was more striking in women than in men. There was also a close relationship between insulin resistance and LV mass, as well as LV wall thickness, in women both with normal and abnormal glucose tolerance [12]. The supraventricular and ventricular arrhythmias are common in chronic obstructive lung disease. The reasons are thought to be due to hypoxia, hypercarbia, pulmonary hypertension, and myocardial ischemia, which are easily provoked by this limited ventilatory condition [13].

Smoking and heavy alcohol intake are also factors in the occurrence of AF. Smoking may harm the heart through causing or aggravating endothelial dysfunction and atherosclerosis as well as causing cardiac rhythm disorders through the combined effects of nicotine, carbon monoxide, and polycyclic aromatic hydrocarbons. Thus, smoking may change the myocardial substrate as well as action potentials, both processes that may provoke and/or facilitate AF [14]. Heavy alcohol drinking is described as the drinking of 5 or more glasses of alcohol on the same occasion on each of 5 or more days in the past 30 days [15]. It is understood that alcohol consumption acutely affects catecholamine release, causes metabolic acidosis and electrolyte disturbances, and increased oxidative distress [16]. In the long term, this results in myocardial fibrosis/dilatation, structural heart disease, metabolic disturbances, and increased sympathetic tone. The combination of these effects contributes to the increase in atrial arrhythmias including AF [16].

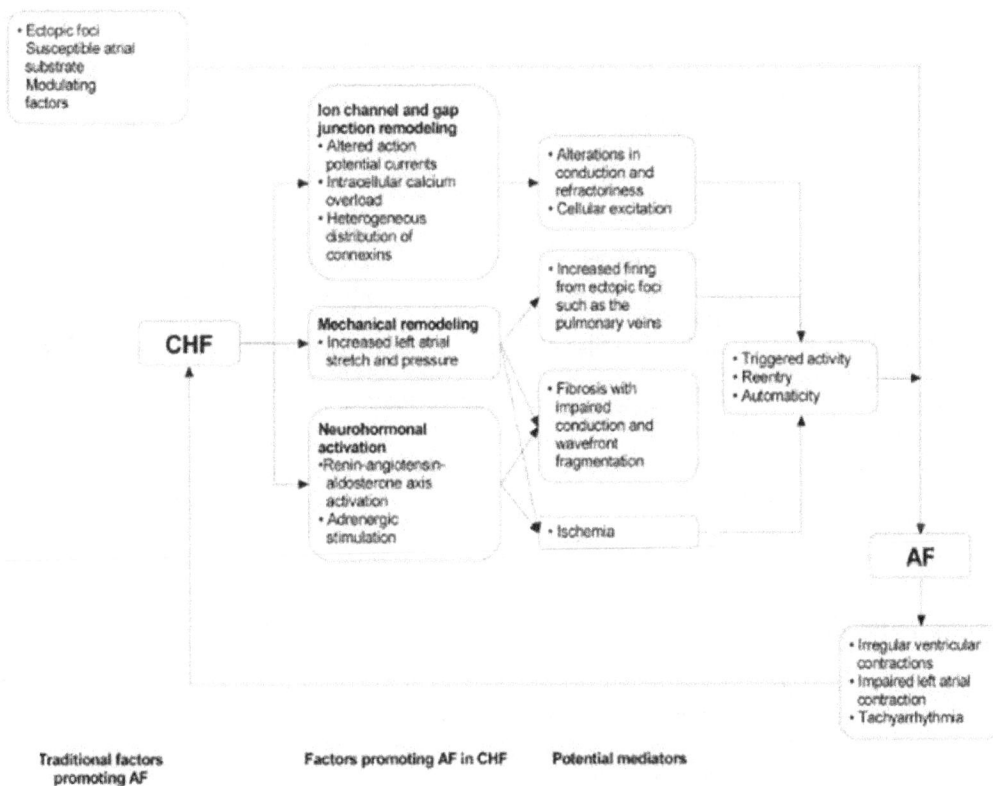

Fig. 1. Pathoetiological inter-relationship between AF and CHF
Source: Lubitz, Benjamin & Ellinor (2010)

2. MATERIALS AND METHODS

This was a hospital based cross-sectional study carried out in adult medical wards at the UTH, a tertiary health centre in Lusaka, Zambia.All known congestive heart failure patients aged 18 years and above who consented to take part in the study were included. However, CHF patients acute patients who were not able to get out of bedwere excluded from the study.

2.1 Data Collection

A structured interview schedule was used to capture data on demographic characteristics, clinical factors and laboratory measurement results. The interview schedule was developed based on the World Health Organization (WHO) stepwise survey (STEPS) instrument [17]. The data on demographic and clinical factors were obtained by interview, review of medical records and anthropometric measurements.

The weight and height of the patients were measured using a ZT-160 adult weighing mechanical scale with a height rod (Wuxi Weigher Factory Co., Ltd, Zhejiang, China) whose values were used to compute the body mass index (BMI) taken as proportion of weight (in kilograms) and square height (in metres). Blood Pressure and pulse rate were measured on the left hand of the patient in a lying position using an Omron HEM 780 automated Blood Pressure machine (Omron HEALTHCARE Co. Ltd, Vietnam). A standard 12-lead Electrocardiogram (ECG) was done using Schiller AT-102 ECG machine on all participants to identify those with and without atrial fibrillation. Then those who had no atrial fibrillation on standard ECG had a holter monitor (DR180+ Digital Recorder, Northeast Monitoring Inc, USA) applied for 24 hours. Data was analysed using IBM®SPSS® version 20.0. The analyses included descriptive statistics and Pearson chi square of independence tests. A 95% confidence interval (CI) and P-value of < 0.05 were set.

3. RESULTS

3.1 Socio-demographic Data

Table 1 shows the socio-demographic characteristics of participants in the study. A total of 49 black African Congestive Heart Failure patients who met the inclusion criterion were enrolled into the study. There were almost equal number of men and women; 49% vs. 51% respectively. Most of the patients (42.9%) were aged 65 years and above. The majority (53.1%) of the patients had a normal BMI (18.5 − 24.9). About 20.4% of the patients were tobacco smokers; and 30.6% of the patients were consumers of alcohol.

Table 1. Socio-demographic characteristics of CHF patients recruited (N=49)

Variable	Frequency	Per cent
Sex		
Female	25	51
Male	24	49
Age		
35 - 44 Years	2	4.1
45 - 54 Years	10	20.4
55 - 64 Years	16	32.7
65 Years and above	21	42.9
Body mass index		
18.5 - 24.9	26	53.1
25 - 29.9	11	22.4
30 and above	12	24.5
Smoking		
No	39	79.6
Yes	10	20.4
Alcohol consumption		
No	34	69.4
Yes	15	30.6

3.2 Clinical Factors Data

Table 2 shows the clinical characteristics of the CHF patients included in the study. The majority of the patients (81.6%) were in the New York Heart failure Association (NYHA) class IV; 26.5% of the patients had hypertension; 18.4% had dilated cardiomyopathy; 14.3% had chronic lung disease; 14.3% had diabetes mellitus; and 6.1% had coronary artery disease.

3.3 Electrodiagnosis of Atrial Fibrillation in CHF Patients

Fig. 2 shows the electrographic modality utilised to diagnose AF. Standard 12-lead ECG showed that 7 (14.3%) participants had atrial fibrillation. The ambulatory ECG monitor revealed atrial fibrillation in another 6 (12.2%) patients, giving a combined prevalence of AF of 26.5% in this study population.

3.4 Association between AF in CHF and the Socio-Demographic Characteristics

Using Pearson chi-square of independence test, the association between atrial fibrillation in congestive heart failure patients and the socio-demographic characteristics. The results obtained are presented in Table 3.

Table 3 shows the cross tabulations of AF by the socio-demographic factors. The incidence of AF was higher in males 8 (33.3%) than in the females 5 (20.0%) although no statistical significance was noted (p>0.05). The presence of AF in CHF patients increased with age from 4 (25%) below 65 years to 9 (42.9%) in those above 65 years. Furthermore, the incidence of AF increased with the increase in the BMI from 3 (27.3%) in the overweight to 10 (83.3) in the obese. 7 (70%) of the 10 smokers in CHF had AF and Fisher's exact test showed that there is a statistically significant association between atrial fibrillation in congestive heart failure and smoking. The majority 12 (80.0%) of the patients who reported taking alcohol had atrial fibrillation.

Table 2. Clinical characteristics of CHF patients (N=49)

Variable	Frequency	Per cent
NYHA class		
Class III	9	18.4
Class IV	40	81.6
Hypertension		
No	36	73.5
Yes	13	26.5
Coronary artery disease		
No	46	93.9
Yes	3	6.1
Dilated cardiomyopathy		
No	40	81.6
Yes	9	18.4
Diabetes mellitus		
No	42	85.7
Yes	7	14.3
Chronic lung disease		
No	42	85.7
Yes	7	14.3

3.5 Association between AF in CHF and the Identified Clinical Factors

Table 4 above shows the Pearson chi-square of independence test of AF in CHF by the clinical factors. While 11 (27.5%) of the 40 patients in NYHA IV had AF, only 2 (22.2%) of the 9 patients in NYHA III had AF. However, this difference did not attain statistical difference. Of the 13 hypertensive patients in the study population, 11 (84.6%) had AF. Only 3 patients were reported to have coronary artery disease. And of these, 2 (66.6%) had AF. Of the nine (9) patients who had Dilated Cardiomyopathy,

7 (77.8%) had AF. Six (6, 85.6%) of the seven patients with diabetes mellitus and similar proportion with chronic lung disease had AF. The results showed that there was a statistically significant association between AF in CHF and hypertension, dilated cardiomyopathy, diabetes mellitus as well as chronic lung disease.

4. DISCUSSION

Atrial fibrillation is said to be the most common arrhythmia seen in clinical practice and is responsible for significant morbidity [18]. The presence of AF is said to confer a five-fold increased risk of stroke [19], a significantly increased risk of dementia [20] and an almost two-fold increased risk of death [21]. The clinical consequences of AF are derived from the loss of organized atrial activity and absence of coordinated atrial mechanical function. Impaired contraction of the atria may cause blood stasis and the potential for thrombus formation, particularly in the left atrial appendage, with a resultant risk of stroke. This risk of stroke is said to be increased in patients with CHF [22]. The concomitant presence of AF and CHF identifies individuals with a higher risk for death than with either condition alone [2].

4.1 Prevalence of Atrial Fibrillation in Congestive Heart Failure

The prevalence of AF in the CHF patients admitted to UTH during the period of the study was 26.5%. This prevalence was quiet high; though almost half of the patients in this group were missed by routine ECG. Indeed this underlines the recommendations that came out of the Cryptogenic Stroke and Underlying Atrial Fibrillation (CRYSTAL-AF) trial [23] and the 30-Day Cardiac Event Monitor Belt for Recording Atrial Fibrillation After Cerebral Ischemic Event (EMBRACE) trial [24] which demonstrated the effectiveness of extended cardiac monitoring. This demonstrates the need for use of ambulatory diagnostic equipment such as ECG Holter monitors and the insertable cardiac monitors (ICM) in the diagnostic investigations for arrhythmias. With prolonged monitoring we may have obtained a higher yield of individuals with AF. However, the prevalence rate recorded on this study is similar to the 30% prevalence rate reported in the Acute Decompensated Heart Failure National Registry [25] in the United States in 2005. The high prevalence rate may be attributed partially to the advancing age of the Zambian population [26] and/or increase in prevalence of the non-communicable diseases [27].

4.2 Socio-demographic Characteristics of the Patients

Although, we did not find any statistical difference (X^2= 1.12, p= 0.291) in the prevalence of AF in CHF between males and females, the majority 8 (61.5%) of patients with AF in CHF were males. Among the male CHF patients, the prevalence of AF was higher (33.3%) compared to 20% among the female CHF patients. Similarly, Lloyd-Jones AM et al. [28] reported that AF after the age of 40 in the United States was 26% for men, and 23% for women and Humphries KH et al. [29] also reported that in all age groups, men have a higher incidence of AF than women.It is postulated that this may be so because males are more exposed to other risk factors for AF like smoking and excessive alcohol intake [3]. However, although women have a lower incidence of AF, studies have shown a worse outcome and a higher rate of recurrence after cardioversion [21,30].

The study also revealed that age 65 years and above was statistically (X^2= 5.03, p< 0.05) associated with AF in CHF. This result was similar to what was reported by Psaty BM et al. [31] and Nazario B [3]. Advancing age is implicated in the development of AF probably because pre-existing alterations, such as autonomic dysbalance, degenerative tissue changes and fibrosis, can provide an electrophysiological and morphological substrate, which increases the likelihood of AF. In

particular, alterations of the interstitial matrix in atrial tissue seem to be significant contributory factors [32].

The majority 26 (53.1%) of the patients in the study had a normal body mass index (18.5 – 24.9) (Table 2). Of the 13 (26.5%) patients who had AF, the majority 10 (76.9%) were obese and 3 (23.1%) were overweight. No case was found among the participants with a normal body mass index. The study also revealed that body mass index is significantly (X^2= 22.59, p<0.001) associated with AF in CHF. Similarly, Guilian L et al. [7] andOvervad TF et al. [33] reported that obesity is associated with the development of AF and may impact AF-related outcomes. However, it is worth noting that it is very difficult to calculate body mass index in CHF patients because of the exaggerated patient's weight resulting from fluid retention.

There were 10 (20.4%) patients who were smokers in the study, and 7 (70%) of them had AF compared to 6 (15.4%) among the 39 non-smokers (X^2= 9.54, p<0.01). This result is in agreement with what was reported by Heeringa J et al. [34] and Chamberlain AM et al. [35] who reported a more than two-fold increased risk of AF attributed to current smoking. Smoking may harm the heart through causing or aggravating endothelial dysfunction and atherosclerosis as well as causing cardiac rhythm disorders through the combined effects of nicotine, carbon monoxide, and polycyclic aromatic hydrocarbons [14]. Thus, smoking may change the myocardial substrate as well as action potentials; of which both processes may provoke and facilitate AF.

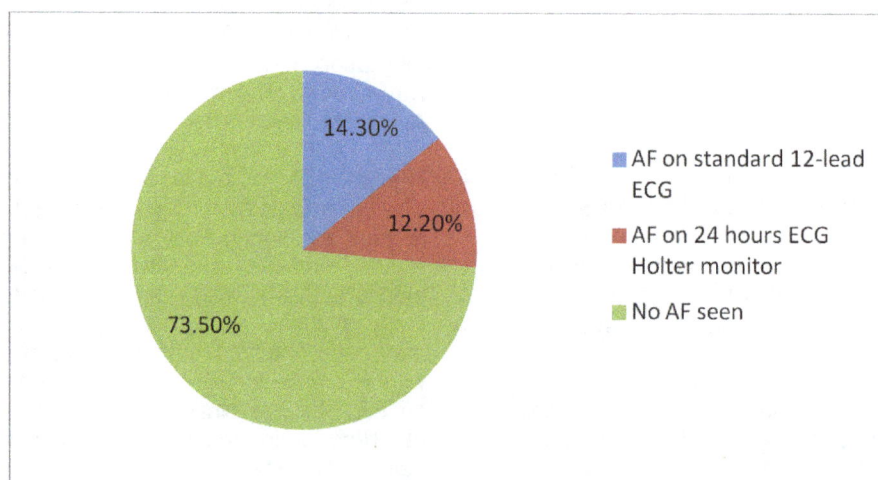

Fig. 2. Electrodiagnosis of atrial fibrillation (N=49)

Table 3. Atrial fibrillation by the socio-demographic factors

Clinical factor	Atrial fibrillation		X^2	P-value
	No AF seen	AF seen		
	N (%)	N (%)		
Sex[a]				
Female	20 (80.0)	5 (20.0)	1.12	NS
Male	16 (66.7)	8 (33.3)		
Age[a]				
35 - 44 Years	2 (100.0)	0 (0.0)		
45 - 54 Years	10 (100.0)	0 (0.0)		
55 - 64 Years	12 (75.0)	4 (25.0)	5.03	<0.05*
65 Years and above	12 (57.1)	9 (42.9)		
Body mass index[a]				
18.5 - 24.9	26 (100.0)	0 (0.0)	22.59	<0.001*
25 - 29.9	8 (72.7)	3 (27.3)		
30 and above	2 (16.7)	10 (83.3)		
Smoking[a]				
No	33 (84.6)	6 (15.4)	9.54	<0.01*
Yes	3 (30.0)	7 (70.0)		
Alcohol intake[a]				
No	33 (97.1)	1 (2.9)	27.88	<0.001*
Yes	3 (20.0)	12 (80.0)		

Indicates significant p-value at $p < 0.05$

Table 4. Atrial fibrillation by the clinical factors

Clinical factor	Atrial fibrillation		X^2	P-value
	No AF seen	AF seen		
	N (%)	N (%)		
NYHA class[a]				
Class III	7 (77.8)	2 (22.2)	0.00	NS
Class IV	29 (72.5)	11 (27.5)		
Hypertension[a]				
No	34 (94.4)	2 (5.6)	26.71	<0.001
Yes	2 (15.4)	11 (84.6)		
Coronary artery disease[a]				
No	35 (76.1)	11 (23.9)	0.90	NS
Yes	1 (33.3)	2 (66.7)		
Dilated cardiomyopathy[a]				
No	34 (85.0)	6 (15.0)	11.81	<0.001
Yes	2 (22.2)	7 (77.8)		
Diabetes mellitus[a]				
No	35 (83.3)	7 (16.7)	11.35	<0.001
Yes	1 (14.3)	6 (85.7)		
Chronic lung disease[a]				
No	35 (83.3)	7 (16.7)	11.35	<0.001
Yes	1 (14.3)	6 (85.7)		

[a]*Fisher's Exact Test. *Indicates significant p-value at $p < 0.05$*

Compared to non-consumers of alcohol where only 1 (2.9%) patient had AF, the majority 12 (80%) of the consumers of alcohol in CHF had AF(X^2= 27.88, p= <0.001). Similarly several case-control studies [36,37,30], reported significantly higher odds of developing AF among heavier drinkers. Furthermore, the risk of developing AF is said to increase with increasing levels of alcohol consumption [38]. There has been much controversy over the exact mechanism by which alcohol induces AF. Mukamal KJ, et al. [38] postulated that alcohol-induced atrial arrhythmias were related to intramyocardial catecholamine release in response to the toxic effects of acetaldehyde. Other studies [39,40], have suggested that an increase in sympathetic reaction could be related to the production of AF based on the increased density of beta-adrenergic receptors in lymphocytes. Balbão CE et al. [16] proposed multiple mechanisms for the acute and long-term consumption of alcohol resulting in AF. Probably a combination of these effects contributes to the increase in atrial arrhythmias.

4.3 Clinical Factors Associated with AF

The patients in this study were in severe CHF (NYHA classes III/IV). Although, there was no statistical difference (X^2= 0.00, p= 1.000) between the two groups, there were more AF cases in NYHA class IV compared to the cases in NYHA class III. Findings from previous studies [8,41-44] have also revealed that the prevalence of AF increases significantly with the increase/severity in the NYHA class. Our small sample size may have influenced the results in this study.

Slightly over a quarter 13 (26.5%) of the patients had hypertension in this study population. The majority 11 (84.6%) of these patients had AF compared to the non hypertensive group where only 2 (5.6%) of 36 patients had AF. Hypertension was strongly associated (X^2= 26.71, p<0.001) with AF in CHF. Similar reports have affirmed this finding [31,45]. Untreated or suboptimally treated hypertension leads to the development of Left Ventricular Hypertrophy (LVH), which is one of the most important expressions of subclinical organ damage, and is an independent risk factor for cardiovascular events, including the development of AF. In the presence of LVH, left ventricular compliance is reduced, left ventricular stiffness and filling pressure increase, coronary flow reserve is decreased, wall stress is increased and there is activation of the sympathetic nervous system and of the renin–angiotensin–aldosterone system. In the atria, proliferation and differentiation of fibroblasts into myofibroblasts and enhanced connective tissue deposition and fibrosis are the hallmarks of this process. Structural remodelling results in electrical dissociation between muscle bundles and in local conduction heterogeneities facilitating the initiation and perpetuation of AF. This electroanatomical substrate permits multiple small re-entrant circuits that can stabilize the arrhythmia. Over time tissue remodelling promotes and maintains AF by changing the fundamental properties of the atria [9].

In this cohort only 3 (6.1%) of the patients had coronary artery disease and out of these 2 (66.8%) had AF. Thakkar S& Bagarhatta R [20]

reported that transient ischemic attack as may be found in coronary artery disease is a risk factor for AF. However, in these patients, systolic heart failure may be more important than atrial ischemia in causing AF [10]. Nevertheless, significant stenosis in the proximal right coronary artery and the circumflex artery prior to the takeoff of the atrial branches increase the likelihood of AF[46].

Only 9 (18.4%) of the patients had dilated cardiomyopathy and the majority 7 (77.8%) of these patients had AF. Dilated cardiomyopathy in CHF was strongly (X^2 = 11.81, p= 0.001) associated with AF. Similar findings have been reported [47,48]. Luchsinger JA & Steinberg JS [49] also reported that Tachycardia-induced cardiomyopathy may be a more common mechanism of LV dysfunction in patients with atrial arrhythmia. Electrophysiological features associated with left atrial dilation in dilated cardiomyopathy include shortening of the refractory period and prolongation of conduction time [11]. Both these alterations may lead to development of multiple reentrant wave fronts starting and possibly perpetuating AF in dilated cardiomyopathy [11].

Diabetes mellitus has been implicated in the initiation and perpetuation of AF [50,51]. In this study 6 (85.7%) of 7 diabetic patients with CHF had AF. Diabetes was strongly (X^2 = 11.35, p< 0.001) associated with AF in CHF. Both dysglycemia and insulin disturbance can directly affect the myocardium in atrium and ventricle, by causing atrial and ventricular hypertrophy leading to AF [12]. In the animal model of diabetes mellitus, the occurrence of AF was enhanced by adrenergic activation. The heterogeneous increase in sympathetic innervations has proved to be associated with the promotion of AF in several studies [52,53].

6(85.7%) of 7 patients with chronic lung disease in CHF had AF. There was a strong association (X^2 = 11.35, p< 0.001). Impaired pulmonary function has been described as an independent risk factor for AF [54]. Indeed, FEV_1%, which represents the severity of airway obstruction, was associated with chronic AF [55] and the greater the pulmonary function impairment, the greater the co-existence with AF. Atrial fibrillation in chronic lung disease is thought to result from changes in blood gases, abnormalities in pulmonary functions, and hemodynamic changes resulting from pulmonary hypertension [56] as well as structural remodelling. Hypoxemia and hypercapnia are associated with over-compensatory fluctuations in autonomic tone, intrathoracic pressures and cardiac haemodynamics, with possible atrial stretch and remodeling, each of which could lead to AF, particularly when hypercapnia causes a significant decrease in pH values [57]. Morphological abnormalities associated with chronic obstructive pulmonary disease (COPD) include signs of right atrial enlargement, and right ventricular hypertrophy. Structural remodeling results in an electrical dissociation between muscle bundles and local conduction heterogeneities, facilitating the initiation and perpetuation of AF. This electro-anatomical substrate allows multiple small re-entrant circuits that may trigger the arrhythmia [57].

5. CONCLUSION

This study objectively evaluated clinical factors associated with AF in CHF patients admitted to UTH, Lusaka, Zambia. AF is quite common in CHF and strongly associated with obesity, smoking, excessive alcohol intake, hypertension, dilated cardiomyopathy, diabetes mellitus and chronic lung disease. AF at UTH is often diagnosed by routine ECG examination, in the course of investigating and/or managing other cardiovascular disorders. However, the ambulatory ECG monitor for 24 hours captured almost as many cases as were missed by the routine ECG.

This study highlights the importance of electrocardiographic evaluation of patients with chronic heart failure and enlightens the physicians to be more vigilant in searching for AF in particular subpopulations. These findings will guide the physicians in risk stratification and in initiating appropriate treatment for prevention and control of AF in CHF thus enhancing the physicians' clinical practice.

ETHICAL APPROVAL

Ethical clearance was obtained from ERES CONVERGE IRB (Reference number 2014-Mar-003) and permission was also sort from UTH Management and the department of Medicine before starting data collection. Participation in this study was voluntary, with participants free to withdraw from the study at any time. Authors further declare that all procedures used to collect data were normal routine procedures done in the routine care of patients, within the patient's natural environment, and nothing was done to the discomfort of the patient. Patients found to have atrial fibrillation were referred to the cardiologist for treatment.

COMPETING INTERESTS

Authors have declared that no competing interests exist.

REFERENCES

1. Caldwell JC, Mamas MA. Heart failure diastolic dysfunction and atrial fibrillation; mechanistic insight of a complex inter-relationship. Heart Failure Review Journal. 2012;17:27-33.

2. Lubitz SA, Benjamin EJ, Ellinor PT. Atrial fibrillation in congestive heart failure. Heart Fail Clin. 2010;6(2):187-200.

3. Nazario B. Atrial fibrillation and stroke – Symptoms of atrial fibrillation. Cardiology Journal. 2013;18(3):356–364.

4. Deedwania PC, Lardizabal JA. Atrial fibrillation in heart failure: A comprehensive review. American Journal of Medicine 2010;123:198-204.

5. Wang TJ, Larson MG, Levy D, Vasan RS, Leip EP, Wolf PA, D'Agostino RB, Murabito JM, Kannel WB, Benjamin E. Temporal relations of atrial fibrillation and congestive heart failure and their joint influence on mortality: The Framingham Heart Study. Circulation. 2003;107:2920–5. [PubMed]

6. Clark DM, Plumb VJ, Epstein AE, Kay GN. Hemodynamic effects of an irregular sequence of ventricular cycle lengths during atrial fibrillation. J Am Coll Cardiol. 1997;30:1039-1045. [PubMed]

7. Guilian L, Jinchuan Y, Rongzeng D, Jun Q, Jun W, Wenqing Z. Impact of body mass index on atrial fibrillation recurrence: A meta-analysis of observational studies. Pacing Clin Electrophysiol. 2013;36(6): 748-56. DOI:10.1111/pace.12106. Epub 2013 Feb 25.

8. Nicol ED, Fittall B, Roughton M, Cleland JGF, Dargie H, d Cowie MR. Heart failure and cardiomyopathy: NHS heart failure survey: A survey of acute heart failure admissions in England, Wales and Northern Ireland. Heart. 2008;94:172-177.

9. Healey JS, Connolly SJ. Atrial fibrillation: Hypertension as a causative agent, risk factor for complications, and potential therapeutic target. Am J Cardiol. 2003; 22;91(10A):9G-14G.

10. Lokshyn S, Mewis C, Kuhlkamp V. Atrial fibrillation in coronary artery disease. Int J Cardiol. 2000;15;72(2):133-6.

11. Lindsay BD, Smith JM. Electrophysiologic aspects of human atrial fibrillation. In: DiMarco JP, ed. Cardiology Clinics. Philadelphia, Pa: WB Saunders. 1996; 483–505.

12. Rutter MK, Parise H, Benjamin EJ, Levy D, Larson MG, Meigs JB, Nesto RW, Wilson PW, Vasan RS. Impact of glucose intolerance and insulin resistance on cardiac structure and function: Sex-related differences in the Framingham Heart Study. Circulation. 2003;28;107(3):448-54.

13. Khokhar N. Cardiac arrhythmias associated with acute respiratory failure in chronic obstructive pulmonary disease. Mil Med. 1981;146(12):856-8.

14. Ambrose JA, Barua RS.; The pathophysiology of cigarette smoking and cardiovascular disease: An update. J Am Coll. Cardiol. 2004;19;43(10):1731-7.

15. Available:http://www.niaaa.nih.gov/alcohol-health/overview-alcohol-consumption/moderate-binge-drinking (Accessed on 25/07/15 11:23 hours).

16. Balbão CE, de Paola AA, Fenelon G. Effects of alcohol on atrial fibrillation: myths and truths. Ther Adv Cardiovasc Dis. 2009;3(1):53–63. [PubMed]

17. World Health Organization. World Health Organization STEPwise approach to chronic disease risk factor surveillance (STEPS) instrument. Version 3. 2007. Geneva. World Health Organization. Google Scholar

18. Fuster V, Rydén LE, Cannom DS, Crijns HJ, Curtis AB, Ellenbogen KA, Halperin JL, Le Heuzey JY, Kay GN, Lowe JE, et al. ACC/AHA/ESC 2006 guidelines for the management of patients with atrial fibrillation: A report of the American College of Cardiology/American Heart Association Task Force on Practice Guidelines and the European Society of Cardiology Committee for Practice Guidelines (Writing Committee to Revise the 2001 Guidelines for the Management of Patients With Atrial Fibrillation): developed in collaboration with the European Heart Rhythm Association and the Heart Rhythm Society. Circulation. 2006;114:e257–e354. [PubMed]

19. Kannel WB, Benjamin EJ. Status of the epidemiology of atrial fibrillation. Med Clin North Am. 2008;92(1):17-40:9. [PMC free article] [PubMed]

20. Thakkar S, Bagarhatta R, Detection of paroxysmal Atrial Fibrillation or Flutter in Patients with Acute Ischemic Stroke or Transient Ischemic Attack by Holter Monitor; Indian Heart Journal. 2014;66(2): 188-192.

21. Benjamin EJ, Wolf PA, D'Agostino RB, et al. Impact of atrial fibrillation on the risk of death: The Framingham Heart Study. Circulation. 1998;98:946-952.

22. Gage BF, Waterman AD, Shannon W, Boechler M, Rich MW, Radford MJ. Validation of clinical classification schemes for predicting stroke: Results from the National Registry of Atrial Fibrillation. JAMA. 2001;285:2864–70. [PubMed]

23. Sanna T, Diener HC, Passman RS, Di Lazzaro, Bernstein RA, Morillo CA et al; CRYSTAL AF Investigators. Cryptogenic stroke and underlying. New England Journal of Medicine. 2014;370:2478-2486.

24. Gladstone DJ, Spring M, Dorian P, Panzov V, Thorpe KE, Hall J, et al. EMBRACE Investigators and Coordinators, Atrial Fibrillation in Patients with Cryptogenic stroke. New England Journal of Medicine. 2014; 370:2467-2477.

25. Adams KF, Fonarow GC, Emerman CL, LeJemtel TH, Costanzo MR, Abraham WT, Berkowitz RL, Galvao M, Horton DP. Characteristics and outcomes of patients hospitalized for heart failure in the United States: Rationale, design and preliminary observations from the first 100,000 cases in the Acute Decompensated Heart Failure National Registry (ADHERE). Am Heart J. 2005;149:209-216. [PubMed]

26. Mapoma CC. Population ageing in Zambia: Magnitude, challenges and determinants, Lusaka, Zambia; 2013.

27. Ministry of Health – Zambia and World Health Organization Country Office (Zambia) STEPS Report Zambia: Prevalence rates of the common non-communicable diseases and their risk factors in Lusaka district, Zambia 2008, Ministry of Health World Health Organization. Survey; 2008.

28. Lloyd-Jones DM, Larson MG, Leip EP, Beiser A, D'Agostino RB, Kannel WB, Murabito JM, Vasan RS, Benjamin EJ, Levy D. Lifetime risk for development of atrial fibrillation: The Framingham Heart Study. Circulation. 2004;31;110(9):1042-6. (Epub 2004 Aug 16).

29. Humphries KH, Kerr CR, Connolly SJ, et al. New-onset atrial fibrillation: Sex differences in presentation, treatment and outcome. Circulation. 2001;103:2365–70.

30. Satoru K, Kazumi S, Shiro T, Chika H, Aki S, Yoriko H, et al. Alcohol consumption and risk of atrial fibrillation: A meta-analysis. J Am Coll Cardiol. 2011; 25;57(4):427-36. DOI:10.1016/j.jacc.2010.08.641.

31. Psaty BM, Manolio TA, Kuller LH, Kronmal RA, Cushman M, Fried LP, White R, Furberg CD, Rautaharju PM. Incidence of and risk factors for atrial fibrillation in older adults. Circulation. 1997;96:2455–2461.

32. Nattel S. New ideas about atrial fibrillation 50 years on. Nature. 2002;415:219–26. [PubMed]

33. Overvad TF, Rasmussen LH, Skjøth F, Overvad K, Albertsen IE, Lane DA, Lip GYH, Larsen TB. Alcohol intake and prognosis of atrial fibrillation patients. Heart. DOI:10.1136/heartjnl-2013-304036.

34. Heeringa J, Kors JA, Hofman A, Van Rooij FJ, Witteman JC. Cigarette smoking and risk of atrial fibrillation: The Rotterdam Study. Am Heart J. 2008;156(6):1163-9. DOI: 10.1016/j.ahj.2008.08.003. Epub 2008 Oct 14. [PubMed]

35. Chamberlain AM, Agarwal SK, Folsom AR, Duval S, Soliman EZ, Ambrose M, Eberly LE, Alonso A. Smoking and incidence of atrial fibrillation: Results from the Atherosclerosis Risk in Communities (ARIC) study. Heart Rhythm. 2011; 8(8):1160-6. DOI:10.1016/j.hrthm.2011.03.038. (Epub 2011 Mar 15). [PubMed]

36. Djoussé L, Levy D, Benjamin EJ, Blease SJ, Russ A, Larson MG, Massaro JM, D'Agostino RB, Wolf PA, Ellison RC. Long-term alcohol consumption and the risk of atrial fibrillation in the Framingham Study. Am J Cardiol. 2004;93(6):710-3. [PubMed]

37. Koskinen P, Kupari M, Leinonen H, et al. Alcohol and new onset atrial fibrillation: A case-control study of a current series. Br Heart Jv. 1987;57(5):PMC1277202.

38. Rich EC, Siebold C, Campion B. Alcohol-related acute atrial fibrillation. A case-control study and review of 40 patients. Arch Intern Med. 1985;145(5):830-3.

39. Mukamal KJ, Tolstrup JS, Friberg J, et al. Alcohol consumption and risk of atrial fibrillation in men and women: The copenhagen city heart study. Circulation.

2005;112(12):1736-42. (Epub 2005 Sep 12).

40. Engel TR, Luck JC. Effect of whiskey on atrial vulnerability and "holiday heart." J Am Coll Cardiol. 1983;1(3):816–818. [PubMed]

41. Wright SP, Verouhis D, Gamble G, Swedberg K, Sharpe N, Doughty RN. Factors influencing the length of hospital stay of patients with heart failure. Eur J Heart Fail. 2003;5(2):201-9.

42. Mwandolela H. Types of cardiac diseases in women presenting with features suggestive of cardiac disease in peripartum period and their pregnancy outcomes in MNH. MMed Thesis, MUHAS; 2007.

43. Rogers A, Julia MA, McCoy ASM, Edmonds PM, Abery AJ, Coats AJS, et al. Qualitative study of chronic heart failure patients, understanding of their symptoms and drug therapy. Eur J Heart Fail. 2002; 4(3):283-7.

44. Fofana M, Toure S, Dadhi Balde M, Sow T, Yassima Camara A, Damby Balde O, Toure A, Conde A. Etiologic and nosologic considerations apropos of 574 cases of cardiac decompensation in Conakry. Ann Cardiol Angeiol (Paris). 1988;37(8):419-24.

45. Hennersdorf MG, Schueller PO, Steiner S, Strauer BE. Prevalence of paroxysmal atrial fibrillation depending on the regression of left ventricular hypertrophy in arterial hypertension. Hypertens Res. 2007;30(6):535-40. [PubMed]

46. Galrinho A, Gomes JA, Antunes E, et al. Atrial fibrillation and coronary disease Rev. Port. Cardiol. 1993;12:1037–1040

47. Aleksova A, et al. Impact of atrial fibrillation on outcome of patients with idiopathic dilated cardiomyopathy: Data from the heart muscle disease registry of Trieste. Clin Med Res. 2010;8(3-4):142–149. DOI: 10.3121/cmr.2010.908

48. Anter E, Jessup M, Callans DJ. Atrial Fibrillation and Heart Failure Treatment Considerations for a Dual Epidemic, Circulation. 2009;119:2516-2525.

49. Luchsinger JA, Steinberg JS. Resolution of cardiomyopathy after ablation of atrial flutter. J Am Coll Cardiol. 1998;32(1):205-10.

50. Murphy NF, Simpson CR, Jhund PS, et al. A national survey of the prevalence, incidence, primary care burden and treatment of atrial fibrillation in Scotland.

Heart. 2007;93(5):606-12. (Epub 2007 Feb 3).

51. Movahed MR, Hashemzadeh M, Jamal MM. Diabetes mellitus is a strong, independent risk for atrial fibrillation and flutter in addition to other cardiovascular disease. Int J Cardiol. 2005;7:105(3):315-8.

52. Schmid H, Forman LA, Cao X, et al. Heterogeneous cardiac sympathetic denervation and decreased myocardial nerve growth factor in streptozotocin induced diabetic rats: Implications for cardiac sympathetic dysinnervation complicating diabetes. Diabetes. 1999; 48(3):603-8.

53. Olgin JE, Sih HJ, Hanish S, et al. Heterogeneous atrial denervation creates substrate for sustained atrial fibrillation. Circulation.1998;98:2608-14.

54. Shibata Y, Watanabe T, Osaka D, Abe S, Inoue S, Tokairin Y, Igarashi A, Yamauchi K, Kimura T, Kishi H, Aida Y, Nunomiya K, Nemoto T, Sato M, Konta T, Kawata S, Kato T, Kayama T, Kubota I. Impairment of pulmonary function is an independent risk factor for AF: The Takahata study. Int J Med Sci. 2011;8(7):514-22. (Epub 2011 Aug 29).

55. Kang H, Bae BS, Kim JH, Jang HS, Lee B, Jung B. The relationship between chronic atrial fibrillation and reduced pulmonary function in cases of preserved left ventricular systolic function. Korean Circ J. 2009;39(9):372-377.

56. Lopez CM, House-Fancher MA. Management of atrial fibrillation in patients with chronic obstructive pulmonary disease. J Cardiovasc Nurs. 2005; 20(2):133-40.

57. Stevenson IH, Roberts-Thomson KC, Kistler PM, Edwards GA, Spence S, Sanders P, Kalman JM. Atrial electrophysiology is altered by acute hypercapnoea but not hypoxiemia: Implications for promotion of atrial fibrillation in pulmonary disease and sleep apnea. Heart Rhythm. 2010;7(9):1263-70. DOI: 10.1016/j.hrthm.2010.03.020. (Epub 2010 Mar 22).

10

Changes of Pre Ejection Period and Left Ventricular Ejection Time during Head up Tilt

Ahlam Kadhim Al Hamdany[1*]

[1]*Department of Physiology, College of Medicine, Babylon University, Iraq.*

Author's contribution

The sole author designed, analyzed and interpreted and prepared the manuscript.

<u>Editor(s):</u>
(1) Francesco Pelliccia, Department of Heart and Great Vessels University La Sapienza, Rome, Italy.
(2) Anonymous
<u>Reviewers:</u>
(1) Andrea Borghini, Institute of Clinical Physiology- CNR, Pisa, Italy.
(2) Anonymous, Ospedale SS Annunziata di Cento (FE), Italy.
(3) Anonymous, Juntendo University, Japan.
(4) Anonymous, Sao Paulo University, Brazil.

ABSTRACT

Objective of the Study: Evaluate changes in Pre ejection period (PEP) and left ventricular ejection time (LVET) during head up tilt (HUT).
Methods: Twenty healthy male subjects were involved in this study, with mean age 29.3 ± 5 years, mean body mass index (BMI) $21.3\pm0.2Kg/m^2$. Measurement of PEP, LVET of Doppler wave form of the aortic flow were done at supine, 30 and 60 degree HUT. Measurement of HR and BP were done at these positions of tilting. Comparison of changes of these variables at different degrees of HUT was done by paired T-Test.
Results: PEP values were significantly higher in 60 degree and 30 degree HUT than PEP values at supine position ($p<0.0001$). PEP values at 60 degree HUT were significantly higher than PEP values at 30 degree HUT ($P=0.05$).
LVET values were significantly lower at 60 degree and 30 degree HUT than values at supine position ($p<0.001$), and LVET values were significantly lower at 60 degree HUT than values at 30 degree HUT ($p<0.001$).
Conclusion: Key findings of PEP and LVET during HUT are progressive prolongation of PEP and shortening of LVET with increasing head up tilting.

Keywords: HUT; LVET; PEP.

*Corresponding author: E-mail: udayjanabia@yahoo.com

ABBREVIATIONS

BMI-body mass index, BP-blood pressure, DBP-diastolic blood pressure, LVET-left ventricular ejection time, PEP-pre ejection period, SBP-systolic blood pressure, TTT-tilt table test.

1. INTRODUCTION

Tilt table test (TTT): TTT, over half a century old, has retained a central place in the investigation of syncope of unknown origin [1-7]. Since the differential diagnosis of syncope of unknown origin is widely spread, there have been many attempts to rationalize and improve the diagnostic procedure [8]. During HUT—or for that matter while standing—a person's cardiovascular system has to adjust itself in order to prevent a significant portion of the blood volume from pooling in the legs.

These adjustments consist of an increase in heart rate, and a constriction of the blood vessels in the legs. These cardiovascular adjustments occur very quickly, and there is no significant drop in the blood pressure [9]. The increase in heart rate of approximately 10-15 beats/min, an elevation of diastolic pressure of about 10mm Hg and little change in systolic pressure [10]. Many previous studies enlighten the changes that occurred in stroke volume, cardiac output, heart rate, and blood pressure during HUT. The aim of this study is to evaluate the changes that occur in LVET and PEP during different degree of tilting.

2. MATERIALS AND METHODS

2.1 Subjects

Twenty healthy male subjects were involved in this study, after having their signed consent and approval of the ethical committee at Kufa faculty of medicine, with mean age 29.3±5 years, BMI 21.3±0.2Kg/m2. The subjects were thoroughly examined clinically to confirm the inclusion criteria (that only healthy subjects were included). Exclusion criteria included hypertension, diabetes mellitus, coronary heart disease and other cardiac problems, renal disease. None was on any medication.

2.2 Apparatus

2.2.1 Tilting table

A motorized tilt table. All TTT were performed in quite air conditioned room, especially equipped for the investigation [11].

2.2.2 Echocardiography equipment

All echocardiographic and Doppler studies were performed using two-dimensional (2D) Philips Sonos 7500 equipment with 2.5 MHZ transducer with tissue harmoni, incorporated ECG, and Doppler facilities for measurement of PEP and LVET.

2.3 Methods

To avoid any possible emotional excitement, reassurance of the subjects were done, of being safe and non invasive procedure.

Participants were examined in a quiet, temperature-controlled room, and were first supine positioned on belt secured tilting table, for at least 10-min to achieve a steady state. A steady state means that heart rate in consecutive minutes changes by less than 3 beats/min [12]. Pulse oximeter (portable battery oximeter-nonin-USA) was fixed on right index so as to digitally follow up the changes in arterial pulse to gain a steady state, and to record the HR. After reaching the steady state, we placed the transducer on the apex to get apical view and we used the continues wave Doppler for aorta. From aortic flow, PEP was estimated from Q-wave in ECG to the opening of aortic valve, estimation of LVET time was done between opening and closure of aortic valve [13]. Several measurements for PEP and LVET were made, then taking the mean for them. After that we raised the subject to 30 degree HUT and wait till reaching steady state by examining the pulseoximeter, then The same parameters were measured again. Returning the subject to supine position followed by raising the subject to 60 degree HUT and same previous measurements were done. Measurement of blood pressure were done at supine, 30 and 60 degree HUT.

2.4 Statistical Analysis

All values were expressed as mean±SD. Comparison between PEP, LVET HR, SBP, DBP and MBP, at supine position and different degrees of HUT were done by paired t-test. p<0.05 was considered statistically significant and P<0.001 was considered statistically highly significant.

3. RESULTS

All hemodynamic parameters were expressed as mean±SD, at different degrees of HUT, at Table 1.

PEP values were significantly higher in 60 degree and 30 degree HUT than PEP values at supine position (p<0.0001), and PEP values at 60 degree HUT were significantly higher than PEP values at 30 degree HUT (P=0.05).

LVET values were statistically lower at 60 degree and 30 degree HUT than values at supine position (p<0.001), and LVET values were significantly lower at 60 degree HUT than values at 30 degree HUT (p<0.001). HR values were significantly higher at 30 degree and 60degree HUT than values at supine position, and HR values at 60 degree HUT were significantly higher than HR values at 30 degree HUT (P<0.001).

There were no statistically significant differences between SBP values at supine and 30 and 60 degree HUT (P>0.05).

DBP and MBP values were significantly higher at 30 degree and 60 degree HUT than values at supine position (p=0.05, p<0.001) respectively. DBP and MBP values at 60 degree were significantly higher at 60 degree HUT than values at 30 degree HUT (P=0.05) Fig. 1.

4. DISCUSSION

The important findings of this study were the progressive reduction of LVET and prolongation of PEP with increasing tilting, which reflect a decline in central blood volume [14-18]. This reduction of central blood volume are due to pooling about 300-800ml of blood to the lower extremities by effect of gravity during HUT [19,20]. Prolongation of PEP and shortening of LVET were more pronounced at 60 degree HUT than 30 degree HUT, this could be explained that increasing tilting leads to more pooling of blood to the lower extremities and reduction of cardiac preload. This is in agreement with other studies like Chan et al. [21] who found that there was a significant increase in PEP at (20-30 degrees) HUT.

Table 1. Hemodynamic parameters at different degrees of HUT (values were expressed as mean±SD)

60 degree HUT	30 degree HUT	Supine	Parameters
90.20±20.5	82.3±16	61.35±14.17	PEP(ms)
240.6±19.1	267.18±20.11	307.5±26.8	LVET(ms)
83.64±9.14	73.11±8.98	69±8.78	HR(beat/min)
126.9±10.88	127.7±7.8	126±7.64	SBP(mmHg)
83.58±8.17	79.47±5.68	77.1±5.4	DBP(mmHg)
98±64±7.59	96.41±41	93±5.51	MBP(mmHg)

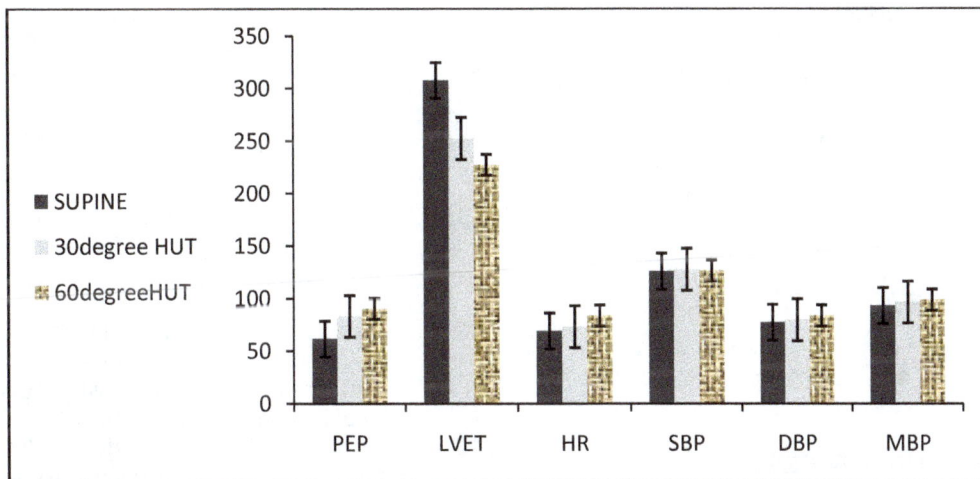

Fig. 1. Hemodynamic parameters during supine, 30 and 60 degree head up tilt

In 2008, Chan et al. [22] found that there was a significant decrease in LVET during HUT. Fucà G et al. [23] in 2011, assessed systolic ejection time as a hemodynamic marker of incipient bradycardiac vasovagal syncope, also found that ET significantly decreased throughout tilt testing.

Pooling of blood during HUT will cause stimulation of baroreceptors and Increase sympathetic activity which will cause increase cardiac contractility, increase HR, and vasoconstriction [24-29]. A 60º HUT maximize passive orthostatic stress on the sympathetic system by blocking the influence of inferior limb musculoskeletal contractions that could increase venous return [30]. For that reason, maximum sympathetic activity are at 60 degree HUT, so HR and diastolic BP and MBP values were significantly higher at 60 degree HUT than values at supine and 30 degree HUT. There were no differences in SBP values at different degrees of tilting due to increased sympathetic activity that compensate for the reduction of cardiac output.

5. CONCLUSION

Key findings of PEP and LVET during HUT are progressive prolongation of PEP and shortening of LVET with increasing HUT.

CONSENT

All authors declare that 'written informed consent was obtained from the patient (or other approved parties) for publication of this case report and accompanying images.

ETHICAL APPROVAL

All authors hereby declare that all experiments have been examined and approved by the appropriate ethics committee and have therefore been performed in accordance with the ethical standards laid down in the 1964 Declaration of Helsinki.

ACKNOWLEDGEMENTS

Special thanks to Dr. Akeel AMH Zwain who support me and helped me during collection of data.

COMPETING INTERESTS

Author has declared that no competing interests exist.

REFERENCES

1. Low PA. Composite autonomic scoring scale for laboratory quantification of generalized autonomic failure. Mayo Clin Proc. 1993;68:748-52.
2. Schondorf R, Low PA. Idiopathic postural orthostatic tachycardia syndrome: An attenuated form of acute pandysautonomia? Neurology. 1993;43:132-7.
3. Kaufmann H. Neurally mediated syncope: Pathogenesis, diagnosis, and treatment. Neurology. 1995;45(suppl 5):12-8.
4. Benditt DG, Ferguson DW, Grubb BP, Kapoor WN, Kugler J, Lerman BB, et al. Tilt table testing for assessing syncope. J Am Coll Cardiol. 1996;28(1):263-75.
5. Grubb BP, Kosinski D. Current trends in etiology, diagnosis, and management of neurocardiogenic syncope. Curr Opin Cardiol. 1996;11:32-41
6. Linzer M, Yang EH, Estes NAM, Wang P, Vorperian VR, Kapoor WN. Diagnosing syncope. Part 1: Value of history, physical examination, and electrocardiography. Ann Intern Med. 1997;126(12):989-96.
7. Kapoor WN. Using a tilt table to evaluate syncope. Am J Med Sci. 1999;317(2):110-6.
8. Brignole M, Alboni P, Benditt D, Bergfeldt L, Blanc J, Bloch Thomsen PE, Van Dijk JG, Fitzpatrick A, Hohnloser S, Janousek J, Kapoor W, Kenny RA. Kulakowskip, Moya A, Raviele A, SuttonR, Theodorakis G, Weilling W. For the task force on syncope. European society of cardiology. Guidelines on management of syncope. European Heart Jour. 2002;22:1256-1306.
9. Richard NF. Tilt table testing. About. com Health's Disease and Condition; 2003.
10. Grubb BP, Kosinski D. Dysautonomic and reflex syncope syndromes. Cardiol Clin. 1997;15(2):257-68.
11. Baron-Esquivias G, Martinez-Rubio AM. Tilt table test: State of the Art. Indian pacing Electrophysiol J. 2003;3(4):239-252.
12. Hainsworth R, AL-Shamma YHH. Cardiovascular responses to stimulation of carotid baroreceptor in healthy subjects. Clinical Science. 1988;75:159-165.
13. Skinner JR, Roy RJ, Heads A, Hey EN, Hunter S. Estimation of pulmonary arterial pressure in the new born: Study of the repeatability of four Doppler

echocardiographic techniques. Pediatr Cardiol. 1996;17:360-369.

14. Stafford RW, Harris WS, Weissler AM. Left ventricular systolic time intervals as indices of postural circulatory stress in man. Circulation. 1970;41:485–492.

15. Geeraerts T, Albaladejo P, Declere AD, Duranteau J, Sales JP, Benhamou D. Decrease in left ventricular ejection time on digital arterial waveform during simulated hypovolemia in normal humans. J Trauma. 2004;56:845–849.

16. Chan GS, Middleton PM, Celler BG, Wang L, Lovell NH. Automatic detection of left ventricular ejection time from a finger photoplethysmographic pulse oximetry waveform: Comparison with Doppler aortic measurement. Physiol Meas. 2007;28:439–452.

17. Chan GS, Middleton PM, Celler BG, Wang L, Lovell NH. Change in pulse transit time and pre-ejection period during head-up tilt-induced progressive central hypovolaemia. J Clin Monit Comput. 2007;21:283–293.

18. Chan GS, Middleton PM, Celler BG, Wang L, Lovell NH. Detecting change in left ventricular ejection time during head-up tilt-induced progressive central hypovolaemia using a finger photoplethysmographic pulse oximetry wave form. J Trauma. 2008;64:390–397

19. Grubb BP, Kosinski D. Dysautonomic and reflex syncope syndromes. Cardiol. Clin. 1997;15(2):257-68.

20. Grubb BP, Kimmels. Head-upright tilt table testing using a safe and easy way to assess neurocardiogenic syncope. Postgrad. Med. 1998;103(1):133-140.

21. Chan GS, Middleton PM, Celler BG, Wang L, Lovell NH. Change in pulse transit time and pre-ejection period during head-up tilt-induced progressive central hypovolaemia. J Clin Monit Comput. 2007;21(5):283-93. Epub 2007 Aug 16.

22. Chan GS, Middleton PM, Celler BG, Wang L, Lovell NH. Detecting change in left ventricular ejection time during head-up tilt-induced progressive central hypovolaemia using a finger photoplethysmographic pulse oximetry wave form. J Trauma. 2008;64:390–397.

23. Fucà G, Dinelli M, Gianfranchi L, Bressan S, Corbucci G, Alboni P. Assessment of systolic ejection time as a hemodynamic marker of incipient bradycardic vasovagal syncope. A pilot study. Pacing Clin Electrophysiol. 2011;34(8):954-62.

24. Hainsworth R, Al-Shamma YMH. Cardiovascular responses to upright tilting in healthy subjects .Clinical Science. 1988;74:17-22.

25. Grubb BP, Kosinski D. Dysautonomic and reflex syncope syndromes. Cardiol Clin. 1997;15(2):257-68.

26. Grubb BP, Kimmels. Head-upright tilt table testing using a safe and easy way to assess neurocardiogenic syncope. Postgrad. Med. 1998;103(1):133-140.

27. Sung RY, Dunz D, Yu GE, Yamme, Fok TF. Cerebral blood flow during vasovagal syncope induce By active standing or hcad up tilt archives of disease in chlldren. 2000;82(2):154-158.

28. Vijayalakshrini P, Veliath S, Moha M. Effect of head-up tilt on cardiovascular responses in normal young volunteers Indian J. Physiol Pharmaco. 2001;44(4): 467-472.

29. AL-Shamma YMH, AL-Khawaja SAM, AL-Abidy JMR. Effect of upright tilting on cardiovascular reflexes using echocardiographic method for estimating cardiac output. Kufa Med J. 2002;5(2):85-96.

30. Lamarre-Cliche M, Cusson J. The fainting patient: Value of head-upright tilt table test in adult patients with orthostatic intolerance. CMA J. 2001;164(3):372-376.

11

Atypical Cardiac Autonomic Neuropathy Identified with Entropy Measures

David J. Cornforth[1,2*] and Herbert F. Jelinek[3,4]

[1]Applied Informatics Research Group, University of Newcastle, Callaghan NSW 2308, Australia.
[2]School of Engineering and Information Technology, University of New South Wales, Australian Defence Force Academy, Canberra, Australia.
[3]Centre for Research in Complex Systems, School of Community Health, Charles Sturt University, Albury, Australia.
[4]Australian School of Advanced Medicine, Macquarie University, Sydney, Australia.

Authors' contributions

This work was carried out in collaboration between all authors. Author DJC designed the study, performed the statistical analysis, and drew the graphs. Author HFJ recruited the participants, collected data and managed the literature searches. All authors contributed to the writing of the manuscript and read and approved the final manuscript.

Editor(s):
(1) Anonymous
Reviewers:
(1) Abdulrahman M. Almoghairi, Adult Cardiology Department, Prince Sultan Cardiac Center, Riyadh, Saudi Arabia.
(2) Iana Simova, Department of Noninvasive Cardiovascular Imaging and Functional Diagnostics, National Cardiology Hospital, Bulgaria.

ABSTRACT

Aims: To identify Cardiac Autonomic Neuropathy (CAN) from a range of measures extracted from Heart Rate Variability (HRV), including higher moments of RR intervals and a spectrum of entropy measures of RR intervals.

Study Design: Analysis of HRV measured from participants at a diabetes screening clinic. Groups were compared using t-tests to identify variables that provide separation between groups.

Place and Duration of Study: Charles Sturt Diabetes Complications Clinic, Albury, NSW Australia.

Methodology: Eleven participants with definite CAN, 67 participants with early CAN, and 71 without CAN had their beat-to-beat fluctuations analyzed using two spectra of HRV: the spectrum of moments of RR intervals and the spectrum of Renyi entropy measures. RR intervals were extracted from ECG recordings and were detrended before analysis.

*Corresponding author: E-mail: David.Cornforth@newcastle.edu.au

Results: Higher moments of RR intervals identified a previously unnoticed sub-group of patients who are atypical within the definite CAN group. Classification of CAN progression was better with Renyi entropy measures than with moments of RR intervals. Significant differences between early and definite CAN were found with the sixth and eighth moments, ($P=.022$ and $P=.042$ respectively), but for entropy measures P values were orders of magnitude smaller.
Conclusion: Identification of early CAN provides the opportunity for early intervention and better treatment outcomes, as well as identifying atypical cases. Our findings illustrate the value of exploring a range of different measures when attempting to detect differences in groups of patients with CAN.

Keywords: Cardiac autonomic neuropathy; cardiac arrhythmia; heart rate variability; entropy measures.

1. INTRODUCTION

Cardiovascular disease (CVD) and sudden cardiac death (SCD) represent a major portion of world-wide morbidity and mortality. In the United States, the incidence of SCD has been reported at 300,000 annually, but may be higher as the exact definition of SCD remains to be clarified [1]. In addition, an aging population and higher rates of obesity and diabetes may lead to an increase in SCD, which is associated with autonomic nervous system dysregulation of the heart [2,3]. Coronary artery disease is a multifactorial disease that is a major contributor to SCD, as are congestive heart failure, left ventricular dysfunction and post-myocardial infarction [4,5]. Accurate, non-invasive, clinical diagnostic tools have the potential to reduce the incidence of SCD in at-risk populations. Autonomic nervous system modulation of the heart leads to variability in the heart rate and in the length of the inter-beat interval. A certain degree of beat-to-beat fluctuation is an important physiological attribute, and a loss of variability in heart rate is associated with pathophysiology and increased risk of adverse cardiac events. Thus an increased heart rate or lowered heart rate variability (HRV) have been validated as markers of increased risk of myocardial infarct [4,6].

Cardiovascular function is under the modulation of the autonomic nervous system. Damage to the parasympathetic or sympathetic part of the autonomic nervous system leads to dysfunction of heart rate control and vascular dynamics, and an increased risk of mortality, as shown in the ACCORD trial [7]. Cardiac Autonomic Neuropathy (CAN) has been described in diabetes, Parkinson's disease, depression, coronary heart disease and congestive heart failure [8-12]. CAN is a disease that involves nerve damage leading to increasingly abnormal control of heart rate, which is especially prominent in people with diabetes. The extent of the loss of sympathetic and parasympathetic involvement in regulating the heart rate can be determined from an ECG recording and analyzed to provide a risk stratification tool.

The standard clinical test for CAN is the Ewing battery, but this has limitations, as one or more of the five tests may be contraindicated due to cardiac or respiratory disease [13-15]. Analysis of the distribution of RR intervals over a selected period such as 20 minutes provides a more robust basis for determining autonomic nervous system function [16]. The simplest characterisation of heart rate variability remains the mean heart rate and standard deviation; however other measures may provide further insight.

1.1 Heart Rate Variability

A common type of ECG signal is shown in (Fig. 1). Such signals have been studied extensively and the diagnostic value of the different features is well established. Letters are used to identify ECG features. The fiducial point or peak of the QRS interval can be identified most easily and is therefore used to obtain an RR interval tachogram, from which the heart rate variability can be obtained. The natural rhythm of the human heart is known to vary in response to sympathetic and parasympathetic signals. Generally, sympathetic activity increases HR and decreases HRV, whereas parasympathetic activity decreases HR and increases HRV [17]. HRV is commonly used in assessing the regulation of cardiac autonomic function [18,10].

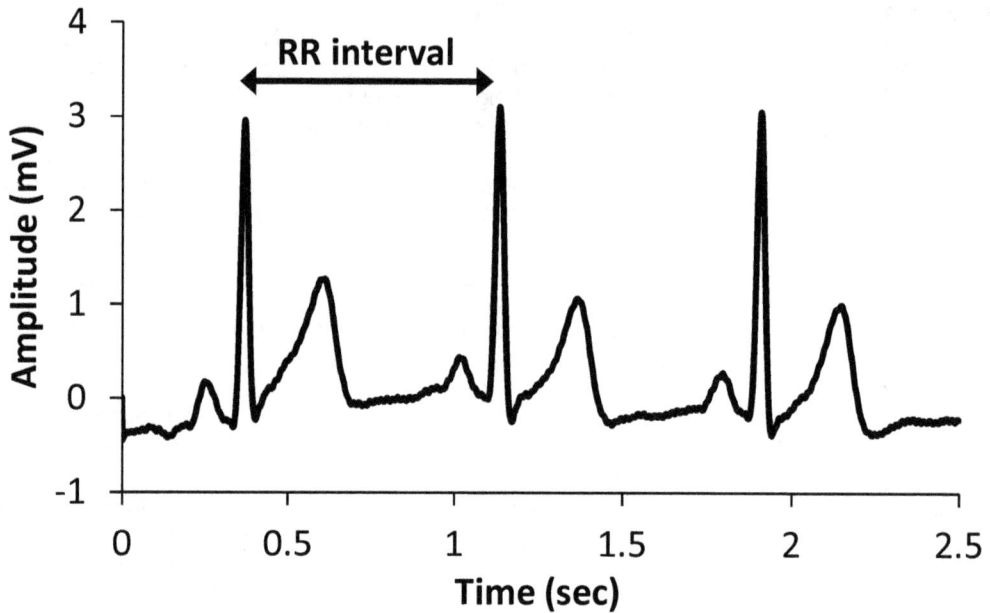

Fig. 1. A typical ECG signal showing the RR Interval

The ECG signal may often be degraded by the presence of noise, so that the most reliable feature that can be obtained from low quality recordings (and therefore the most easily obtained measurement) is the interval between successive R peaks, the RR interval, which is the inverse of the heart rate. A typical adult heart rate is 60-80 beats per minute, with typical RR interval lengths between 750 and 1000 milliseconds. RR intervals can be subjected to further analysis through a variety of algorithms in order to provide measures with good discriminant power, based on the difference of RR interval variability. HRV provides information only on the changes in the interval length, is non-invasive and easy to obtain from an ECG recording.

Cardiac Autonomic Neuropathy (CAN) leads to arrhythmias and may precipitate SCD. An open question is to what extent this condition is detectable by measures based on HRV. An even more desirable option is to detect CAN in its early, preclinical stage, to improve treatment and treatment outcomes.

1.2 Multi-scale Moments

Moments are measures of distribution such as mean, median, mode, skewness and kurtosis. The various moments from RR intervals provide a numeric value by which the distribution can be characterized. The familiar arithmetic mean and variance of RR intervals can be informally viewed as moments of order 1 and 2 respectively, where order refers to the exponent used in calculating these values. Higher order moments can be defined as:

$$m_k = E[(X - \mu)^k] \qquad (1)$$

where $E[x]$ is the expectation of X, and μ is the arithmetic mean of the variable X. Expectation is commonly interpreted as the sum of observations on X in a sample of size n, divided by n, so that for example the second moment or variance is defined as:

$$s^2 = \frac{1}{n}\sum_{i=1}^{n}(x_i - \bar{x})^2 \qquad (2)$$

which calculates deviation in observations x_i in the sample of size n from the mean. The third and fourth moments have a known interpretation, as the Skewness and Kurtosis respectively, although m_3 and m_4 are usually subject to corrections in order to address statistical bias and magnitude. Skewness describes the amount of asymmetry of the distribution, so can reveal whether the distribution is leaning to the left or right, and consequently whether the tails are larger on the lower or upper sides of the distribution. A negative value indicates a larger tail for values lower than the mean, while a positive value indicates a larger tail above the mean. Kurtosis measures the flatness of the distribution. A flat or platykurtic distribution has a negative value for kurtosis, while a peaked or leptokurtic distribution has a sharp peak. The former indicates that the variance of the distribution is due to unusually large deviations from the mean, when compared to a Gaussian distribution. The latter indicates that the variance is due to frequent small deviations.

Higher moments have more difficult interpretations, but provide different measures of the distribution of RR intervals, so can be used to compare different groups of patients. It is usual to normalize these moments to provide a scale invariant spectrum:

$$\mu_k = \frac{m_k}{\sigma^k} \tag{3}$$

where μ_k is the standardized moment, and σ^k is the standard deviation raised to the power of k.

1.3 Multiscale Renyi Entropy

In the context of the analysis of heart rate variability, various entropy measures can estimate the variability of the HRV. An entropy measure is typically of the form:

$$H(X) = -\sum_{i=1}^{n} p(x_i) log_b p(x_i) \tag{4}$$

where $p(x_i)$ is the probability of the random variable x, and b is the base of the logarithm, commonly 2. Renyi entropy H is a generalization of the Shannon entropy:

$$H_\alpha(X) = \frac{1}{1-\alpha} log_2 \left(\sum_{i=1}^{n} p_i^\alpha \right) \tag{5}$$

where p_i is the probability that $X=x$ and α is the order of the entropy measure. This is the parameter that is varied to produce the multi-scale entropy. The probability can be estimated in a number of ways. In this work we estimate the probability of a *sequence* of RR intervals of length π by comparing the sample i with all other samples of length π in the recording, using methods similar to those used to estimate sample entropy, and as outlined by Lake [19]. This involves measuring the distance between

sample i and all other samples j, then estimating p_i using a Gaussian (normal) kernel:

$$p_i = \sum_{j=0}^{n} exp \left(\frac{-dist_{ij}^2}{2\sigma^2} \right) \tag{6}$$

where σ is a parameter controlling the width of the density function and $dist_{ij}$ is a distance measure, in this case Euclidean, in π dimensions:

$$dist_{ij} = \sum_{k=0}^{\pi} \left(x_{i+k} - x_{j+k} \right)^2 \tag{7}$$

This yields a probability estimate for each sample of length π, with the desirable property that its value lies between 0 and 1.

2. METHODOLOGY

Anthropometric and clinical data were obtained from patients reviewed at the Charles Sturt Diabetes Complications Screening Group (DiScRi), Australia [20]. Participants attending the screening clinic had their lead II ECG recorded for 20 minutes and RR intervals analysed. The subjects were comparable for age, gender, and heart rate, and the same physical conditions were used for each subject. ECGs were recorded using a Maclab Pro with Chart 7 software (AD Instruments, Sydney). Initial screening of participants led to the exclusion of those with heart disease, presence of a pacemaker, kidney disease or polypharmacy including multiple anti-arrhythmic medications. The study was approved by the Charles Sturt University Human Ethics Committee and written informed consent was obtained from all participants. CAN was defined using the Ewing battery criteria, and so participants were separated into early CAN, definite CAN, or no CAN [13,21,22].

Eleven participants with definite CAN, 67 participants with early CAN, and 71 without CAN attending the screening clinic participated. From the 20-minute recording, a 15-minute segment was taken from the middle of the original recording to remove start-up artefacts and movement artefacts at the end of the recording. Only the RR intervals were retained, and no other information from the ECG were utilised in this study. The baseline was removed by subtracting the mean value of the RR interval from the RR data. The trend was removed after analysis by linear correlation. For each detrended series the mean, variance, and higher moments were calculated as described above.

The multi-scale Renyi Entropy was calculated from $-5 < \alpha < +5$, where α represents the scaling exponent and $\alpha=1$ is the Shannon entropy. For all calculated measures, a student's t-test was performed to compare the means of every variable. For all variables from the moments and the Renyi spectra, histograms were calculated and smoothed using a filter of:

$$f_i^* = \frac{1}{9}(f_{i-2} + 2f_{i-1} + 3f_i + 2f_{i+1} + f_{i+2}) \qquad (8)$$

Frequency values for all histograms were then normalised, by dividing by the number of patients in each class. A selection of these histograms is presented below.

3. RESULTS AND DISCUSSION

Results for the spectrum of moments are shown in (Table 1). Column headings are given for each calculated moment. The first two columns provide the mean and variance. Under these headings, the *P*-value results of t-tests are provided, comparing the means of the three patient groups for each moment. Any value below $P=.05$ is regarded as significant at the 95% confidence interval level, and is indicated by shading.

(Table 1) shows there is evidence for a difference between the mean of RR intervals ($P \leq 4.99E\text{-}6$), and evidence of a difference between variance of RR intervals ($P \leq 8.53E\text{-}4$). These results are well known and agree with the findings of previous studies [23]. Also of clinical interest is the significant difference between Early and Normal CAN groups for the sixth and eighth moments ($P=.022$ and $P=.042$ respectively).

The values of mean and variance for the three patient groups are illustrated using smoothed histograms in (Figs. 2 and 3). Patients in the Normal group (controls) have lower mean RR interval (Fig. 2) and higher variance (Fig. 3), while patients in the Definite group (confirmed CAN) have a higher mean and lower variance. The values of the 6th and 8th moments are illustrated similarly in (Figs. 4 and 5). Examination of these two figures reveals a hitherto unnoticed outlier sub-group in the Definite CAN group, which is apparent in both (Figs. 4 and 5). This outlier sub-group consists of two patients who have elevated values, apparent in higher even moments including the 4th moment (not shown) but not apparent from any of the odd moments analysed. This difference is due to the fact that moments calculated using even exponents treat both positive and negative deviations from the mean as equivalent. Moments calculated using odd exponents on the other hand, treat deviation from the means differently, depending on whether they are positive or negative. These outliers were not detected by the mean or variance, but became apparent when higher moments were examined. This highlights the value of exploring higher moments associated with the RR interval distribution for analysis of HRV.

The results for Renyi entropy are shown in (Table 2). Column headings identify the Renyi entropy calculated for different values of the exponent α. As in the previous table, the *P*-values resulting from t-tests are provided below these headings. An examination of significant results, in shaded cells, reveals very different results for negative and positive values of α. Nearly all the significant values correspond to $\alpha<0$. There is little difference resulting from the actual value of α chosen, but in general the negative part of the Renyi spectrum appears to provide superior discrimination between patient groups.

Table 1. *P* values comparing mean value of moments for each of the 3 classes: D: Definite CAN, E: Early CAN and N: Normal (controls). Skewness is closely related to $\mu3$, while kurtosis is closely related to $\mu4$. Shaded cells indicate significance at $P = .05$ or better

T-test	Mean	Vari	$\mu3$	$\mu4$	$\mu5$	$\mu6$	$\mu7$	$\mu8$	$\mu9$
D vs. E	5.0E-6	8.5E-4	.63	.89	.17	.83	.16	.53	.15
E vs. N	5.6E-7	9.1E-6	.74	.063	.29	.022	.23	.042	.28
N vs. D	4.7E-10	1.8E-7	.84	.32	.41	.24	.44	.22	.055

Table 2. *P* values comparing mean of renyi entropy for each of the 3 classes: D: Definite CAN, E: Early CAN and N: Normal (controls). Shaded cells indicate significance at *P*=.05 or better

T-test	H(-5)	H(-4)	H(-3)	H(-2)	H(-1)	H(1)	H(2)	H(3)	H(4)	H(5)
D vs. E	.15	.16	.17	.18	.22	.27	.25	.22	.21	.20
E vs. N	7.7E-5	7.0E-5	6.1E-5	5.3E-5	7.2E-5	.09	.19	.22	.21	.20
N vs. D	8.9E-5	1.0E-4	1.3E-4	2.2E-4	7.4E-4	.057	.066	.060	.054	.050

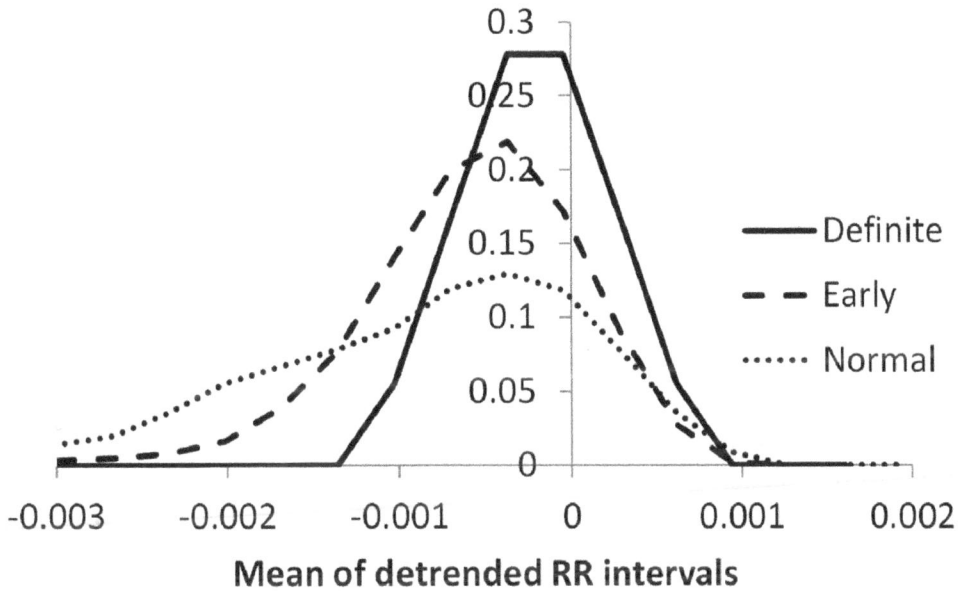

Fig. 2. Smoothed histogram comparing the three patient groups for mean RR interval

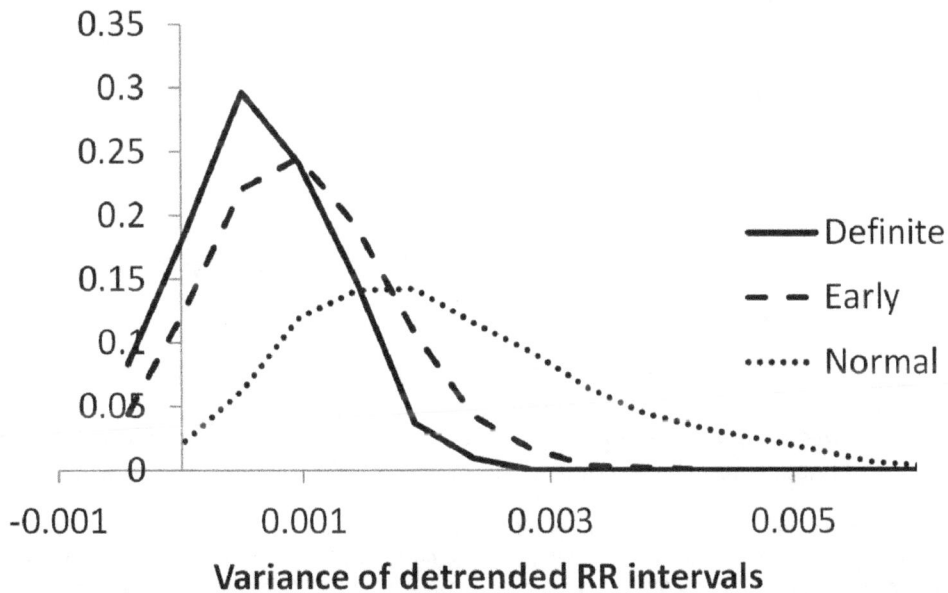

Fig. 3. Smoothed histogram comparing the three patient groups for variance of RR interval

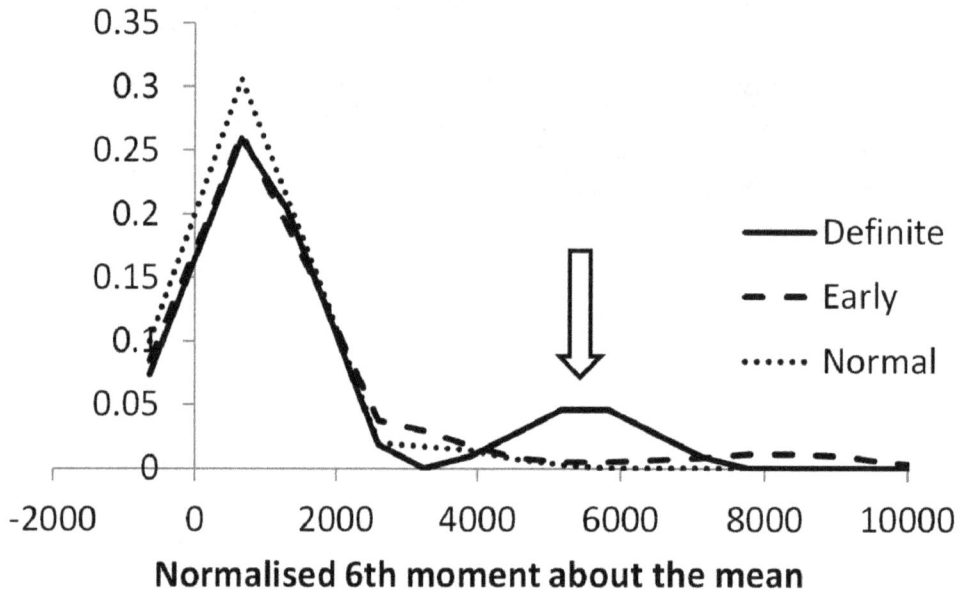

Fig. 4. Smoothed histogram comparing the three patient groups for the 6th moment. This reveals a previously undetected outlier sub-group (indicated with arrow) in the definite group

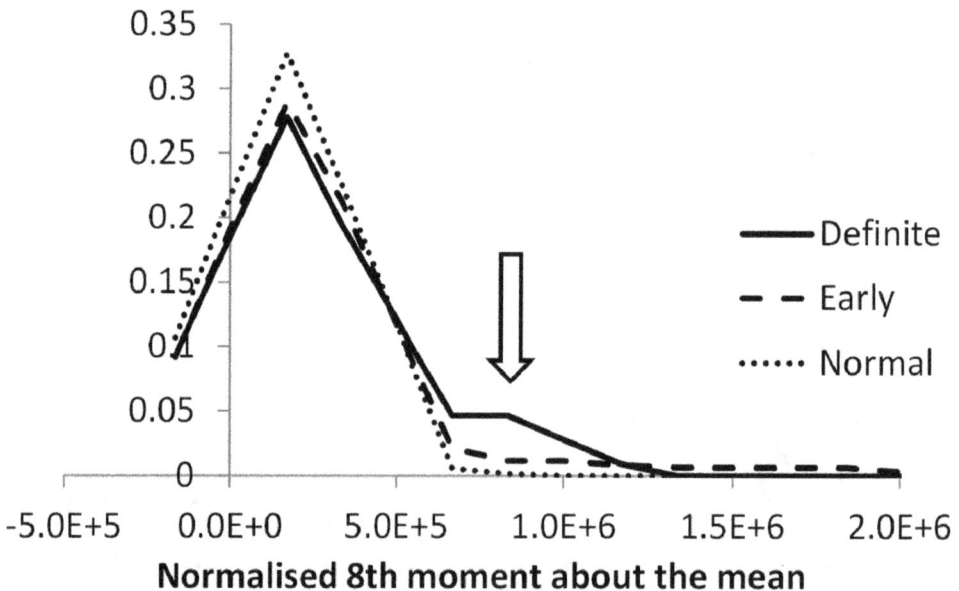

Fig. 5. Smoothed histograms comparing the three patient groups for the 8th moment. The previously undetected outlier sub-group is indicated with an arrow

The smoothed histogram for Renyi entropy with $\alpha=-5$ is shown in (Fig. 6). The differences are readily observed, with patients from the Definite group providing, on average, a higher value of Renyi entropy (mean of 2.14), followed by patients from the Early group (mean of 2.06).

The lowest values for $H(-5)$ were obtained from patients in the Normal CAN group, with a mean value of 1.88. Compare this with the smoothed histogram for the Shannon entropy $H(1)$ shown in (Fig. 7). Here the three patient groups cannot be distinguished from each other. It is clear that the

Shannon entropy is unable to distinguish between the three groups of patients, whereas the Renyi entropy with negative exponents is able to separate these groups.

In this study, we have examined two spectra of measures. The spectrum of moments is obtained by extending the variance using exponents greater than 2. These moments include skewness and kurtosis, but form part of a spectrum, which extends further to include moments of order 8 and higher. For instance the third moment (or skewness) indicates whether the variance is due to fewer, larger deviations on one side of the distribution compared to the other. In definite CAN when the sympathetic component of autonomic regulation starts to predominate or parasympathetic withdrawal is occurring, a skewed distribution favouring shorter RR intervals can be expected. The current work indicates that the distributions are fairly symmetrical, as shown by relatively low values for the third moment (skewness) and values that were similar across all three patient groups. Kurtosis describes the flatness of the distribution relative to the normal distribution. RR interval time series with high kurtosis have a distinct peak near the mean, decline rather rapidly, and have heavy tails. In this case the relatively large values for the 4th moment indicate a distribution with a high peak around the mean, indicating that

most of the variance is due to many relatively small deviations of the RR interval size from the mean, and very few large deviations.

The spectrum of moments higher than of order 4 for RR intervals suggested that higher odd numbered moments do not afford a measure to assist in distinguishing the three groups. However, the higher even moments drew attention to a sub-group of patients who are atypical within the group with definite CAN. Moments with even exponent treat positive and negative deviations from the mean in a similar way, so may group together values that may not be associated using odd moments. This sub-group requires further investigation. However it is not uncommon to misclassify a patient using the Ewing battery, especially if only one or two of the required five tests are used. For the current study, only those ECGs were analysed where results for the complete Ewing battery of tests was available. In spite of this, some misclassification is possible. In addition, patients with cardio respiratory disorders, those that are frail or obese may have difficulty in performing the required tests. Therefore passive testing for CAN, as is the case by interpreting the RR intervals obtained from an ECG recorded at rest, may provide more robust results for assessment of CAN progression.

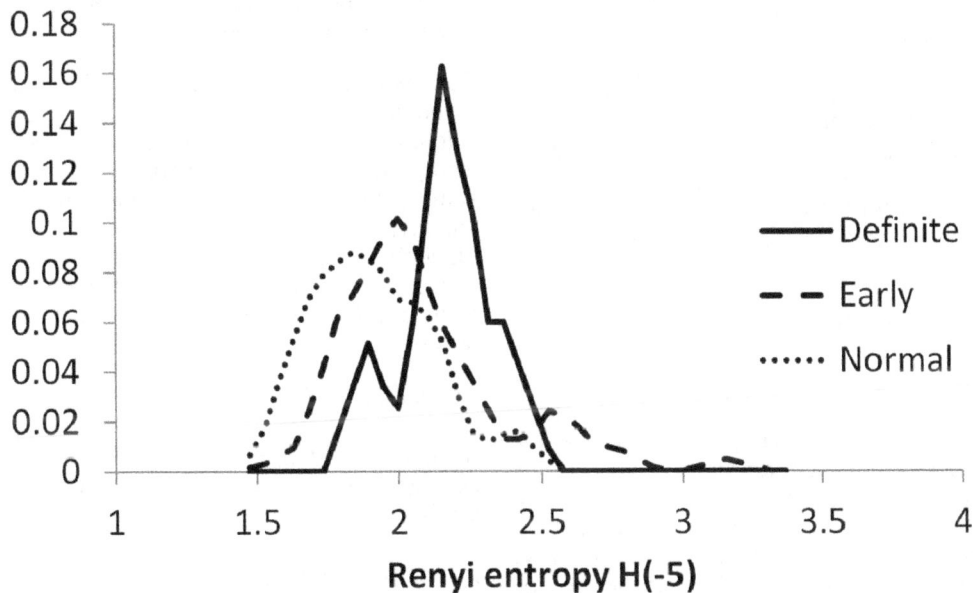

Fig. 6. Smoothed histograms comparing the three patient groups for renyi entropy with α=-5

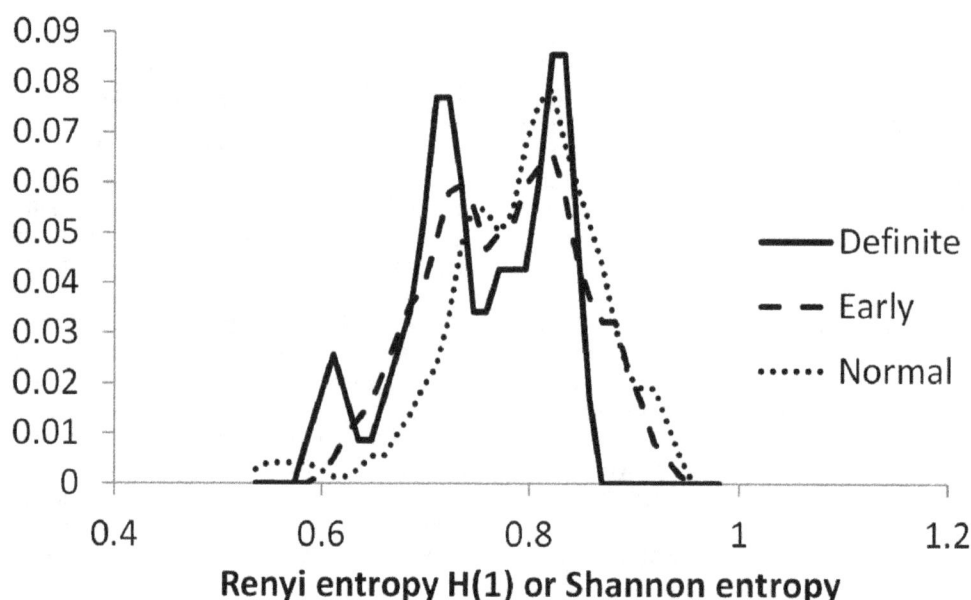

Fig. 7. Smoothed histograms comparing the three patient groups for Renyi entropy with α=1 (equivalent to Shannon entropy)

The spectrum of Renyi entropy was much more successful in distinguishing patient groups, showing highly significant differences in means for the three groups (*P<.0001*). However, the use of a spectrum of measures revealed that these differences could not be detected using the Shannon entropy (*α=1*). It was necessary to explore more fully the range of possible exponents in order to discover a suitable entropy measure that could distinguish patient groups. One drawback of the study was that groups such as those with diabetes or obesity often have prescribed medication, which may directly or indirectly affect cardiac function and therefore rhythm analysis. Our data reflect this, as the number of participants identified with definite CAN is rather small due to the exclusion criteria applied.

4. CONCLUSION

Risk stratification of sudden cardiac death is an important component in clinical practice, especially in patients with diabetes, where the risk is much higher and an asymptomatic stage associated with Cardiac Autonomic Neuropathy (CAN) often occurs. It is desirable to find a relatively non-invasive method to identify CAN, and this work explores the feasibility of identification based on measures of Heart Rate Variability (HRV). In this work, we have examined the use of two spectra of measurements to identify CAN: the spectra of

moments and the spectra of Renyi entropy, both calculated from RR intervals.

The mean and variance of the RR interval are useful discriminators, but higher moments did not provide any additional discriminating power, except that some moments were able to detect outliers. However the Renyi spectrum, in particular the negative part, was consistently successful in identifying groups of patients.

Our findings illustrate the value of exploring a range of measures when attempting to detect differences in groups of patients. Although measures such as mean, variance and Shannon entropy may be more well-known than Renyi entropy, these measures may not provide the required discrimination. An exploration of multiscale measures as demonstrated in this study provides new insights into cardiovascular disease.

CONSENT

All authors declare that written informed consent was obtained from the patients for publication of the study.

ETHICAL APPROVAL

All authors hereby declare that all experiments have been examined and approved by the Charles Sturt University Human Ethics

Committee and have therefore been performed in accordance with the ethical standards laid down in the 1964 Declaration of Helsinki.

ACKNOWLEDGEMENTS

The authors would like to thank Bev de Jong for technical assistance and Roche Australia Pty for providing consumables for blood glucose measurements. The study was funded in part by a Compacts Funding from Charles Sturt University. Roche Australia Pty and Charles Sturt University played no role in the design, data collection, analysis and interpretation of the study.

COMPETING INTERESTS

Authors have declared that no competing interests exist.

REFERENCES

1. Myerburg RJ. Sudden cardiac death: Exploring the limits of our knowledge. J Cardiovasc Electrophysiol. 2001;12(3):369-381.

2. Friedman GD, Klatsky AL, et al. Predictors of sudden cardiac death. Circulation. 1975;52(6):164-169.

3. Sexton PT, Walsh J, et al. Risk factors for sudden unexpected cardiac death in Tasmanian men. Aust NZ J Med. 1997;27:45-50.

4. Priori SG, Aliot E, et al. Task force on sudden cardiac death of the European society of cardiology. Eur Heart J. 2001;22(16):1374-1450.

5. Zheng ZJ, Croft JB, et al. Sudden cardiac death in the United States, 1989 to 1998. Circulation. 2001;104(18):2158-2163.

6. La Rovere MT. Heart rate and arrhythmic risk: Old markers never die. Europace. 2010;12(2):155-157.

7. Pop-Busui R, Evans GW, et al. The ACCORD study group. Effects of cardiac autonomic dysfunction on mortality risk in the action to control cardiovascular risk in diabetes (ACCORD) trial. Diabetes Care. 2010;33(7):1578-1584.

8. Kemp AH, Quintana DS, et al. Heart rate variability in unmedicated depressed patients without comorbid cardiovascular disease. Plos ONE. 2012;7(2):e30777.

9. Voss A, Schroeder R, et al. Segmented symbolic dynamics for risk stratification in patients with ischemic heart failure. Cardiovascular Engineering and Technology. 2010;1(4):290-298.

10. Vinik AI, Erbas T, et al. Diabetic cardiac autonomic neuropathy, inflammation and cardiovascular disease. Journal of Diabetes Investigation. 2013;4(1):4-8.

11. Salvi V, Hingorani P, et al. Prediction of mortality using measures of cardiac autonomic dysfunction in the diabetic and non diabetic population: The MONICA/KORA Augsburg Cohort Study. Diabetes Care. 2008;31(10):e74.

12. Siddiqui MF, Rast S, et al. Autonomic dysfunction in Parkinson's disease: A comprehensive symptom survey. Parkinsonism & Related Disorders. 2002;8(4):277-284.

13. Ewing DJ, Martyn CN, et al. The value of cardiovascular autonomic functions tests: 10 years' experience in diabetes. Diabetes Care. 1985;8(5):491-498.

14. Jelinek HF, Kelarev AV, et al. Rule-based classifiers and meta-classifiers for identification of cardiac autonomic neuropathy progression. International Journal of Information Science and Computer Mathematics. 2012;5(2):49-53.

15. Stranieri A, Abawajy J, et al. A decision tree approach for ewing test selection to support the clinical assessment of cardiac autonomic neuropathy. Australian Datamining Conference Aus DM; 2012.

16. TFESC/NASPE. Heart rate variability. Standards of measurement, physiological interpretation, and clinical use. Task Force of the European Society of Cardiology and the North American Society of Pacing and Electrophysiology. European Heart Journal. 1996;17(3):354-381.

17. Berntson GG, Bigger JT Jr, Eckberg DL, et al. Heart rate variability: Origins, methods, and interpretive caveats. Psychophysiol. 1997;34(6):623-48.

18. Flynn AC, Jelinek HF, Smith MC. Heart rate variability analysis: A useful assessment tool for diabetes associated cardiac dysfunction in rural and remote areas. Aust J Rural Health. 2005;13:77-82.

19. Lake DE. Renyi entropy measures of heart rate Gaussianity, IEEE Transactions on Biomedical Engineering. 2006;53(1).

20. Jelinek HF, Wilding C, Tinley P. An innovative multi-disciplinary diabetes complications screening programme in a rural community: A description and preliminary results of the screening.

Australian Journal of Primary Health. 2006;12:14-20.

21. Javorka M, Trunkvalterova Z, Tonhajzerova I, et al. Short-term heart rate complexity is reduced in patients with type 1 diabetes mellitus. Clin. Neurophysiol. 2008;119:1071-81.

22. Khandoker AH, Jelinek HF, Palaniswami M. Identifying diabetic patients with cardiac autonomic neuropathy by heart rate complexity analysis. Biomed Eng Online. 2009;8:3.

23. Goldberger JJ, Challapalli S, Tung R, et al. Relationship of heart rate variability to parasympathetic effect. Circulation. 2001;103(15):1977-1983.

12

Correlation of Left Atrial Septal Pouch with the Prevalence of Patent Foramen Ovale: A Retrospective Review

Silanath Terpenning[1*], Loren H. Ketai[1], Stacy M. Rissing[2] and Shawn D. Teague[2]

[1]Department of Radiology, University of New Mexico, Albuquerque, NM, 87131, USA.
[2]Department of Radiology, Indiana University, School of Medicine, 550 N University Blvd, Indianapolis, IN 46202, USA.

Authors' contributions

This work was carried out in collaboration between all authors. Author ST designed the study, co-interpreted the studies and wrote the first draft of the manuscript. Author LHK managed the literature searches, analyses of the study and performed the final manuscript editing. Author SMR co-interpreted the studies and performed the initial manuscript editing and author SDT wrote the protocol and performed the initial manuscript editing. All authors read and approved the final manuscript.

Editor(s):
(1) Francesco Pelliccia, Department of Heart and Great Vessels University La Sapienza, Rome, Italy.
(2) Fatih Yalcin, School of Medicine, Department of Cardiology, Johns Hopkins University, USA.
(3) Gen-Min Lin, Division of Cardiology, Hualien-Armed Forces General Hospital, National Defense Medical Center, Taiwa.
Reviewers:
(1) Anonymous, Spain.
(2) Anonymous, Brasil.
(3) Anonymous, Switzerland.

ABSTRACT

Purpose: To determine the prevalence of Left Atrial Septal Pouch (LASP) and assess the association with Patent Foramen Ovale (PFO).

Materials and Methods: We retrospectively reviewed 275 cardiac-gated CT examinations at Indiana University from January 2010 to June 2012, 160 cardiac CTs performed prior to pulmonary vein ablation, 115 for evaluation of coronary artery evaluation. Consensus readings were performed by two readers on a PACS workstation using the Multiplanar Reformat software to identify the presence or absence of LASP and PFO. PFO was diagnosed by the presence of a contrast jet extending from the left atrium to the right atrium.

Results: Overall prevalence of LASP was 24.7% (68 LASPs out of 275 patients). There was no

*Corresponding author: E-mail: natsawadee@yahoo.com

significant difference regarding the gender and age between patients with and without LASP, p-values 0.054 and 0.63 respectively. The overall prevalence of PFO in both groups is low 2.2% (6 PFOs out of 275 patients). The prevalence of PFO in patients with LASP was 5.9% (4 out of 68 patients) and was 1.0% (2 PFOs out of 207 patients) in patients without LASP. There was a significant difference in prevalence of PFO between patients with and without LASP, p-value 0.035. **Conclusions:** LASP is a common finding on cardiac CT, its prevalence not affected by age or gender. Patients with LASP have statistically greater prevalence of PFO than patients without LASP, but the prevalence remains low.

Keywords: Left atrial pouch; left atrium septal pouch; patent foramen ovale.

1. INTRODUCTION

Left atrial septal pouch (LASP) and patent foramen ovale (PFO) are both manifestations of interatrial septal developmental abnormalities. PFO is the sequelae of an unfused septum primum and septum secundum while LASP is the product of incomplete fusion, the residual unfused septum primum and septum secundum forming a flap in the left atrium. The prevalence of LASP was as high as 44.7% in the largest autopsy series [1] and its detectable prevalence on cardiac CT is between 11.5 to 40% [2,3]. The prevalence of PFO has been reported up to 25% of Transesophageal Echocardiography (TEE) [4] and between 22.6% and 23.5% on 64 Multidetector CT scan [2,5].

Our observation was that Atrial Fibrillation (AF) patients who underwent cardiac CT for pre-ablation mapping had high prevalence of LASP, a form of atrial septal abnormalities. Since PFO is also an atrial wall anomaly, we hypothesized that presence of LASP is associated with higher prevalence of PFO. Accordingly we sought to determine both the prevalence of LASP on cardiac CT and the strength of its association with CT detectable PFO.

To our knowledge, no publications in the literatures have investigated the co-existence of LASP and PFO.

2. MATERIALS AND METHODS

This retrospective study was approved by Institutional Review Board (IRB). The need for inform consent was waived.

A total of 275 cardiac CT examinations were performed. These included 160 pulmonary vein CT exams prior to pulmonary vein ablation and 115 coronary CTA exams for coronary artery evaluation. Studies were performed at Indiana University between January 2010 and June 2012.

2.1 CT Techniques

For CT of the pulmonary vein, a retrospective technique was applied with a Phillips 64 Brilliance (Philips Medical Systems, Cleveland, OH) multidetector CT scanner. We performed prospective or step and shoot technique on a Philips 256 iCT (Philips Medical Systems, Cleveland, OH) multidetector CT scanner based on rhythm, when possible, for pulmonary vein evaluation. No premedication was given. Intravenous contrast bolus tracking protocol was applied to optimize contrast enhancement in the left atrium. Images were reconstructed at 78% of the R-R interval. 3D images were created and stored on PACS for later evaluation. Multiplanar reformat software (MPR) was used for each study to better visualize the pulmonary vein ostium.

Coronary CTA protocol was tailored to each patient's cardiac history. In all cases, the target heart rate was less than 60 BPM. Retrospective, or prospective ECG gating techniques or occasionally a step and shoot technique by a Phillips 64 Brilliance or a Philips 256 iCT (Philips Medical Systems, Cleveland, OH) multidetector CT scanners were used with premedication by 5-25 mg intravenous Metoprolol for heart rate control and 2 tablets (0.4 mg) sublingual Nitroglycerin for coronary artery vasodilation (if not contraindicated). Cardiac-gated CT cathode tube modulation was used to reduce radiation exposure. The images were acquired 5-6 minutes after sublingual Nitroglycerin, if administered. Radiation technique, premedical-tion, and the amount and rate of contrast injection were under radiologists' supervision. Cardiac function calculation was post processed by radiologists at the Philips EBW workstations (Philips Medical Systems, Cleveland, OH).

For both groups, Isovue 370 was administered intravenously at the rate of 5 ml/s followed by saline flush. The amount of contrast was calculated based on the scan time, post threshold trigger delay, and location of tracker trigger region of interest in the ascending, descending aorta or left atrium. Image acquisition extended from the carina to the diaphragms.

The CT parameters were adjusted according to the patient's conditions (heart rate, age, BMI), clinical indications, available CT scanners (64 or 256 detector CT scanners), ECG gating technique and reconstruction techniques. We used 100-150 kV, 100-1050 mAs, 0.9 mm thickness with 0.45 increment and the fastest available rotation time (0.4s on 64 detector scanners and 0.27s on 256 detector scanners).

2.2 Image Analysis

Two radiologists reviewed the images retrospectively and reported the presence of PFO by consensus (ST, SMR). The studies were reviewed on a PACS workstation (Fuji Medical, Stamford, CT) using the MPR software. Radiologists were blinded to patient's clinical history any prior echocardiographic results.

Presence or absence of LASP and PFO was identified for individual patients. The imaging criteria of PFO, independent of the presence of LASP are based on the work from Kim et al [6]. We chose the most specific criteria for PFO, independence of a flow jet traversing the internal septum.

For atrial fibrillation patients, we measured LA size in the maximal transverse dimension on the axial plane.

2.3 Statistics

Demographic data and the presence or absence of both LASP and PFO on cardiac CTs were recorded. Statistical analysis was performed by Pearson Chi-Square test, ANOVA table and Fisher-Exact test depending on the quality and quantity of the variables. Presence of PFO, mean age and gender were analyzed by Fisher-Exact test, ANOVA table and Pearson Chi-Square test, respectively.

The difference in LA size between patients with and without LASPs was analyzed by student's t Test.

3. RESULTS

A total of 383 exams (203 Pulmonary Vein CT exams and 180 Coronary CTA exams) were performed between January 2010 and June 2012. One hundred and eight exams were excluded (43 exams from Pulmonary Vein CT and 65 exams from Coronary CTA) due to suboptimal diagnostic exams, known congenital heart disease, known prior pulmonary vein ablation, known coronary artery disease, prior coronary artery stent placement, or coronary artery bypass grafts.

A total of 275 exams (153 CT examinations of pulmonary veins and 122 CT Coronary angiogram) with adequate diagnostic quality were included, 68 patients with LASP and 207 patients without LASP, 118 female and 157 male. Patients with LASP had a mean age of 53.4±14 years (range of 22-82 years) and did not differ statistically from patients without LASP, mean age of 56.8 ±12.years (range 58-83 years), (p >.05). Neither did patients with and without LASP differ in gender, (p>.05).

The prevalence of LASP and PFO in atrial fibrillation patients were 24.8% and 1.9% respectively (39 LASPs and 3 PFOs out of 153 patients). Normal sinus rhythm patients showed similar trend. The prevalence of LASP and PFO were 23.8% and 2.5% respectively (29 LASPs and 3 PFOs out of 122 normal sinus rhythm patients).

Overall prevalence of LASP was 24.7% (68 out of 275 patients) and the prevalence was PFO was 2.2% (6 PFOs out of 275 patients). The prevalence of PFO in patients with LASP was 5.9% (4 PFOs out of 68 patients) and in patients without LASP was 1.0% (2 PFOs out of 207 patients) (Table 1).

There is significant difference in the prevalence of PFO between patients with and without LASP (p<0.05)

The size of LA in AF patients was not affected by presence of absence of LASPs. LA size in AF patients with and without LASPs was 4.3 cm (SD=0.9) and 4.2 cm (SD=0.8), respectively and did not differ significantly (p-value=0.37).

4. DISCUSSION

There are 2 possible theories for the existence of an LASP. The LASP may be the remnant of the embryologic left venous valve from the sinus venosus or, alternatively, it may be derived from an abnormal duplication or persistence septum primum or secundum [7]. Our hypothesis is that LASP and PFO are within the spectrum of developmental defects of the interatrial septum (Figs. 1-2). We propose that the LASP is the remnant of incompletely fused septum primum and septum secundum, while PFO is the sequel of unfused septum primum and septum secundum (Figs. 3-4).

Our study shows that the prevalence of LASP is high and that there is a significant association between LASP and PFO. The prevalence of PFO in the setting of LASP, however, remains relatively low, approximately 6%.

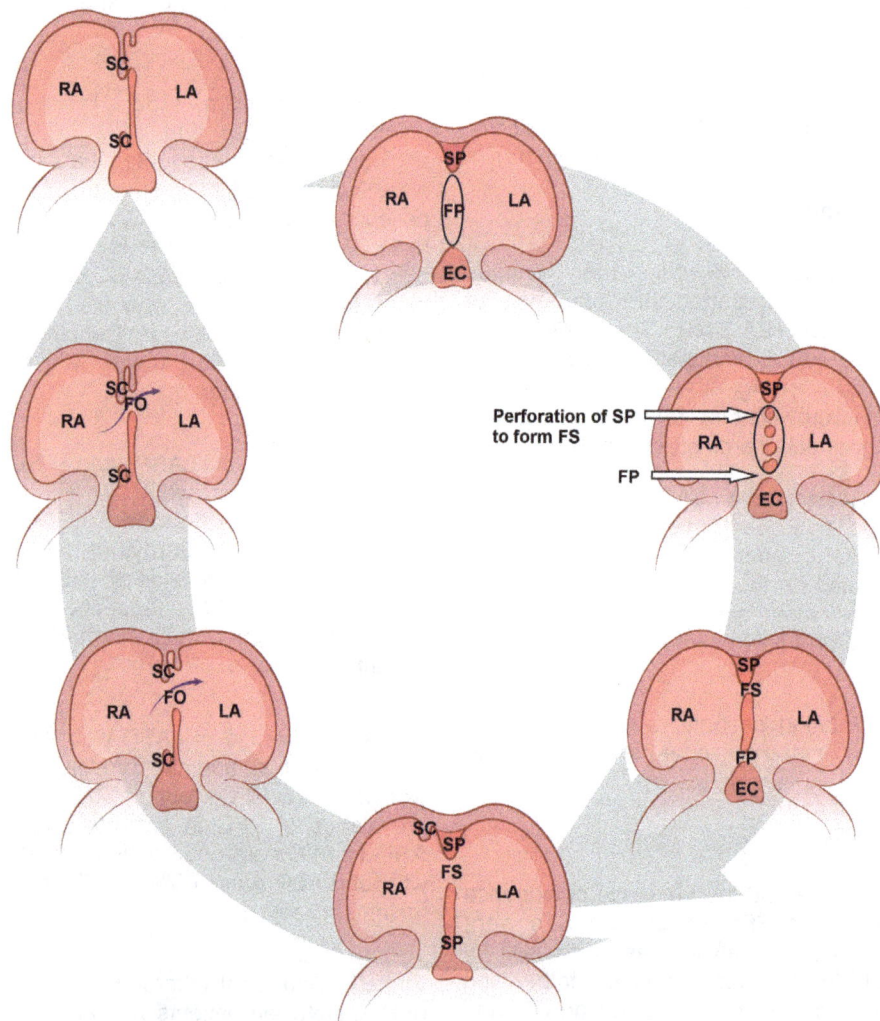

Fig. 1. The illustration shows the embryologic development of IAS in coronal plane. The septum primum is formed and expands, resulting in a smaller foramen; primum. The foramen secumdum is created by perforation of the septum primum followed by fusion of the small defects. At the same time, the endocardial cushion fuses with the septum primum becoming the lower part of IAS and upper part of IVS and creating separated atria. The septum secundum is formed and extended inferiorly to seal the foramen ovale. The 2 atria are finally completely separated by IAS. This illustration was modified from The Developing Human: Clinically Orientated Embryology, 8th edition, the cardiovascular System, page 299-300, copyright Elsevier (2008) with permission

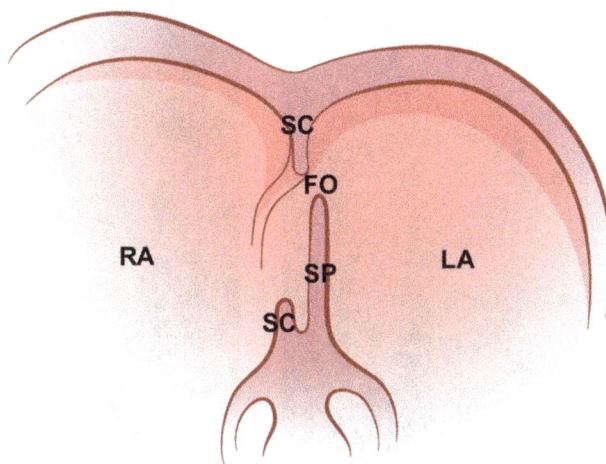

Fig. 2. The illustration shows the embryologic development of the Patent Foramen Ovale (PFO). If the septum secundum is not completely fused with the septum primum and persists as a flap against the foramen ovale, PFO, a persistent valve between RA and LA, occurs. This illustration was modified from The Developing Human: Clinically Orientated Embryology, 8th edition, the cardiovascular System, page 300, copyright Elsevier (2008) with permission

Table 1. A table demonstrated the results of statistical analysis of patients with LASP and without LASP with PFO, age and gender

	Present LASP N=68	Absent LASP N=207	p-value
PFO	4	2	0.035a
Gender Female	29	89	0.054b
Male	38	119	0.054b
Mean age (years)	53.41	56.75	0.063c
SD	14.48	12.19	0.063c

a: calculated by Fisher-Exact test , b: calculated by Pearson Chi-Square test, c: calculated by ANOVA test

We recognize that our study methods may have minimized the apparent association between PFO and LASP. The prevalence of these entities varies among studies and is dependent on the investigative approaches and patient population. Proposed CT criteria for the diagnosis of PFO have included visualization of the contrast jet from the left atrium to the right atrium, subjective recognition of LA enhancement before pulmonary vein enhancement, and software detection of early 1st peak of LA enhancement > of the maximal LA enhancement [3,5,8,9]. Williamson et al used 3 CT criteria to establish PFO: 1) presence of a distinct "flap" in the left atrium at the expected location of the septum primum (equivalent to an LASP), 2) a continuous column of contrast between septum primum and septum secundmum and 3) the presence of contrast jet into the right atrium [3]. Purvis et al reported 4.6% prevalence of PFO using the presence of a jet alone, and Kim et al found 2.1%

on his series (2,6). Kim also demonstrated that presence of a jet alone was 98% specific and 73% sensitive for PFO (9) (Fig. 2). Our definition of PFO relied on this highly specific but only moderately sensitive finding, and accordingly we recognize that some PFOs that were present could have been missed. Accordingly we consider our observed co-occurrence of LASP and PFO to be a lower limit of the association.

Although Tugca et al. [10] did not find the association of LASP or Atrial Septal Pouch (ASP) or Double Atrial Septum or Left Atrial Roof pouch with ischemic or cryptogenic strokes, other investigators have suggested that LASP is a potential site of thrombus formation. Case reports have demonstrated LSAP as a potential cause of either cryptogenic stroke, other thromboembolic events such as a coronary embolus or a false positive diagnosis of atrial myxoma [11-17].

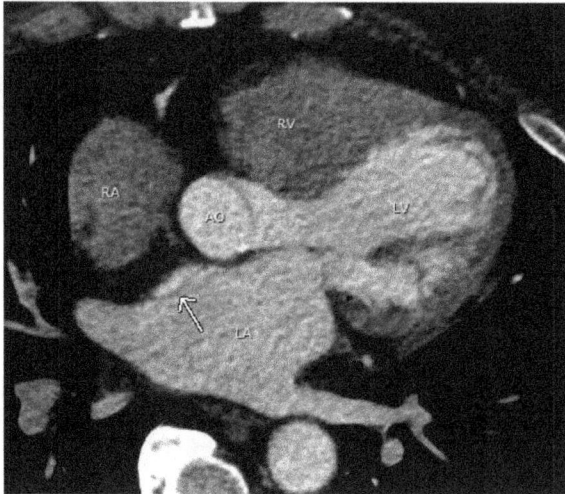

Fig. 3 A

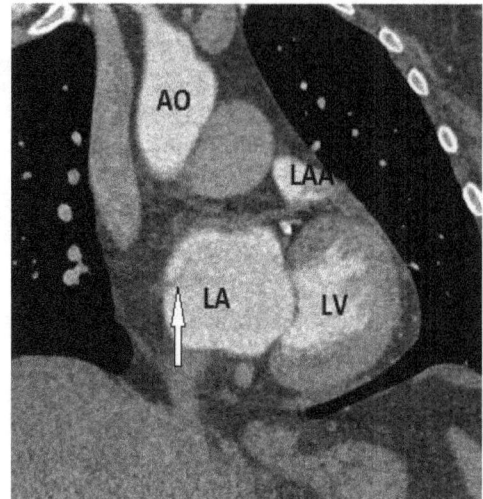

Fig. 3B

Fig. 3A-B: 59 year-old female with Atrial Fibrillation. Pre-ablation mapping for pulmonary ablation shows a slit-like structure in the right anterior left atrium on axial (arrow in Figure 3A) and coronal (arrow in Figure 3B), compatible with Left Atrial Septal Pouch (LASP). RA=Right Atrium, RV=Right Ventricle, LA=Left Atrium, LV=Left Ventricle and Ao=Aorta, LAA = Left Atrial Appendage

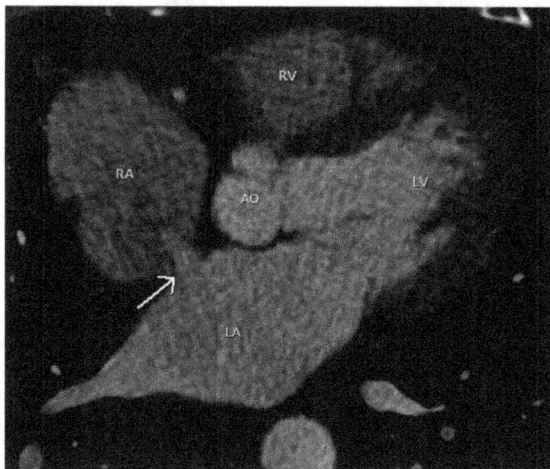

Fig. 4A

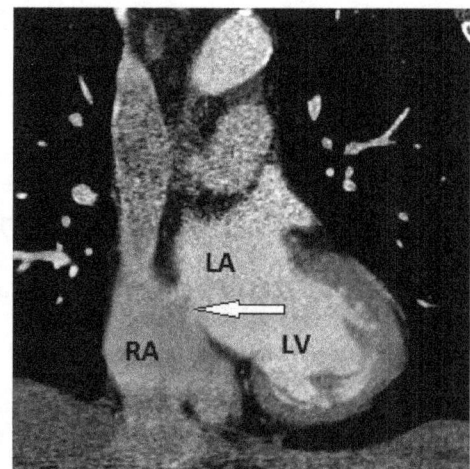

Fig. 4B

Fig. 4A-B: 68 year-old female with Atrial Fibrillation. Pre-ablation mapping shows a jet of contrast from the left atrium to the right atrium via the small defect, suggestive of Patent Foramen Ovale (PFO) (arrows in Figure 4A and 4B). RA=Right Atrium, RV=Right Ventricle, LA=Left Atrium, LV=Left Ventricle and Ao=Aorta

The proposed etiology of stroke due to PFOs is different from that hypothesized for LASP, and is usually attributed to passage of paradoxical emboli during right to left shunting. Left to right shunting may predominate, with the pathogenic right to left shunt only being present episodically [18]. Regardless of mechanism, controversy also remains regarding the correlation of PFO and cryptogenic stroke. Some studies showed a positive correlation in young population (patients < 40 years old and a separate study of patients < 55 years old) [19,20]. At least one study has shown this correlation persists in older population (older than 55 years old) [20]. Some investigators did not find this association [2], however there is consensus among investigators that presence of Atrial Septal Aneurysm (ASA) may increase the risk of stroke.

The clinical relevance of the co-occurrence of LASP and PFO remains to be determined. Answering this question would require a larger population based study in which both abnormalities are specifically evaluated by CT. In such a study additional co-variables that could independently increase the risk of embolic stroke via increasing left atrial stasis or augmenting right to left shunt would need to be included in the analysis. Assessment of left atrial size, atrial arrhythmias, evidence of elevated right heart pressures and possibly quantitation of PFO size could therefore be important.

Our study is limited by selection bias the lack of the gold standard for diagnosis such as TEE. In addition, our stringent definition of PFO resulted in a small number of positive cases of PFO, limiting the power of the study. Fortunately this limitation was not sufficient to confound our results.

5. CONCLUSION

LASPs are frequently detectable on cardiac CTA. PFOs are statistically more common among patients who demonstrate a LSAP but the prevalence remains relatively low. The potential significance of combined LASP and PFO on the incidence of embolic stroke is unknown and warrants further investigation.

COMPETING INTERESTS

Authors have declared that no competing interests exist.

REFERENCES

1. Krishnan SC, Slazar M. Septal pouch in the left atrium: a new anatomical entity with potential for embolic complications. J Am Coll Cardiol. 2010;3:98-104.

2. Purvis JA, Morgan DR, Hughes SM. Prevalence of patent foramen ovale in a consecutive cohort of 261 patients undergoing routine "coronary" 64-multi-detector cardiac computed tomography. Ulster Med J. 2011;80:72-75.

3. Williamson EE, Kirsch J, Araoz PA, Edminster WB, Borgeson DD, Glockner JF, et al. ECG-gated cardiac CT angiography using 64-MDCT for detection of patent foramen Ovale. Am J Radool. 2008;190:929-933.

4. Meissner I, Khandheria BK, Heit JA, Petty GW, Sheps SG, Schwartz GL, et al. Patent foramen ovale: innocent or guilty? Evidence from a prospective population-based study. J Am Coll Cardiol. 2006;47:440-445.

5. Saremi F, Channual S, Raney A, Gurudevan SV, Nurula J, Fowler S, et al. Imaging of patent foramen ovale with 64-section multidetector CT. Radiology. 2009;249:483-92.

6. Kim YJ, MD, Hur J, Choe KO, Choi BW, Shim C, Choi E, et al. Interatrial shunt detected in coronary computed tomography angiography: differential features of a patent foramen ovale and an atrial septal defect. J Comput Assist Tomogr. 2008;32:663-667.

7. Roberson DA, Javois AJ, Cui W, Mandronero LF, Cuneo BF, Muangmingsuk S. Double atrial septum with persistent interatrial space: echocardiographic features of a rare atrial septal malformation. J Am Soc Echocardiogr. 2006;19:1175-1181.

8. Revel MP, Faivre JB, Letourneau T, Henon H, Leys D, Delannoy-Deken V, Remy-Jardin M, Remy J. Patent foramen ovale: detection with non-gated multidetector CT. Radiology; 2008.

9. Kim YJ, Hur J, Shim CY, Ha JW, Choe KO, Heo JH, Choi EY, Choi BW. Patent fpramen ovale: diagnosis with multidetector CT-comparison with transesophageal echocardiography. Radiology; 2009.

10. Tugcu A, Okajima K, Jin Z, Rundek T, Homma S, Sacco R, et al. Septal pouch in the left atrium and risk of ischemic stroke: a case-control study. J Am Coll Cardiol. 2010;3:1276-1283.

11. Gurudevan AV, Shah H, Tolstrup K, Siegel R, Krisnan SC. Septal thrombus in the left atrium: is the left atrial septal pouch the culprit? J Am Coll Cardiol. 2010;3:1284-1286.

12. Elsokkari I, Reyneke E, William M. Left atrial septal pouch causing an ischemic stroke in association with aortic coarctation. Eur J Echocardiogr. 2011;12:916.

doi: 10.1093/ejechocard/jer224.

13. Kuwaki H, Takeuchi M, Kaku K, Haruki N, Yoshitani H, Tamura M, et al. Thrombus attached to the left atrial septal pouch assessed on 3-dimensional transeso-phageal echocardiography. Circulation. 2011;75:2280-2281.

14. Buchholz S, Robaei D, Jacobs NH, O'Rourke M, Fenel MP. Thromboembolic stroke with concurrent left atrial appendage and left atrial septal pouch thrombus. Int J Cardiol. 2012;162:e16-e17.

15. Strachinaru M, Wauthy P, Sanossi A, Morissens M, Costescu I, Catez E. The left atrial septal pouch as a possible location for thrombus formation. J Cardiovasc Med. 2013;14:000-000.

16. Shimamoto K, Kawagoe T, Dai K, Inoue I. Thrombus in the left atrial septal pouch mimicking myxoma. J Clin Ultrasound. 2014;42:185-188.

17. Breithardt OA, Papavassiliu T, Borggrefe M. A coronary embolus originating from the interatrial septum. Eur Heart J. 2006;27:2745.

18. Saremi F, Emmanuel N, Wu PF, Ohde L, Shavelle D, Go JL, Sanchez-Quintana D. Paradoxical embolism: role of imaging in diagnosis and treatment planning. Radiographics. 2014;34:1571-92.

19. Webster MWI, Smith HJ, Sharpe DN, Chancellor AM, Swift DL, Bass NM, et al. Patent foramen ovale in young stroke patients. The Lancet.1988;2:11-12.

20. Handke M, Harloff A, Olschewski M, Hetzel A, Geibel A. Patent foramen ovale and cryptogenic stroke in older patients. N Engl J Med. 2007;357 :2262-8.

13

Congestive Heart Failure among the Libyan Population (North Africa); A Community Based Survey of Risk Factors and Complication

Mohamed Kaled A. Shambesh[1*], Taher Mohamed Emahbes[1],
Zeinab Elmehdi Saleh[1], Iman Mohamed Shambesh[2]
and Malik Abdurrazag A. Elosta[3]

[1]Department of Community Medicine, Faculty of Medicine, University of Tripoli, Libya.
[2]Department of English, Faculty of Education, University of Tripoli, Libya.
[3]CELTA, American Star Books, Headquartered in Frederick, Maryland, USA.

Authors' contributions

This work was carried out in collaboration between all authors. Author IMS designed the study, wrote the protocol. Authors MKAS and ZES wrote the first draft of the manuscript. Author TME managed the literature searches and help in discussion writing. Author MKAS done the analyses of the study with help of statisticians. Authors MAAE and IMS was done the English editing. All authors read and approved the final manuscript.

Editor(s):
(1) Obinna Ikechukwu Ekwunife, Department of Clinical Pharmacy and Pharmacy Management, Nnamdi Azikiwe University Awka, Anambra State, Nigeria.
Reviewers:
(1) Dmitry Napalkov, Moscow State Medical University, Russia.
(2) Alexander Berezin, Medical University, Zaporozhye, Ukraine.

ABSTRACT

Congestive Heart failure (CHF) is a very common medical disorder and a major health problem in Libya. CHF is associated with an increase in the risk of stroke and hospitalization.
Objectives: To estimate and describe the main risk factors and complications of CHF among people with a particular interest in Libyan community.
Methodology: This project is classified as a community based descriptive cross-sectional study using the CHADS2 questionnaire as well as the local Libyan classification called the Community Stroke Risk Classification (CSRC).
Area; North Africa (North of Libya, the capital Tripoli).
Time; five years from 2010-2014

Corresponding author: E-mail: mkshambesh@yahoo.com

Population: Convenient sampling was done from a large cohort of individuals living in the Libyan community. 7497 individuals were screened for risk factors of stroke. CHF was one such factor which was studied in detail among the sample population and was diagnosed by taking detailed histories (including treatment), medical examinations and previous hospital confirmations.

Results: The prevalence of CHF among our participants (7497 individuals) was 15.2% (1139 patients) among the sample population as a total with males and females being 51.2% and 48.8% respectively (P=0.87). Among different age groups, females had higher rates than the males except for age interval from 60 to 79 where males had higher rates. The male to female ratio among the total population screened for CHF was 7.8%: 7.4% (583:556 respectively with males being higher). CHF prevalence increased with the progress of age, with higher rates among age groups of over 40 (P <0.0001).

68.3% of CHF patients had hypertension (778 patients), 54.3% had DM (618 patients), 38.7% had transient ischemic attach (TIA) (441 patients), 27.2% had atrial fibrillation (AF) (310 patients), 25.9% had prior stroke (PS) (295 patients), All of these risk factors accompanying CHF increased with age (P<0.0001).

99.92% of CHF patients had risk points of stroke in CHADS2 scores (0.08% had no risk points), from whom 27.1% had intermediate scores (1-2 Risk Points) and 72.9% had high scores (≥3 risk points) (P<0.0001).

Results of the CSRC scores showed that 99.91% had risk factors of stroke (0.09% had no risk factors), from whom 29.5% had intermediate scores (1-2 Risk Factors) and 70.5% had high scores (≥3 risk factors) (P<0.0001).

Conclusion: CHF is a major risk factor of stroke among the Libyan population in North Africa of whom had very high CHADS2 risk scores. These scores are defined as a combination of six different risk points; 0 points being low risk, 1-2 being intermediate, and a score of 3 or more risk points is defined as being high risk. CHF appeared to dominate the high scores (≥3 risk points). Almost all CHF patients had risk factors of stroke on the CSRC scoring system of whom expressed intermediate and high scores with a significant proportion of high scores (≥3 risk factors of stroke). Hypertension, DM, AF and being aged of over 40 years were very important risk factors contributing to CHF. Both genders of male and female had similar chances of developing CHF in the Libyan community. CHADS2 & CSRC classification scores are very useful and simple tools to be used to classify and describe the risk factors of stroke in populations living within a community.

Keywords: CHF; stroke; prevalence; risk factors; risk points; classification; community; CHADS2; CSRC; Africa; Libya.

ABBREVIATIONS

AF   : *Atrial Fibrillation*
HT   : *Hypertension*
DM   : *Diabetes Mellitus*
CHF   : *Congestive Heart Failure*
TIA   : *Transient Ischemic attack*
PS   : *Prior Stroke*
WHO : *World Health Organization*
CDC   : *Centers of Disease Control*
CSRC : *Community Stroke Risk Classification*
RF   : *Risk Factor*
RP   : *Risk Points*

1. INTRODUCTION

Congestive Heart failure is a common, costly, and potentially fatal condition [1]. In developed countries, around 2% of adults have heart failure and in individuals over the age of 65, this risk increases to 6–10% [1,2]. In the following year after diagnosis of CHF, the risk of death is about 35% after which it decreases to below 10% each year afterwards [2]. This is similar to the risks with a number of types of cancer [3]. In the United Kingdom, this illness is the reason for 5% of emergency hospital admissions [3].

Common causes of heart failure are usually comprised of coronary artery disease including a previous myocardial infarction (heart attack), high blood pressure, atrial fibrillation, valvular heart disease, and cardiomyopathy [1,3].

Men have a higher incidence of heart failure than women, but the overall prevalence rate is similar in both sex, since women survive longer after the onset of heart failure [4]. Women tend to be older when diagnosed with heart failure (after menopause), they are more likely than men to have diastolic dysfunction, and seem to experience a lower overall quality of life than men after diagnosis [4].

Heart failure is associated with high health expenditures, mostly because of the cost of hospitalizations; costs have been estimated to amount to 2% of the total budget of the National Health Service in the United Kingdom, and more than $35 billion in the United States [5,6].

Heart failure is the leading cause of hospitalization in people older than 65 years of age [7]. In developed countries, the mean age of patients with heart failure is 75 years old. In developing countries, two to three percent of the population have heart failure but the rate rises dramatically to 20-30% in those 70 to 80 years old [7].

More than 20 million people have heart failure worldwide [8,9]. The prevalence and incidence of heart failure is increasing, mostly because of increasing longer life spans, but also because of a higher prevalence of risk factors (hypertension, diabetes, dyslipidemia, and obesity) and improved survival rates from other types of cardiovascular disease (myocardial infarction, valvular disease, and arrhythmias) [9,10].

In the United States, heart failure affects 5.8 million people, and each year 550,000 new cases are diagnosed [8]. In 2011, congestive heart failure was the most common reason for hospitalization for adults aged 85 years and older, and the second most common for adults aged 65–84 years [11].

Heart failure is much higher in African Americans, Hispanics, Native Americans and recent immigrants from the eastern bloc countries like Russia. This high prevalence in these ethnic minority populations in the U.S. has been linked to an increasing incidence of diabetes and hypertension. In many new immigrants to the U.S., the high prevalence of heart failure has largely been attributed to lack of preventive health care or substandard treatment [12].

Nearly one out of every four patients (24.7%) hospitalized In the U.S. with congestive heart failure are readmitted within 30 days [12]. Additionally, more than 50% of patients seek re-admission within 6 months after treatment and the average duration of hospital stay is 6 days.

Congestive heart failure is the leading cause of hospital readmissions in the U.S. In a study of 18 States, Medicare patients aged 65 and older were readmitted at a rate of 24.5 per 100

admissions in 2011. In the same year, Medicaid patients were readmitted at a rate of 30.4 per 100 admissions, and uninsured patients were readmitted at a rate of 16.8 per 100 admissions. These are the highest readmission rates for both patient categories. Notably, congestive heart failure was not among the top ten conditions with the most 30-day readmissions among the privately insured [13].

In 2011, non-hypertensive congestive heart failure was one of the ten most expensive conditions seen during inpatient hospitalizations in the U.S., with aggregate inpatient hospital costs of more than $10.5 billion [14].

In tropical countries, the most common cause of HF is valvular heart disease or a type of cardiomyopathy. As underdeveloped countries have become more affluent, there has also been an increase in the incidence of diabetes, hypertension and obesity, which have in turn raised the incidence of heart failure [13].

As CHF research studies in Libya are seldom, this study was done to find the most important risk factors of CHF and to describe the role of CHF as one of the most important conditions associated with cerebovascular accidents among populations living in a community.

2. OBJECTIVES

This study was done to find the most important risk factors of CHF and to describe the role of CHF as one of the most important conditions associated with Cerebovascular accidents among a population living in a community by using both CHADS2 and the Community Stroke Risk Classification (CSRC) scoring systems.

3. METHODOLOGY

Study was a community based descriptive, cross-sectional study.

3.1 Populations

Individuals who are 16 years old or above.

3.2 Population Sample

Sampling was done from a large cohort of individuals living in a community. 7497 individuals were screened by Shambesh et al. [15] looking for risk factors of stroke.

3.2.1 Sample size calculation

Results were obtained by Epi-Info statistic package USA version-6, calculating the sample size of the descriptive cross section survey for convenient sampling; using the Tripoli population size of 2.000.000 and an expected CHF frequency of 20% [13], the calculated sample size by this system was 7.000 which was used in our sampling model (7497) (with an 80% confidence level).

3.3 Area

North Africa, Mediterranean area of Libya (Tripoli the Capital).

3.4 Time

Five years from 2010-2014.

3.5 Method of Survey

3.5.1 Using CHADS2 questionnaire

Individuals were interviewed using CHADS2 questionnaires which is usually used to assess stroke risk in patients with atrial fibrillation [16], and was adapted in this study to be used among a population without AF as it had been used in other studies elsewhere [17]. Additionally, the local Libyan classification of stroke risk factors was also used in this study (known as the Community Stroke Risk Classification-CSRC which was created to be used for the first time in Libya by Shambesh et al. [15]. CHADS2 scores are derived from the sum of point values of individual stroke risk factors {congestive heart failure (CHF), hypertension (HT), age≥ 70, diabetes (DM) (1 point each), and prior stroke or transient ischemic attack (2 points) (Table 1). The CHADS2 scoring table which, shown below, adds together the points that correspond to the condition, representing the result as a CHADS2

score which is used to estimate stroke risk as follows:

Score Zero points = No risk = Low Risk Score
Score 1 & 2 points = Intermediate Risk Score
Score ≥3 points = High Risk Score

Table 1. Showing CHADS2 score questionnaire used in the study

Condition	Points
C: Congestive heart failure	1
H: Hypertension	1
A: Age ≥70	1
D: DM	1
S: Prior Stroke or TIA	2

3.5.2 Community stroke risk classification-CSRC

This classification depends on a calculation on a number of risk factors (RF), each risk factor used in the study (age ≥ 70, DM, Hypertension, CHF, TIA and prior stroke) was given a value (number) for each condition and applied to each individual who participated. The score is a result of summation of those risk factors as shown in Table 2.

3.6 Field Survey

The sampling method was convenient, doctors working in the community and family medicine department were trained by professionals to collect data using CHADS2 questionnaires and CSRC scores by interviewing individuals about their families and relatives, by taking a detailed history (present, past, medical, hospital admission), checking of any available investigations, discharge letters and medical reports as well as doing medical examinations. Known cases of DM, hypertension, CHF, AF, TIA and prior strokes had been established by previous medical diagnoses by hospital specialists. CHF was diagnosed through histories (treatments taken), medical examinations and previous hospital confirmations.

Table 2. Showing CSRC score used in the study

Level	Score	No. of Risks
Low risk score	Score of zero	No risk factors
Intermediate risk score-1	Score of one	One risk factor
Intermediate risk score-2	Score of two	Two risk factors
High risk with a score 3. Subdivided to:		
High risk score-3	Score three	Three risk factors
High risk score-4	Score four	Four risk factors
High risk score-5	Score five	Five risk factors
High risk score-6	Score six	Six risk factors

3.7 Statistical Analysis

This step was done by statisticians who scored the CHADS2 and CSRC grades by the statistical package of social sciences (SPSS) version 19-USA. Data was calculated and described by using mean, mode, standard deviation, cross tabulations and graphical presentations. "T" student test for independent samples of numerical data were used with Chi-square analysis for categorized data.

4. RESULTS

4.1 Congestive Heart Failure (CHF) Prevalence

The prevalence of CHF among our participants (7497 individuals) in this study done by Shambesh et al. [15] was 15.2% (1139 patients). Males and females expressed a similar prevalence in individuals known to have CHF in this study (51.2% and 48.8% respectively) (P=0.87). Among different age groups, females had higher rates than males except for age interval from 60 to 79 where males had higher rate as shown in Table 3 and Fig. 1.

Males had a slightly higher rate of prevalence than females but was not considered to be significant among the total population screened (P=0.51). (7.8%:7.4%, 583:556 respectively). CHF prevalence increased with the progress of age, with higher rates among age groups of over 40 (P <0.0001) Fig. 1.

4.2 CHF and Hypertension

68.3% of CHF patients had hypertension (778 patients), of whom 48.9% were males and 51% female (P=0.87) with the rate of CHF increasing with the progress of age (P<0.0001).

4.3 CHF and Diabetes Mellitus (DM)

54.3% of CHF patients had DM (618 patients), of whom 50.6% were males and 49.4% female (P=0.87) with the rate of CHF increasing with the progress of age (P<0.0001).

Table 3. Showing CHF age/sex structure

Sex	10-19	20-29	30-39	40-49	50-59	60-69	70-79	>80
Male	2	10	24	58	86	158	159	86
Female	0	21	27	64	97	108	148	91
Total	2 (0.17%)	31 (2.7%)	51 (4.5%)	122 (10.7%)	183 (16%)	266 (23.4%)	307 (27%)	177 (15.5%)

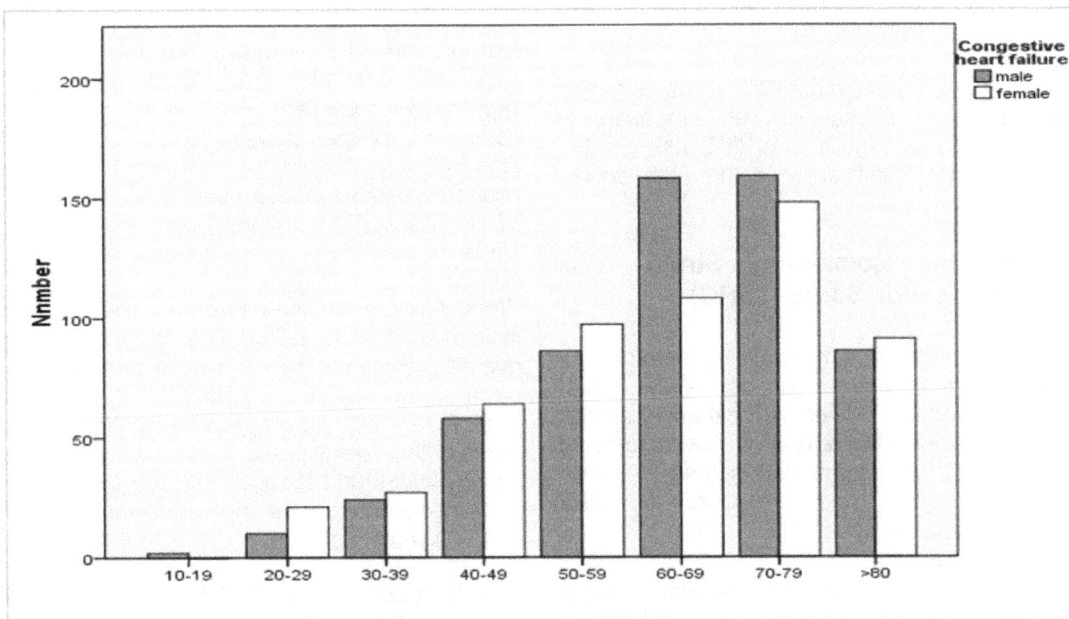

Fig. 1. Showing CHF age/sex structure

4.4 CHF and Atrial Fibrillation (AF)

27.2% of CHF patients had AF (310 patients), of whom 50.3% were males and 49.7% female (P=0.87) with the rate of CHF increasing with the progress of age (P<0.0001).

4.5 CHF and Transient Ischemic Attack (TIA)

38.7% of CHF patients had TIA (441 patients), of whom males displayed a significantly higher proportion (56.7%) than females (43.3%) (P<0.0001), with the rate of TIA increasing with the progress of age (P<0.0001).

4.6 CHF and Prior Stroke (PS) (Embolic or Hemorrhagic)

25.9% of CHF patients had PS (295 patients) of whom 50.2% were males and 49.8% female (P=0.87) with the rate of CHF increasing with the progress of age (P<0.0001).

4.7 CHF and CHADS2 Scores

The CHADS2 scores work with points; the higher the points (P) the higher the risk (R) score for stroke. CHF patients showed that 99.92% had risk points of stroke (0.08% had no risk points), of whom 27.1% had intermediate scores (1-2 Risk Points) and 72.9% had high scores (≥3 Risk Points) (Table 4 and Fig. 2).

These results found almost all CHF patients had risk factors of stroke with an emphasis in intermediate and high scores (1-6 risk points), with particular significance in the high scores (P<0.0001).

4.8 CHF and Community Stroke Risk Classification Score (CSRC)

CSRC works with a number of risk factors (RF), the higher the number of risk factors, the higher the stroke risk. 99.91% of CHF patients had risk factors of stroke (0.09% had no risk factors), of whom 29.5% had intermediate scores (1-2 Risk Factor) and 70.5% had high scores (≥3 Risk Factors) (Table 5 and Fig. 3).

These results found that almost all CHF patients had risk factors of stroke with an emphasis in intermediate and high scores (1-6 risk points), with particular significance in the high scores (P<0.0001).

Table 4. Showing CHADS2 score among CHF patients

Score	No.	%
Low	2	0.08
Intermediate-1	91	8
Intermediate-2	217	19
High-3	262	23
High-4	261	23
High-5	220	19
High-6	86	8

Table 5. Showing CSRC score among CHF patients

Score	No.	%
low risk NF	1	0.01
intermediate risk 1F	91	7.9
intermediate risk 2F	245	21.5
high risk 3F	336	29.5
high risk 4F	272	23.9
high risk 5F	149	13.1
high risk 6F	45	3.9

5. DISCUSSION

This study confirms that CHF is a very important public health problem among the Libyan population. The prevalence of CHF was found to be very high (15.2%) which agreed with very few studies done previously in Libya [18,19].

Congestive Heart failure is a common and potentially fatal condition [1]. In developed countries, around 2% of adults have heart failure and in those over the age of 65, this proportion increases to 6–10% [1,2], These numbers in developed countries are very low when compared to the prevalence of CHF in this present study could be attributed to socio-economic status differences and low public health services in developing countries like Libya.

Worldwide reports show that men have a higher incidence of heart failure than women, but the overall prevalence rate is similar in both sexes since women survive longer after the onset of heart failure [4]. Our results showed the same in terms of the overall prevalence which was similar among males and females with the exception of males dominating over the age group between 50 to 79 years old.

This study confirmed that CHF increases with the progress of age. Hence, the increase in stroke prevalence among older ages was also reported by other studies done in USA [11].

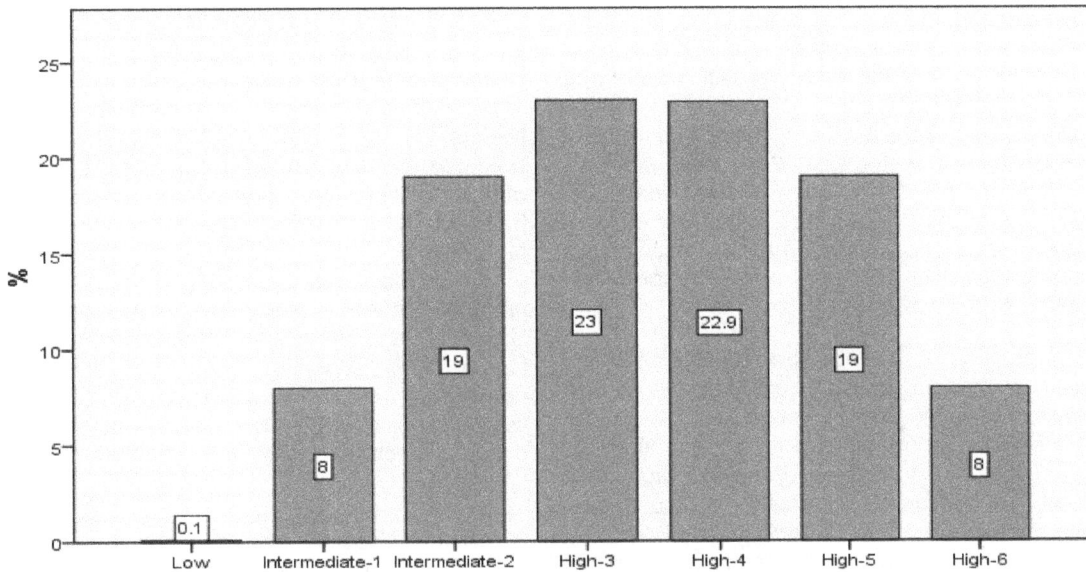

Fig. 2. Showing CHADS2 score among CHF patients

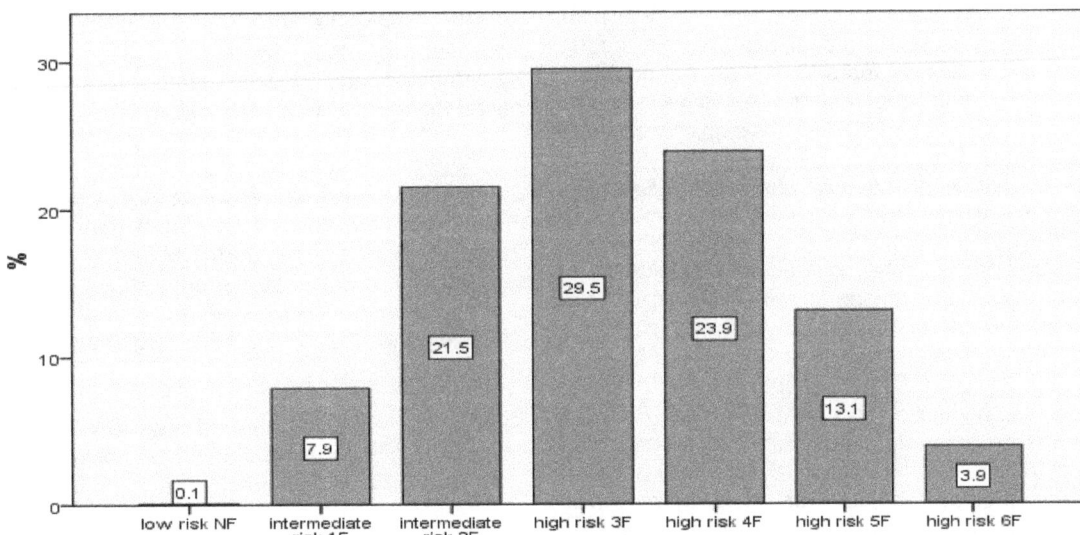

Fig. 3. Showing CSRC score among CHF patients

The prevalence and incidence of heart failure are increasing in Libya and other parts of the world, mostly because of increasing longer life spans, but also because of an increased prevalence of risk factors (hypertension, diabetes, dyslipidemia, and obesity) and improved survival rates from other types of cardiovascular disease (myocardial infarction, valvular disease, and arrhythmias) [9,10].

In developed countries, the mean age of patients with heart failure is 75 years old. In developing countries, two to three percent of the population have heart failure, but in those demographics of 70 to 80 years of age, occurrence dramatically increases to 20–30 percent [7], all these findings were confirmed to be present among the Libyan population and confirmed by results of the present study.

Risk factors of stroke in Libya are multiple and complex. Libyan population surveys done in 2001, showed obesity prevalence at 32.7%, only 18% of the study population were performing exercise and 45% were smokers of whom 99.3% were male [18]. A survey done in 2009 showed that only 12.4% of the study population as having a daily healthy diet, only 22.6% of the population having daily exercise, 63.5% were obese, 20% having high cholesterol and 25% were smokers [19]. These reports in Libya showed that such risk factors may play a role in the increase of CHF prevalence and hence accelerated cerebrovascular accidents rates among the Libyan population.

Hypertension, ischemic heart disease, diabetes mellitus, smoking and hypercholesterolemia are well-known risk factors for stroke [20]. The Oxfordshire community stroke project study in the United Kingdom showed that risk factors for cerebral infarction were present in 80% of cases, hypertension in 52%, ischemic heart disease in 38%, peripheral vascular disease in 25%; cardiac lesions resulting in a major potential source of emboli to the brain in 20% and diabetes mellitus in 10% [20]. Our study results also confirmed such reports that CHF is a major risk factor for stroke but the stroke prevalence in Libya among CHF (15.2%) was more than that of the United Kingdom, and this may be explained by the increase in rates of CHF in developing countries in Africa like Libya following the trend of urbanization and lifestyle changes, including a "Western-style" diet [21].

Several articles have reported stroke incidence in Arab and North African countries: Kuwait, Saudi Arabia, Qatar, Libya and Bahrain. The incidence varied from the lowest of 27.5 per 100,000 population per year in Kuwait to highest of 63 per 100,000 population in Libya. The most frequent stroke type is ischemic. Stroke increased with age affecting older patients, with males being more affected than females. Hypertension was the most frequent risk factor, followed by DM, hyperlipidemia, cardiac diseases and cigarettes smoking [22]. Our study results confirmed that all these stroke results were reviewed in previous Arab articles with particular relation to CHF as one of the leading factors. Also these reports imply that Arab countries constitute populations with similar lifestyles and diet that may influence CHF risk and stroke risk, type and survival after stroke [22,23].

Mortel et al. [24] reported that CHF is the third risk factor for stroke, followed by hypertension, DM and smoking, which were also shown by the results of this study and by Shambesh et al. [15], where DM & hypertension are leading risk factors followed by CHF.

CHF and stroke among patients in Libya is high and this can be explained by reports done in the United states, which showed that heart failure is much higher in African Americans, Hispanics, Native Americans and recent immigrants to the U.S. from the eastern bloc countries like Russia and Africa. The high prevalence of heart failure in these ethnic populations has been linked to a high incidence of diabetes and hypertension which were also confirmed by the results of this study. In regards to many new immigrants to the U.S., the high prevalence of heart failure has largely been attributed to lack of preventive health care or substandard treatment [12] which could be a major cause of CHF and stroke prevalence presented by this study among the Libyan population.

As Libya is located near the tropical countries where the most common cause of CHF is valvular heart disease or some type of cardiomyopathy and is classified as an underdeveloped country, it has become more affluent, therefore has also witnessed an increase in the incidence of diabetes, hypertension and obesity, which has in turn raised the incidence of heart failure [13].

This study confirmed that Hypertension, DM, AF and being of over 40 years of age were very important risk factors of CHF and that CHF is third to hypertension and DM as the most frequent risk factor of stroke among Libyans and this was also found to be true in other studies in Arab countries [22], in the Middle East and North Africa [23].

Finally, this study confirmed that CHF widely affects the Libyan population which constitutes a very important public health problem.

6. CONCLUSION

This study concluded that CHF is indeed a major public health problem in Libya. CHF is a major risk factor associated with stroke. Moreover, stroke risk factors such as Hypertension, DM and previous history of stroke or transient ischemic attack are higher among CHF patients. Hypertension, DM, AF and being of over 40 years of age were very important risk factors of CHF. CHF prevalence was similar among males and females but increased significantly with the progress of age.

Additionally, both CHADS2 & CSRC classification scores are very useful, easy to use and simple tools which are used to estimate, describe and classify the risk factors of stroke in a population living in a community based on studies of having CHF or not.

7. STRENGTHS & LIMITATIONS OF THE STUDY

It is the first Libyan community based study to use CHADS2 & CSRC questionnaires to assess stroke risk factors among those who have hypertension. The limitations of this type of study as being a cross-sectional descriptive one explore associations, not causation. But as it uses a large sample size, the results produced thus should reflect the real situation in the Libyan community. Also because data was used on a huge scale and took a long time to be collected (more than five years), the study was affected by the loss of follow up from physicians working in the field of research and also by the loss of interest of residents in some areas.

8. RECOMMENDATIONS

To do other studies in order to measure CHF risk factors by using laboratory investigations and other medical diagnostic procedures. In conclusion, to estimate the most accurate and true rates especially in other parts of Libya like the North-East and South.

CONSENT

All authors declare that 'written informed consent was obtained from the patient (or other approved parties) for publication of this paper and accompanying images.

ETHICAL APPROVAL

All authors hereby declare that all research steps have been examined and approved by the appropriate ethics committee and have therefore been performed in accordance with the ethical standards laid down in the 1964 Declaration of Helsinki.

COMPETING INTERESTS

Authors have declared that no competing interests exist.

REFERENCES

1. McMurray JJ, Pfeffer MA. Heart failure. Lancet. 2005;365(9474):1877–89.

2. Dickstein K, Cohen-Solal A, Filippatos G, et al. ESC Guidelines for the diagnosis and treatment of acute and chronic heart failure 2008: the task force for the diagnosis and treatment of acute and chronic heart failure 2008 of the European Society of Cardiology. Developed in collaboration with the Heart Failure Association of the ESC (HFA) and endorsed by the European Society of Intensive Care Medicine (ESICM). Eur. Heart J. 2008;29(19): 2388–442.

3. Chronic Heart Failure: National Clinical Guideline for Diagnosis and Management in Primary and Secondary Care: Partial Update. National Clinical Guideline Centre: 2010;19–24. PMID 22741186.

4. Strömberg A, Mårtensson J. Gender differences in patients with heart failure. Eur. J. Cardiovasc. Nurs. 2003;2(1):7–18.

5. Stewart S, Jenkins A, Buchan S, McGuire A, Capewell S, McMurray JJ. The current cost of heart failure to the National Health Service in the UK. Eur. J. Heart Fail. 2002; 4(3):361–71.

6. Rosamond W, Flegal K, Furie K, et al. Heart disease and stroke statistics-2008 update: A report from the American Heart Association Statistics Committee and Stroke Statistics Subcommittee. Circulation 117. 2008;4:e25–146.

7. Krumholz HM, Chen YT, Wang Y, Vaccarino V, Radford MJ, Horwitz RI. Predictors of readmission among elderly survivors of admission with heart failure. Am. Heart J. 2000;139(1 Pt 1):72–7.

8. Bui AL, Horwich TB, Fonarow GC. Epidemiology and risk profile of heart failure. Nature Reviews Cardiology. 2011; 8(1):30–41.

9. Mann DL, Chakinala M. Harrison's principles of internal medicine: Chapter 234. Heart Failure and Cor Pulmonale. (18th ed.). New York: McGraw-Hill; 2012. ISBN 978-0071748896.

10. Goldman Lee. Goldman's Cecil Medicine: Heart Failure (Ch 58, 59) (24th ed.). Philadelphia: Elsevier Saunders. 2011; 295–317. ISBN 1437727883.

11. Pfuntner A, Wier LM, Stocks C. Most Frequent Conditions in U.S. Hospitals. HCUP Statistical Brief #162. September 2013. Agency for Healthcare Research and Quality, Rockville, MD; 2011.

12. Elixhauser A, Steiner C. Readmissions to U.S. Hospitals by Diagnosis, 2010. HCUP Statistical Brief #153. Agency for Healthcare Research and Quality; 2013.

13. Hines AL, Barrett ML, Jiang HJ, and Steiner CA. Conditions With the Largest Number of Adult Hospital Readmissions by Payer, 2011. HCUP Statistical Brief #172. Rockville, MD: Agency for Healthcare Research and Quality; 2014.

14. Torio CM, Andrews RM, Rockville MD. National Inpatient Hospital Costs: The Most Expensive Conditions by Payer, 2011. HCUP Statistical Brief #160. Agency for Healthcare Research and Quality; 2013.

15. Shambesh M, Emahbes T, Saleh Z, Franks E, Bosnena O. Community based study of cerebrovascular risk factors in Tripoli-Libya (North Africa). Journal of Scientific Research and Reports. 2015; 6(6):451–60.

16. Skanes A, Healey J, Cairns J, Dorian P, Gillis A, McMurtry M, et al. Focused 2012 update of the Canadian Cardiovascular Society atrial fibrillation guidelines: recommendations for stroke prevention and rate/rhythm control. Can J Cardiol. 2012;28:125–36.

17. Morillas P, Pallarés V, Fácila L, Llisterri JL, et al. The CHADS2 score to predict stroke risk in the absence of atrial fibrillation in hypertensive patients aged 65 years or older. Rev Esp Cardiol (Engl Ed). 2014; 1-7.

18. Bony AM, Sasi AA, Bacuch MM, Elmshergy A. Risk factors of hypertension in Libya. National Research Institute. 2001;1-32

19. Tamer HE, Al-Shref EA, Imsalem OR, et al. Survey of risk factors of non-communicable diseases in Libya. Ministry of Health Report. 2009;1-48

20. Sandercock PA, Warlow CP, Jones LN, et al. Predisposing factors for cerebral infarction: the Oxfordshire community stroke project. BMJ. 1989;298:75-80.

21. Wild S, Roglic G, Green A, Sicree R, King H. Global prevalence of diabetes: Estimates for the year 2000 and projections for 2030. Diabetes Care. 2004; 27(5):1047–53.

22. Benamer HT, Grosset D. Stroke in Arab countries: A systematic literature review. J Neurol Sci. 2009;(jns-10981):1-6.

23. Tran J, Mirzaei M, Anderson L, et al. The epidemiology of stroke in the Middle East and North Africa. J Neurol Sci. 2010;(jns-11401):1-3.

24. Mortel KF, Meyer JS, Sim PA, et al. Diabetes mellitus as a risk factor for stroke. South Med J. 1990;83:904-11.

14

Hammock Bridge on Fire: Complete AV Block in a Patient with Congenitally-corrected Transposition of the Great Arteries and Wolff-Parkinson-White Pre-excitation Pattern

Jorge A. Brenes-Salazar[1*] and Paul A. Friedman[1]

[1]Department of Medicine, Division of Cardiovascular Diseases, 200 First St SW, Rochester, MN 55901, Mayo Clinic Rochester, USA.

Authors' contributions

Both authors designed, analyzed and interpreted and prepared the manuscript.

Editor(s):
(1) Francesco Pelliccia, Department of Heart and Great Vessels University La Sapienza, Rome, Italy.
Reviewers:
(1) Anonymous, Centre Cardiologique du Nord, St. Denis, France.
(2) Alexander Berezin, Internal Medicine Department, Medical University, Zaporozhye, Ukraine.
(3) Massimo Slavich, Division of Cardiology, San Raffaele University Hospital, Via Olgettina 58, 20100 Milan, Italy.

ABSTRACT

Aims: To recognize heart block as a complication associated with congenitally-corrected transposition of the great arteries (CCTGA).
Presentation of the Case: A healthy 36 year old male with CCTGA presented with syncope as a manifestation of heart block. A unique feature of this case was the presence of an accessory pathway that served as the atrio-ventricular conducting structure for more than 3 decades.
Discussion: rationale for a cardiac resynchronization device (CRT) as opposed to a simple pacemaker system is emphasized in this case.
Conclusion: clinicians must be aware of heart block a frequent complication of CCGTA. CRT appears as a more favorable option than a single systemic ventricular pacemaker in such patients.

Keywords: Congenitally-corrected transposition; complete heart block; wolff-parkinson-white; cardiac resynchronization therapy.

*Corresponding author: E-mail: brenessalazar.jorge@mayo.edu

1. INTRODUCTION

Congenital heart disease is the most common group of birth defects. Advances in detection, medical and surgical treatment have allowed infants and children with inborn cardiac structural defects to reach adulthood. As a consequence, physicians face the challenge of taking care of a growing number of survivors, and thus, must be familiar with the long-term complications of congenital heart disease, whether related or not to prior surgical interventions. We discuss the unusual case of a patient with congenitally-corrected transposition of the great arteries associated with an electrical accessory pathway, presenting with a relatively common complication of this congenital abnormality: complete heart block.

2. CASE PRESENTATION

A 36-year old active male with a history of congenitally-corrected transposition of the great arteries (CCTGA), situs solitus type (normal position of thoraco-abdominal structures) presented with complaints of weakness, fatigue and an episode of syncope. He was known to have a Wolff-Parkinson-White (WPW) pattern without evidence of spontaneous supra ventricular dysrhythmias (Fig. 1).

At an outside institution, he had undergone an EP study a decade prior which revealed no

antegrade conduction through the AV node, as impulses travelled through a left postero-septal accessory pathway. Additionally, he had a long-standing non-ischemic cardiomyopathy on maximum medical therapy, with an estimated EF of 25% for his systemic ventricle. Initial assessment revealed an athletic gentleman in no acute distress, with a blood pressure of 90/60 mmHg and a pulse of 40 beats per minute. Cardiovascular examination was significant for prominent, intermittent venous pulsations of the neck, variable S1 and a 2/6 systolic ejection murmur best heard at the left lower sternal border. A 12-lead ECG at the office is shown in Fig. 2.

3. INTERPRETATION OF ECG FINDINGS

His baseline ECG (Fig. 1) indicates sinus brady-cardia at a rate of 55 bpm, a wide QRS complex with slurred-onset (delta wave) and a short PR interval consistent with a pre-excitation pattern of WPW. In contrast, his ECG on presentation (Fig. 2) shows atrio-ventricular dissociation, with an atrial rate of 68 bpm and a junctional escape rhythm at lower rate of 39 bpm, consistent with complete heart block. Occasional premature atrial complexes (third and last QRS complexes) are conducted through the failing accessory pathway. The junctional escape complexes utilize the His-Purkinje system and not the bypass tract, resulting in narrow complexes that lack the delta wave.

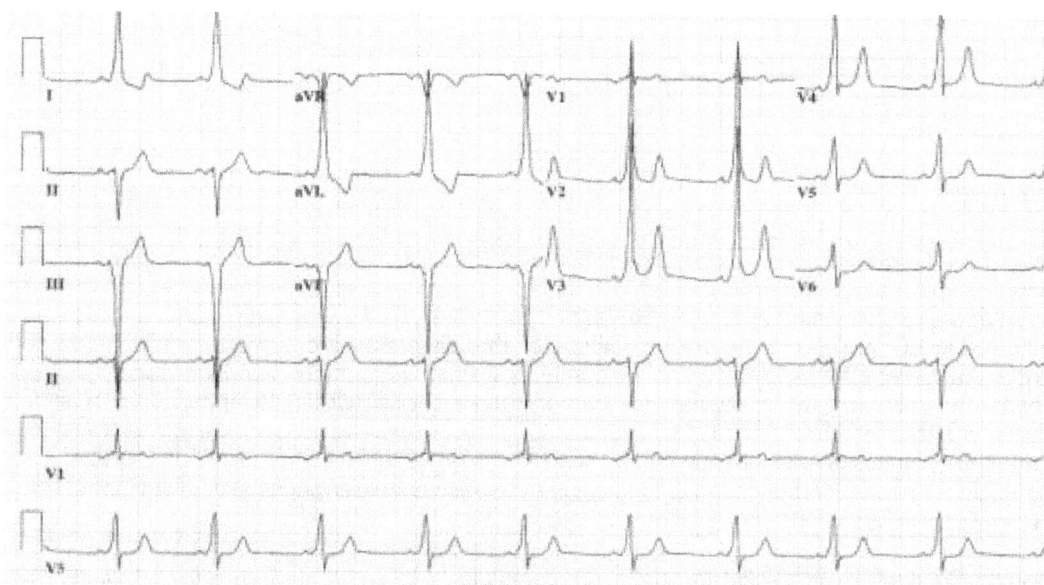

Fig. 1. Baseline electrocardiogram with normal sinus rhythm prior to presentation

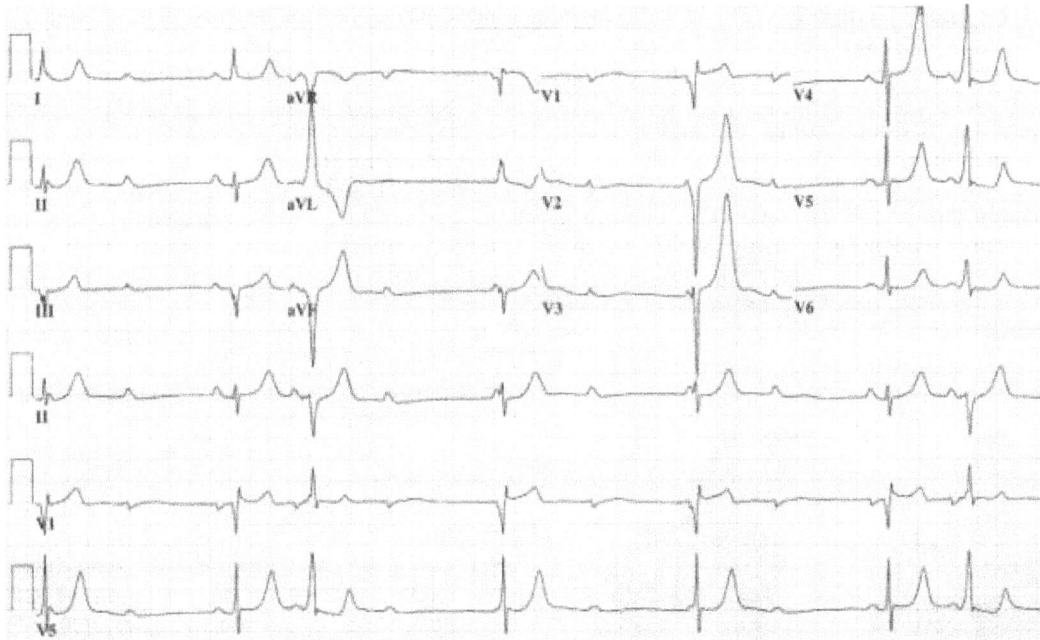

Fig. 2. Electrocardiogram on presentation, displaying complete AV dissociation, consistent with complete heart block

4. CLINICAL COURSE

Dual chamber pacemaker was clearly indicated, but decision making regarding other components of his device was more challenging. Given his depressed systemic ventricular function on adequate medical therapy, as well as impending high frequency of ventricular pacing, a cardiac resynchronization (CRT) system was highly recommended to the patient. A typical CRT system includes a left ventricular lead that is placed into a coronary sinus branch vein to pace the LV epicardially in addition to the standard right a trial and right ventricular leads. While use of CRT systems in CCTGA has been described, the diminutive venous system of the morphologic right ventricle can make LV systemic lead placement difficult [1]. Prophylactic defibrillator implantation was also offered to the patient, but he declined. He underwent placement of a standard CRT-P, with RA, RV and LV leads with no peri-procedural complications. During the procedure, there was evidence of intermittent retrograde conduction through the accessory pathway, but no pacemaker-induced tachycardia could be elicited, thus, ablation of the accessory pathway was deferred. Repeat echocardiogram at 3 months indicated an improvement in ejection fraction to 35%, and at 9-months of follow up, he remained asymptomatic, with normal device function and no dysrhythmias noted.

5. DISCUSSION

In the 1950's, only 1 out of 5 children with congenital heart disease (CHD) was expected to survive through infancy; medical advances have been able to reverse those statistics, and nowadays only 1 out of those 5 children will not reach adulthood [2]. Familiarity of health-care providers with long-term cardiovascular complications of individuals with CHD becomes crucial in this context.

CCTGA is relatively rare, and represents less than 1% of all cases of congenital heart disease [3]. In the setting of situs solitus (normal position of thoraco-abdominal organs), the left ventricle lies to the right and the right ventricle to the left. The mitral valve then lies to the right and the tricuspid valve to the left. The left ventricle is usually slightly posterior or inferior to the right ventricle. In addition to the atrio-ventricular and ventriculo-arterial discordance (Fig. 3), patients may have other associated anomalies such as a ventricular septal defect, pulmonary stenosis or abnormalities of the systemic (tricuspid) valve, including the presence of a supravalvular left a trial ring. Furthermore, the position of the AV node and His bundle in these patients is abnormal, with a more anterior orientation that makes it prone to fibrosis and degeneration [2].

It is estimated that at least 13% of individuals with CCTGA will have developed complete AV block at the time of diagnosis [4], and roughly 30% on long-term follow-up [5], at a rate of 2% per year [3]. Although complete heart block is thus a well-recognized long-term complication in patients with CCTGA, to the best of our knowledge this is the first case description of a concomitant accessory pathway, which served as the atrio-ventricular conducting structure for almost 4 decades, given the presence of a non-functional native AV node, but eventually this tenuous system collapsed.

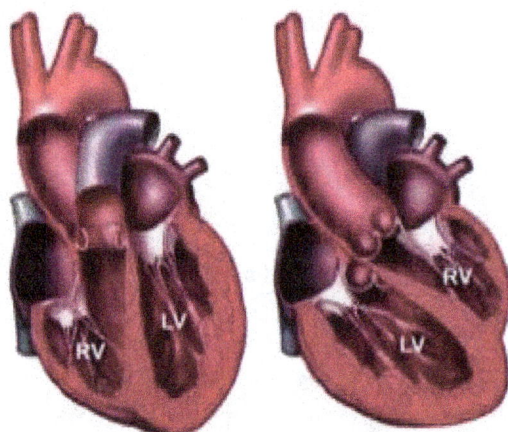

Fig. 3. Comparison of normal cardiac anatomy (left) to congenitally-corrected transposition of the great arteries (right). RV= right ventricle, LV= left ventricle

The clinical manifestations of complete heart block can be quite variable. In a classic clinical series of 251 patients [6], Samuel Levine and colleagues described that palpitations or self-perceived bradycardia were common complaints, as well as weakness, extreme fatigue and dizziness. Syncope was recognized as the gravest presentation in terms of morbidity and mortality. These authors described that the most useful physical finding, almost pathognomonic, is the changing intensity of the first heart sound in the setting of marked, regular bradycardia.

The noxious effects of isolated right ventricular pacing have been well established in structurally normal hearts with complete AV block: dyssynchronous contraction, increased oxygen consumption and adverse remodeling amongst others [7]. Patients with CHD and a systemic right ventricle have a limited ability to cope with dyssynchrony, due to inherent structural

abnormalities, lack of torsion and presence of fibrotic areas [8]. Therefore, a high burden of non-systemic ventricular pacing can have catastrophic consequences in these patients, including development of congestive heart failure [3]. Long-term pacing of the non-systemic ventricle in patients with atrial switch for TGA has been associated with significantly impaired functional status, exercise capacity and overall systemic ventricular performance [9].

Thus, we strongly recommended implantation of a cardiac resynchronization therapy (CRT) device instead of a standard pacemaker. From a pathophysiologic standpoint, this approach appears prudent, as ventricular dyssynchrony appears to be a major mechanism for systemic ventricular failure in patients with CHD; it is estimated that more than 25% of patients with CHD will eventually progress to symptomatic heart failure [10]. Based on the landmark CRT trials, about 10% of patients with a systemic RV would qualify for such a device according to commonly accepted criteria [11]. In a limited retrospective series of 7 patients with TGA, dyssynchrony and systemic ventricular dysfunction, CRT improved both NYHA functional class and peak oxygen consumption [12].

Our patient declined implantation of an ICD lead as part of the CRT system. Indeed, our ability to predict sudden cardiac death in patients with TGA is limited [13], and the evidence to support implantation of an ICD in patients with CHD is rather scarce. In a single-center experience from the Mayo Clinic [14], which included 73 patients with complex CHD, more than one-quarter of the devices were placed in patients with TGA; for all patients, the rate of appropriate shocks was 19%. However, ICD implantation in patients with CHD can be associated with considerable morbidity, including high rates of inappropriate shocks (30%) and procedure-related complications [15].

6. CONCLUSIONS

Physicians should be aware of the long-term complications of CHD in adult survivors. A significant proportion of patients with CCTGA will develop complete heart block at some stage in their lives. Syncope (Stokes-Adams syndrome) is one of the various manifestations of complete heart block, but weakness, fatigue and palpitations are also described by patients. Isolated pacing of the non-systemic ventricle is associated with adverse long-term consequences; CRT appears to be a more attractive option than mono-ventricular non-systemic pacing in patients with CCTGA and heart block, particularly those with ventricular dysfunction at baseline. There is conflicting and limited data at the present time about the risks and benefits of ICDs in patients with CHD.

CONSENT

It is not applicable.

ETHICAL APPROVAL

It is not applicable.

ACKNOWLEDGMENTS

The authors wish to thank Dr. Jeff Goldberger and the organizing committee of the 12th International Dead Sea Symposium (Tel Aviv, Israel, March 2014) for allowing a brief discussion of this clinical case.

COMPETING INTERESTS

Authors have declared that no competing interests exist.

REFERENCES

1. Bottega NA, Kapa S, Edwards WD, Conolly HM, Munger TM, Warnes CA, et al. The cardiac veins in congenitally-corrected transposition of the great arteries: delivery options for cardiac devices. Heart Rhythm. 2009;6(10):1450-1456.

2. Reid GJ, Webb GD, Barzel M, McCrindle BW, Irvine MJ, Siu SC. Estimates and life expectancy by adolescents and young adults with congenital heart disease. J Am Coll Cardiol. 2006;48(2):349-355.

3. Warnes CA. Transposition of the great arteries. Circulation. 2006;114:2699-2709.

4. Kafali G, Elsharshari H, Ozer S, Celiker A, Ozme S, Demircin M. Incidence of dysrhythmias in congenitally corrected transposition of the great arteries. Turk J Pediatr. 2002;44(3):219-223.

5. Daliento L, Corrado D, Buja G, John N, Nava A, Thiene G. Rhythm and conduction disturbances in isolated, congenitally corrected transposition of the great arteries. Am J Cardiol. 1986;58(3):314-318.

6. Penton GB, Miller H, Levine SA. Some clinical features of complete heart block. Circulation. 1956;13(6):801-824.

7. Tse HF, Lau CP. Long-term effect of right ventricular pacing on myocardial perfusion and function. J Am Coll Cardiol. 1997;29(4):744-749.

8. Giardini A, Lovato L, Donti A, Formigari R, Oppido G, Gargiulo G, Picchio FM, Fattori R. Relation between right ventricular structural alterations and markers of adverse clinical outcome in adults with systemic right ventricle and either congenitally complete or congenitally corrected transposition of the great arteries. Am J Cardiol. 2006;98:1277-1282.

9. Horovitz A, De Guillebon M, Van Geldorp IE, Bordachar P, Roubertie F, Iriart X, et al. Effects of Nonsystemic ventricular pacing in patients with transposition of the great arteries and atrial redirection. J Cardiovasc-Electrophys. 2012;23(7):766-770.

10. Piran S, Veldtman G, Siu S, Webb GD, Liu P. Heart failure and ventricular dysfunction in patients with single or systemic ventricles. Circulation. 2002;105:1189-1194.

11. Diller GP, Okonko D, Uebing A, Ho SY, Gatzoulis MA. Cardiac resynchronization for adult congenital heart disease patients with a systemic right ventricle: analysis of feasibility and review of early experience. Europace. 2006;8:267-272.

12. Jauvert G, Rousseau-Paziaud J, Villain E, Iserin L, Hidden-Lucet F, Ladouceur M, Sidi D. Effects of cardiac resynchronization therapy on echocardiographic indices, functional capacity and clinical outcomes of patients with a systemic right ventricle. Europace. 2009;11:184-190.

13. Wheeler M, Grigg L, Zentner D. Can we predict sudden cardiac death in long-term survivors of atrial switch surgery for transposition of the great arteries? Congenit Heart Dis. 2013;9(4):326-332.

14. Khanna AD, Warnes CA, Phillips SD, Lin G, Brady P. Single-center experience with implantable cardioverter-defibrillators in adults with complex congenital heart disease. Am J Cardiol. 2011;108:729-734.

15. Koyak Z, De Groot JR, Van Gelder IC, Bouma BJ, Van Dessel P, Budts W, et al. Implantable cardioverter defibrillator therapy in adults with congenital heart disease: Who is at risk of shocks? Circ Arrhythm Electrophysiol. 2012;5:101-110.

15

Cardiac Computed Tomographic Angiography: Clinical Applications

Haliah Z. Al Shehri[1], Yahya S. Al Hebaishi[2] and Abdulrahman M. Al Moghairi[2*]

[1]Adult Cardiology Department, Prince Salman Heart Center, King Fahad Medical City, Riyadh, Saudi Arabia.
[2]Adult Cardiology Department, Prince Sultan Cardiac Centre (PSCC), Prince Sultan Military Medical City, Riyadh, Saudi Arabia.

Authors' contributions

This work was carried out in collaboration between all both authors. The authors proposed the article format, reviewed the literature and wrote the first draft of the manuscript. The team joined again to make the second review and link the information together and select the appropriate figures and tables in the related sections. All both authors read and approved the final manuscript.

<u>Editor(s):</u>
(1) Anonymous.
<u>Reviewers:</u>
(1) Alexander E Berezin, Internal medicine Department, State Medical University, Zaporozhye, Ukraine.
(2) Anonymous, Fanfani Clinical Research Institute, Italy.
(3) Mojtaba Jafari Tadi, Department of clinical physiology and nuclear medicine, University of Turku, Finland.

ABSTRACT

Cardiovascular disease is the leading cause of morbidity and mortality worldwide. Cardiac imaging plays an important role in diagnosis and risk stratification of various cardiac diseases. Cardiac computed tomography added a major diagnostic value and led to reducing the need for invasive cardiac measures in many cardiac conditions. Cardiac computed tomography has emerged as an accurate anatomic method for detection of coronary artery disease. The negative predictive value to exclude significant coronary artery stenosis approaches 100%. Advances in multidetector computed tomography technology improved coronary arteries imaging during a single breath hold in a wide range of coronary pathologies. Appropriate patient preparation, image acquisition, and post processing techniques to detect coronary artery stenosis and plaque are prerequisites to achieving diagnostic image quality. Cardiac computed tomography applications also include assessment of cardiac structure and function, post myocardial infarction complications, electro anatomical mapping, and delineation of the pericardium.

Corresponding author: E-mail: aalmoghairi@pscc.med.sa, Almoghairi@gmail.com

Keywords: Coronary CT angiography; coronary MDCT; coronary artery stenosis; coronary heart disease.

1. INTRODUCTION

Cardiac computed tomography (CCT) has been increasingly used in the diagnosis of coronary artery disease (CAD) due to significant technological developments that led to improved spatial and temporal resolution [1]. High diagnostic accuracy has been achieved with multidetector computed tomography (MDCT) scanners (64 slice and higher). Furthermore, coronary CT angiography (CCTA) is considered as a reliable alternative to invasive coronary angiography [2-21]. Image quality must be ensured through multiple steps, including patient preparation, the actual protocol, and the synchronization of raw image data with electrocardiography (ECG) (Table 1). Additionally, some attention must be given to the potential risks associated with the ionizing radiation received during CT examinations. Various methods for reducing radiation dose have been implemented [22-25].

Table 1. Recommendations for patients undergoing computed tomography coronary angiography

• In sinus rhythm
• Heart rate <65 beats per minute
• Able to take B-blockers or alternative medication
• Able to hold breath for 10 seconds.
• Normal renal function
• No history of contrast allergy
• Able to hold arms above head during scan
• Sublingual nitroglycerin for coronary vasodilatation

2. CORONARY CT ANGIOGRAPHY

In the current American College of Cardiology Foundation appropriateness criteria guidelines for cardiac CT and (magnetic resonance) MR, CCTA is deemed to be appropriate in the evaluation of intermediate risk patients presented with chest pain whose ECG cannot be interpreted or who are unable to exercise. Although noncontract-enhanced CT can detect calcific coronary atherosclerosis in its early stages, it cannot accurately predict coronary stenosis. On the other hand, contrast-enhanced CTA can detect subclinical atherosclerosis and coronary stenosis and this has proven to be of diagnostic and prognostic value, incremental to traditional risk stratification methods.

2.1 Diagnostic Value of Coronary CT Angiography in Coronary Artery Disease

Coronary artery calcification (CAC) detected by non-contrast enhanced CT is pathognomonic for atherosclerosis [26-28] (Fig. 1). The original calcium score developed by Agatston et al. [29]. Standardized categories for the calcium score have been developed with scores of 1–10 considered minimal, 11–100 mild, 101–400 moderate, and >400 severe. While the presence of CAC is nearly 100% specific for atherosclerosis, it is not specific for obstructive disease since both obstructive and nonobstructive lesions have calcification [30-32] (Fig. 2). However the likelihood of significant coronary stenosis increases with the total CAC score [33,34]. CAC alone is not justified in the symptomatic population since noncalcified plaques and even obstructive disease may present in many young adults [35]. CCTA should perform in symptomatic patients even with 0 CAC (Fig. 3).

Clinical applications of CCTA depend mainly on its accuracy for detection of significant coronary artery stenosis. Numerous studies have evaluated the accuracy of CCTA for stenosis detection in comparison to invasive coronary angiography [2-21] (Fig. 3). The sensitivity for the detection of coronary artery stenosis has ranged from 86 to 100% and specificity has been reported between 91 and 98%. Several trials have demonstrated that high heart rates and extensive coronary calcification negatively influence accuracy [19-21,36-38]. Meijboom et al. correlate the diagnostic accuracy of CCTA to the clinical presentation and pretest likelihood of coronary artery disease [39]. It was demonstrated that the diagnostic value of CCTA was highest in patients with a relatively low pretest likelihood of disease and lowest in patients with a high likelihood of disease based on the clinical presentation.

The "ACCURACY" trial studied 230 patients with suspected CAD [37]. Prevalence of disease was 25%, and per patient sensitivity and specificity for detecting individuals with at least one stenosis ≥ 50% were 95 and 83%. In addition to that the negative predictive value was 99%.

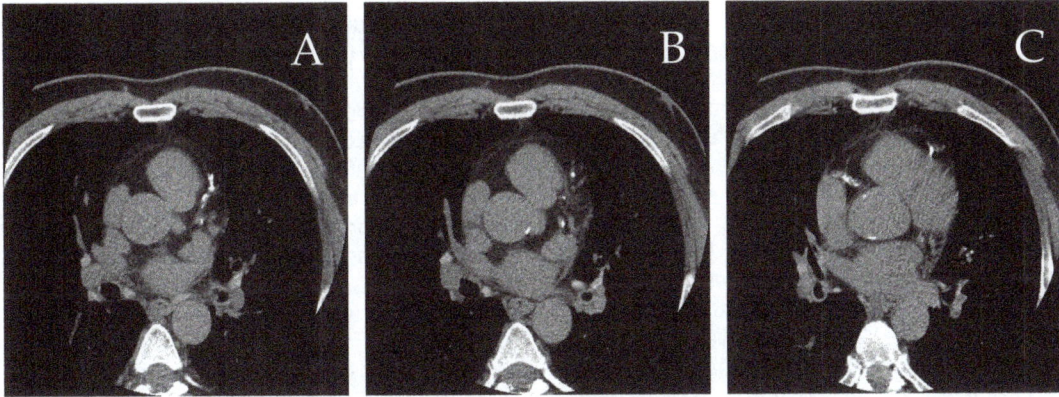

Fig. 1. A non contract-enhanced cardiac CT revealed significant calcifications in all coronary arteries and the ascending aorta

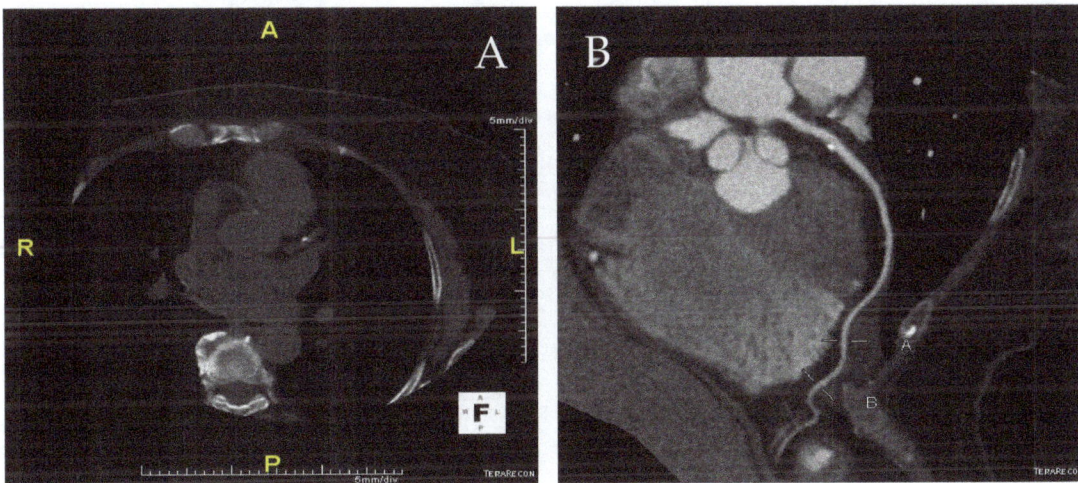

Fig. 2. Coronary CT angiography of the left descending coronary artery showing non-obstructive calcified plaque

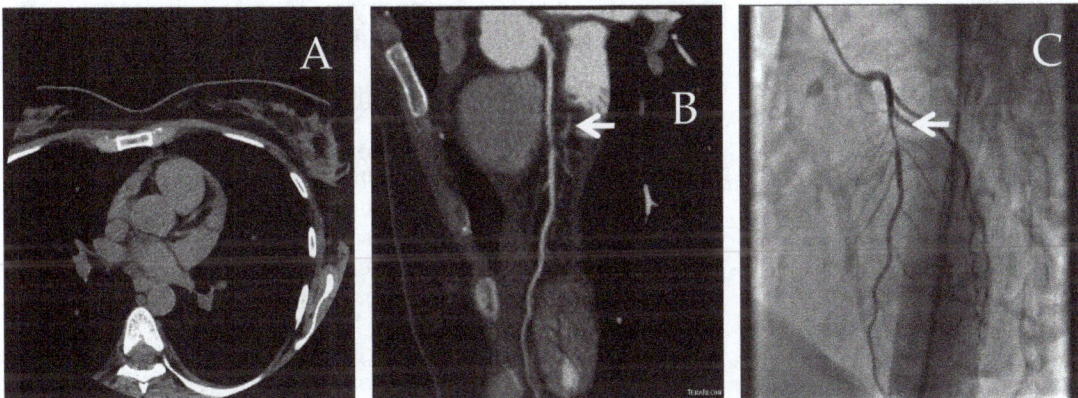

Fig. 3. A 45-year-old woman with hypertension presents with chest pain. (A) No coronary artery calcification was seen on the non contrast CT. (B) A severe left descending coronary artery stenosis was seen with CT coronary angiography (arrow). (C) Stenosis confirmed with invasive coronary angiography (arrow)

Several observational trials have demonstrated that symptomatic patients, when high quality CCTA scan was negative, had a very favorable clinical outcome even without further additional testing [40-42]. Another clinical situation in which noninvasive imaging is indicated to rule out coronary stenosis is the setting of acute chest pain particularly if the ECG and cardiac biomarkers were non diagnostic [43]. CTA has been shown to be accurate and safe to stratify patients with acute chest pain and absence of ECG changes as well as cardiac biomarkers elevation [44-48]. In addition to that Triple-rule-out (TRO) CTA can provide a cost-effective evaluation of the coronary arteries, aorta, pulmonary arteries, and adjacent extra cardiac structures for the patient with acute chest pain. It is most appropriate for the patient who is judged to be at low to intermediate risk for acute coronary syndrome (ACS) and whose symptoms may also be attributed to acute pathologic conditions of the aorta or pulmonary arteries. CCTA has emerged as the standard of reference for identification and characterization of coronary artery anomalies [49] (Table 2). CCTA offers superior definition of the ostial origin and proximal path of the anomalous coronary artery compared with conventional angiography [50-56] (Fig. 4).

Table 2. Classification of coronary artery anomalies

Anomalies of origin
High takeoff
Multiple ostia
Single coronary artery
Anomalous origin of coronary artery from pulmonary
artery (ALCAPA) Origin of coronary artery or branch
from oppositeor noncoronary sinus and an anomalous
(retroaortic, interarterial, prepulmonic, septal) course

Anomalies of course
Myocardial bridging
Duplication of arteries

Anomalies of termination
Coronary artery fistula
Coronary arcade
Extracardiac termination

Greenberg MA, Fish BG, Spindola-Franco H: Congenital anomalies of the coronary arteries. Classification and significance.Radiologic clinics of North America 1989, 27(6): 1127-1146.

2.2 Prognostic Value of CCTA in Coronary Artery Disease

CAC is superior to conventional risk factors in predicting outcomes [57,58]. Use of noncontract CT for calcium scoring was rated as appropriate within intermediate- and selected low-risk patients according to American College of Cardiology Foundation appropriateness criteria guidelines for cardiac CT and MR for risk stratification and primary prevention in a symptomatic individuals [43]. The prognostic value of extensive CAC was demonstrated in a meta-analysis of 3,924 symptomatic patients with a 3.5 year follow-up, the cardiac event rate was 2.6% per year in those with CAC > 0 and 0.5% per year in 0 CAC patients [59].

Recent data suggest that CCTA had incremental prognostic value over traditional risk factors [60]. Prognosis is predicted by coronary anatomy such as left main stenosis ≥ 50%, 3 vessel disease and 2-vessel disease including proximal LAD. The absence of CAD on CCTA conveys an excellent prognosis for symptomatic patients being evaluated for suspected CAD. Werkhoven et al. demonstrated that in patients with suspected CAD and intermediate pretest likeli-hood, CTA could efficiently make a distinction between patients at low or at high risk for future events [61]. Recently, Chow et al. verified that incremental prognostic value of CCTA could be achieved by the addition of the left ventricular ejection fraction (LVEF) and the total plaque score to CAD severity as determined by CCTA [62].

2.3 Coronary CT Angiography after Revascularization

2.3.1 Bypass grafts

CCTA is increasingly used as a noninvasive modality for the assessment of bypass graft patency and stenosis. Grafts and the anastomosis region of venous and arterial grafts can be analyzed with increased diagnostic yield [63-71] (Fig. 5). Recently published studies have demonstrated a negative predictive value for ruling out high-grade bypass graft stenosis ranging between 96 and 99% [70,71]. However, the distal anastomosis can still be challenging and the degree of stenosis tends to be overestimated [70] (Fig. 6). Additionally the native coronary circulation can be assessed with high diagnostic yield despite previous bypass surgery [71].

2.3.2 Coronary stents

The vast majority of coronary interventions are performed in association with placement of a coronary stent. Most coronary stents are made of stainless steel. Coronary stents usually measure 2.5–4 mm in diameter and are constantly subjected to cardiac motion. Nearly all coronary stents are made of metal and produce typical blooming ("thickening") of the stent struts with an apparent reduction of the visible stent lumen [72].

Detailed analysis of the inner-stent lumen is essential to detect intimal hyperplasia, which is the major mechanism of in-stent restenosis (Fig. 7). Complete stent occlusion could be reliably detected, while high-grade and even subtotal stenosis is frequently not identified. This can be explained by the observation that even vessels with subtotal stenosis often show unimpeded contrast flow or due to retrograde filling via collaterals.

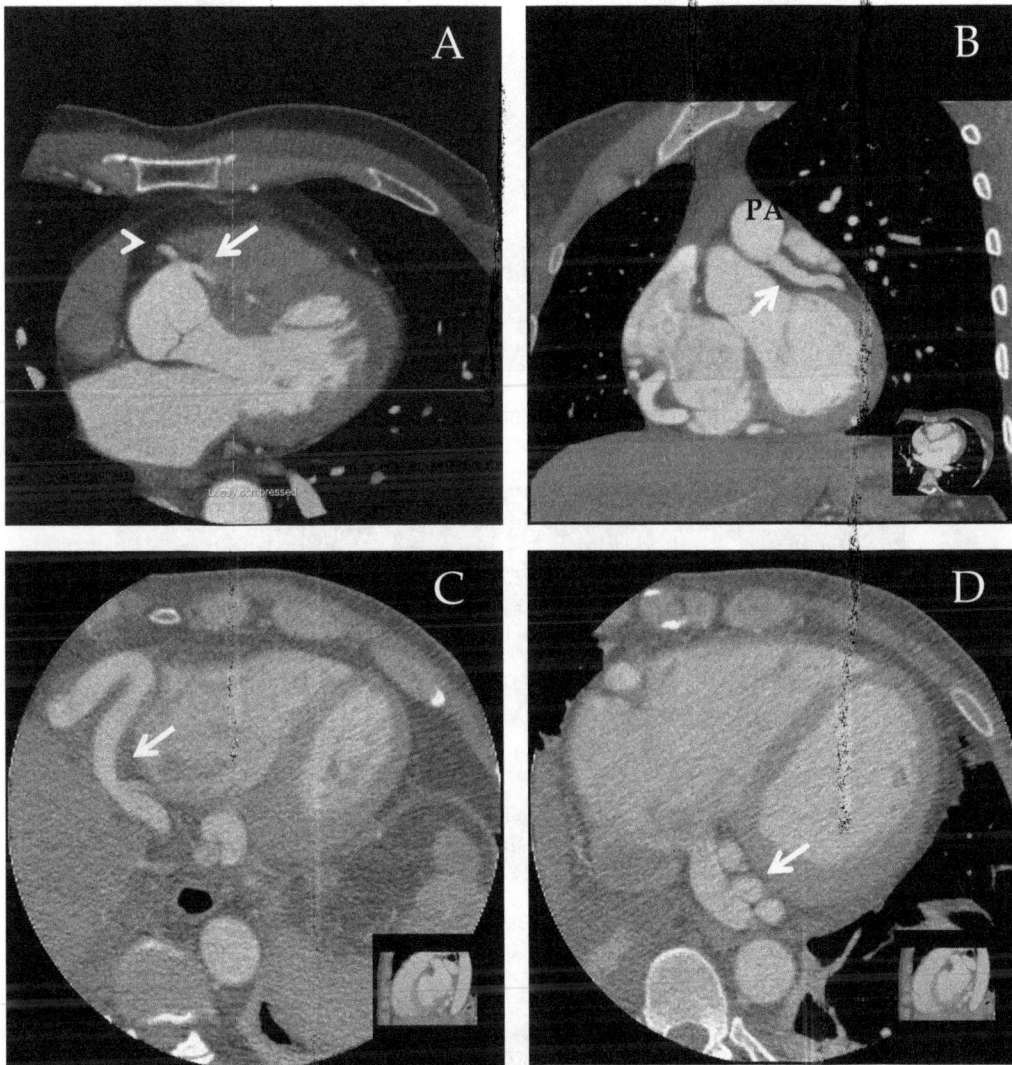

Fig. 4. Coronary artery anomalies. (A) Axial CT image shows a transseptal left descending artery (arrow) that arises from the right coronary artery (arrowhead). (B) Left coronary artery (arrow) arises from pulmonary artery (ALCAPA). Coronary artery fistula in a 44-year-old woman with palpitations (C) CT images show a tortuous and dilated right coronary artery (arrows) terminates into coronary sinus (D)

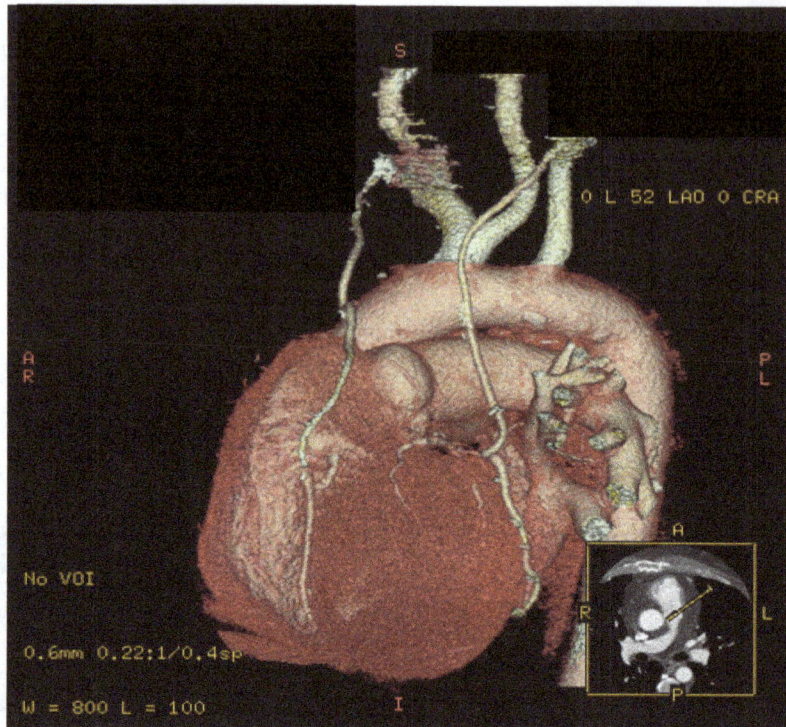

Fig. 5. 64-row MDCT 3D image reconstruction shows two patent arterial grafts coursing to the left anterior descending coronary artery and an obtuse marginal branch

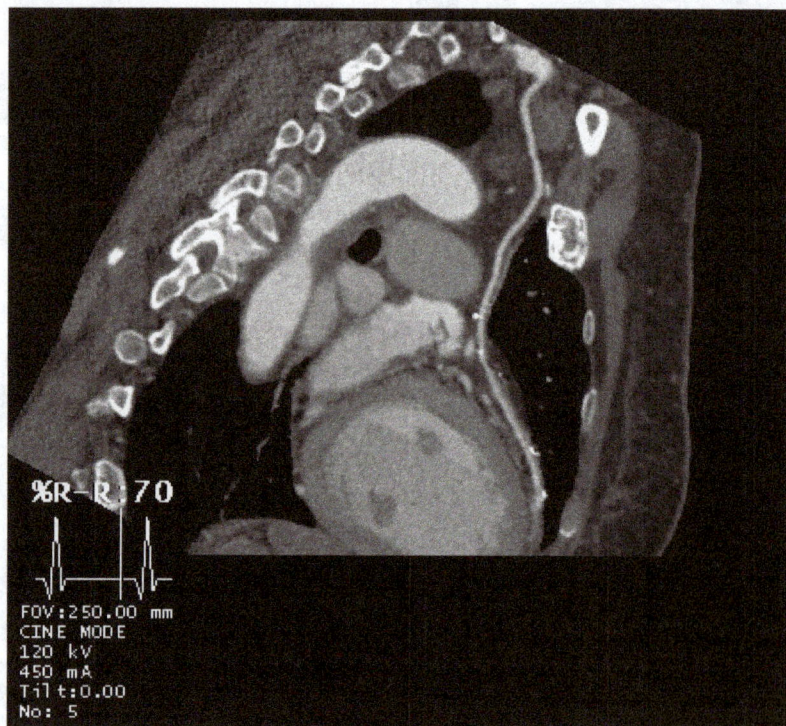

Fig. 6. 64-row MDCT 3D image shows a patent left internal mammary graft to the left anterior descending coronary artery

Recently, two meta-analyses of 16- and 64-row MDCT studies of coronary stents have been published regarding the diagnostic efficiency after stent implantation [73,74]. Overall sensitivity was 91%, specificity was 91% with a positive predictive value of 68%, and a negative predictive value of 98% [74]. Stent material, strut thickness and stent diameter are important factors influencing the ability to achieve diagnostic images. In fact, stents with a diameter ≥4.0 mm can be evaluated with fairly good diagnostic accuracy [75]. The thinner the struts of the usual metal stents are, the fewer artifacts hamper image quality.

2.4 Is Clinical Utility of Cardiovascular CT Limited to CAD?

CCT clinical utility is not limited to the assessment of coronary vasculature, but can yield information about other causes of chest pain such as aortic dissection, or pulmonary embolism. Other applications include assessment of cardiac structure and function, post myocardial infarction complications, and delineation of the pericardium. CT angiography is a useful modality in imaging the aorta and peripheral arterial tree. Furthermore, cardiac CTA became standard of care in pre procedural assessment of trans catheter aortic valve implantation and atrial fibrillation ablation procedures. In addition to that non-contrast studies allow for accurate quantification of coronary calcification, which provides important prognostic information.

2.5 Cardiac CT Angiography Assessment for Cardiac Pathology

Retrospective ECG-gating protocols can provide quantitative data on global and regional left ventricle (LV) and right ventricle (RV) systolic function with excellent correlation to echocardiography and CMRI [76,77]. It can also assess myocardial thickness, cardiac chamber sizes and volumes. Reproducibility of CT in performing right and left ventricular volume and function measurements has been established [78,79]. Further, CCT can effectively evaluate various myocardial diseases, including post myocardial infarction complications (Fig. 8) and other cardiomyopathies [80-82] (Fig. 9). CCT is extremely sensitive to the detection of pericardial thickening and calcification, a finding that can be associated with constrictive pericarditis [83,84]

(Fig. 10). Additional applications include assessment of intracardiac shunts, masses, and congenital defects [85-87] (Fig. 11). CCT has a limited role for the evaluation of valvular heart disease (VHD) but CCTA for preoperative evaluation in VHD is increasingly used, and high accuracy for the detection of significant coronary stenosis has been reported [88-90].

3. MYOCARDIAL VIABILITY

The ability to distinguish dysfunctional but viable myocardium from nonviable tissue after acute or chronic ischemia is a potentially important component in the evaluation of patients with CAD and LV dysfunction. Patients with viable myocardium have excellent prognosis after revascularization [91]. Fluorine-18 (fluoro-deoxy-glucose) FDG (positron emission tomography) PET in conjunction with resting perfusion images (N-13 ammonia, rubidium-82 or (single-photon emission computed tomography) SPECT using technitium-99m agents) is one of the established and accurate metabolic imaging techniques used for myocardial viability assessment [92]. The assessment of myocardial viability and infarct morphology with delayed contrast-enhanced MRI has been well validated over the past several years [93]. The recent advent of MDCT technology has expanded its potential for a more comprehensive evaluation of cardiovascular diseases. Delayed MDCT myocardial imaging can accurately identify and characterize morphological features of acute and healed myocardial infarction, including infarct size, transmurality, and the presence of micro vascular obstruction and scar [94,95]. Well-delineated hyper enhanced regions characterize infarcted myocardial tissue by prospective ECG-gated MDCT at lower radiation dose and good resolution [96], whereas regions of micro vascular obstruction by MDCT are characterized by hypo-enhancement on imaging early after MI [94,95]. The mechanism of myocardial hyper-enhancement and hypo-enhancement in acutely injured myocardial territories after iodinated contrast administration is similar to that proposed for delayed gadolinium-enhanced MRI [97]. The better spatial resolution of MDCT as compared to (cardiac magnetic resonance image) CMRI may influence the accuracy of viability assessment, but no study so far has tested this hypothesis.

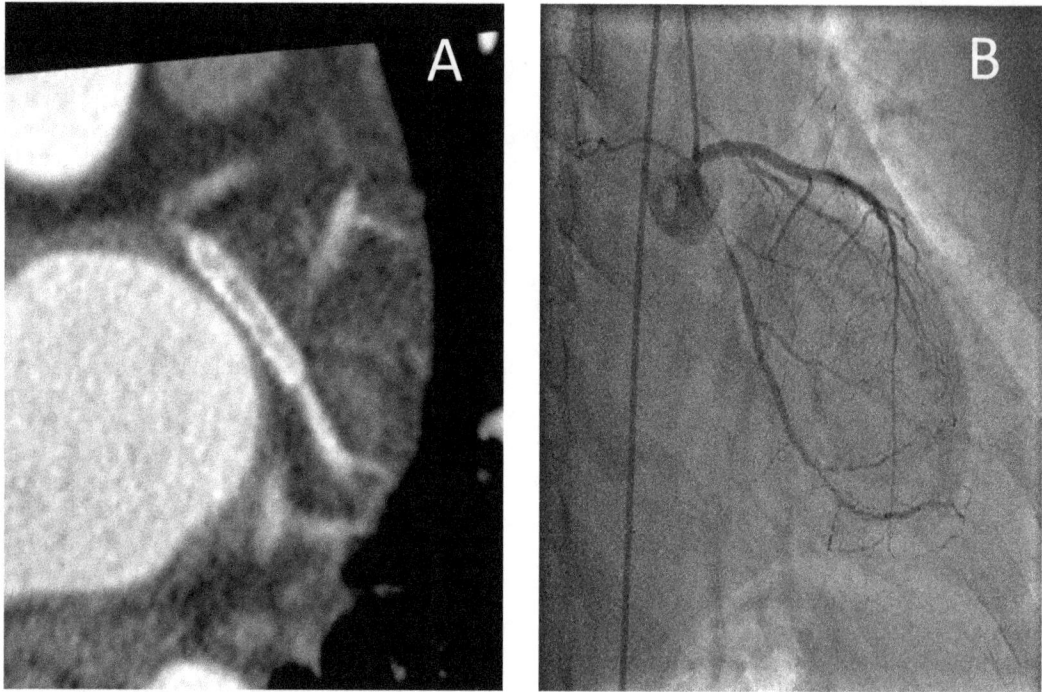

Fig. 7. In-stent stenosis proximal and distal left circumflex coronary artery. (A) 64-row MDCT. (B) Invasive coronary angiography

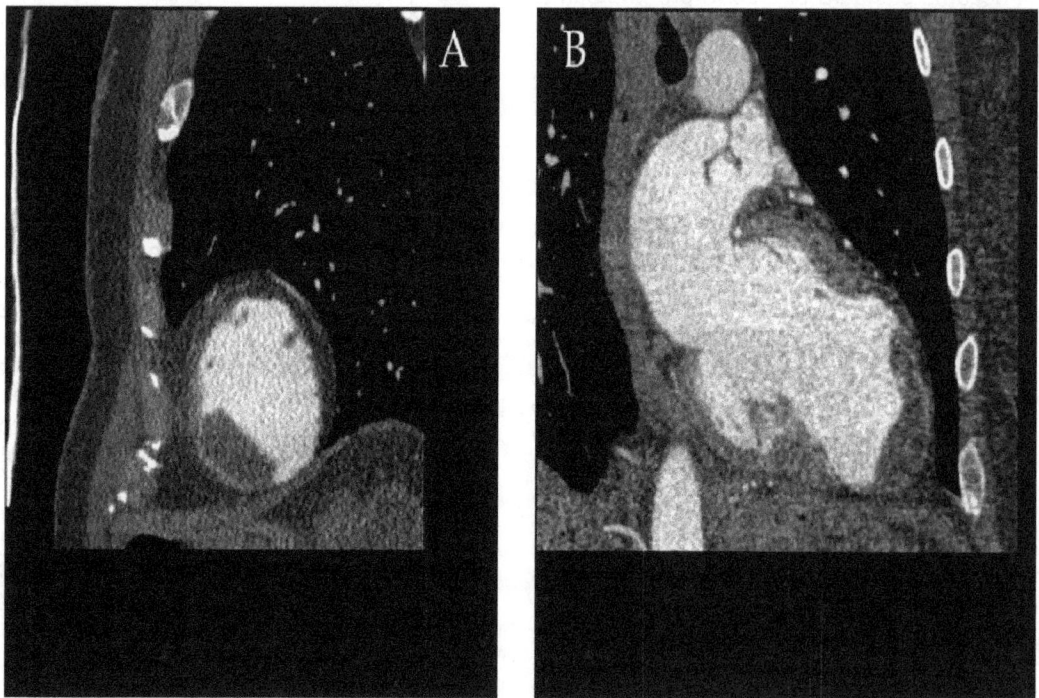

Fig. 8. Fortyfive-year-old woman with a recent myocardial infarction. Short axis (A) and two-chamber (B) views show a left ventricular apical aneurysm with thrombus

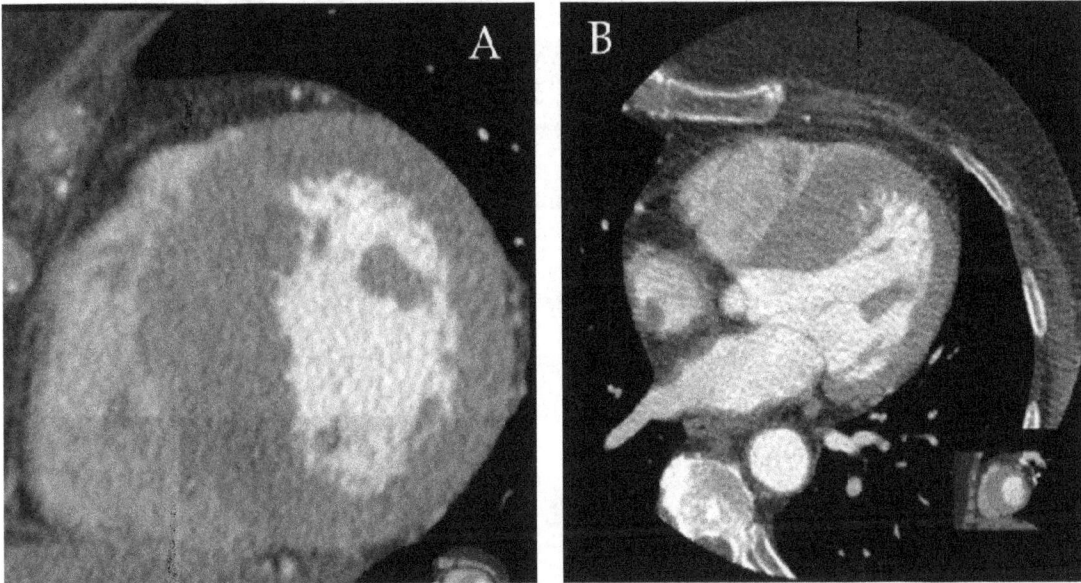

Fig. 9. Short axis and five-chamber view demonstrates abnormal thickening of the mid-and basal interventricular septum. The most common form of hypertrophic cardiomyopathy with or without obstruction

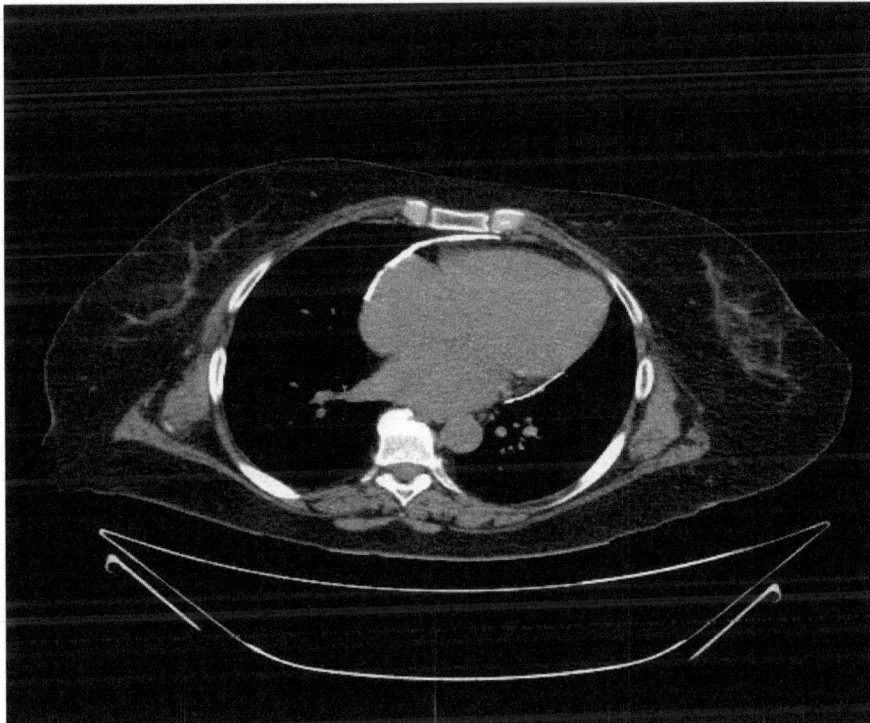

Fig. 10. Non-enhanced contrast CT demonstrates concentric, densely calcified pericardium in a patient with constrictive pericarditis

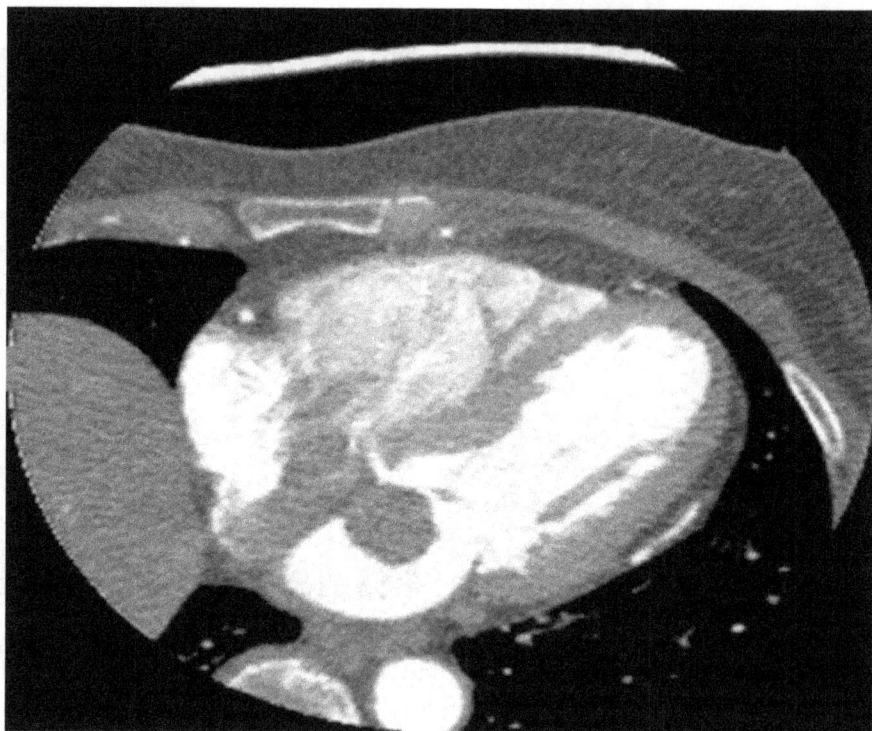

Fig. 11. Fifty two-year-old male with a left atrial mass. The post contrast study shows non-enhancement of the pedunculated mass arises from the region of the fossa ovalis, consistent with left atrial myxoma

4. ISCHEMIA DETECTION

The combination of coronary angiogram with stress-induced myocardial perfusion assessment had to wait until spiral CT technology progressed sufficiently to enable the acquisition of 64 slices simultaneously [98]. Current generation 64-detector scanners still have limited coverage of the heart, resulting in the base of the heart being scanned earlier in time than the apex, making comparisons in signal intensities between the two areas problematic. The greatest limitations to CCTA are the presence of severely calcified coronary segments, stents, or other artifacts that limit luminal visualization. The possibility of quantifying epicardial coronary plaque while also assessing microvascular disease during maximal vasodilatation enables coronary MDCTA to characterize macrovascular atherosclerosis as well as microvascular dysfunction.

5. ELECTROPHYSIOLOGICAL MAPPING AND RADIOFREQUENCY CATHETER ABLATION

Atrial fibrillation ablation requires a detailed understanding of cardiovascular anatomy through 3-D characterization of the relationships between the left atrium, the adjacent cardiac structures, and extra-cardiac structures [99] (Fig. 12). Cardiac CT study serves as a preprocedure roadmap for procedural planning, a 3-D data set for intraprocedure electro anatomic mapping and ablation. CTA characterization of the left atrium and pulmonary veins is achieved through multiple modalities of evaluation including multiplane 2-D views, 3-D volumetric reconstructions, virtual endocardial views, and volumetric quantification of the atria. Workstation software can be used for assessment of pulmonary veins anatomy and ostial diameter. Additionally, atrial anatomy, left atrial appendage thrombus and the relationship of the esophagus and aorta to the posterior left atrium and pulmonary veins can be defined [99,100]. Electro anatomic mapping with CCTA image integration has revolutionized catheter-based therapies by allowing for electrical mapping and ablation to occur on a 3 D map of the patient's individual endocardial left atrial anatomy.

6. LIMITATIONS and CHALLENGES

High-quality images are the most important requirement for the diagnostic assessment of CCTA. Image quality must be ensured through multiple steps, including patient preparation, the actual CCTA scan protocol, and the synchronization of raw image data with ECG information. Motion artifacts occur in patients with high heart rates, heart rate variability, and the presence of irregular or ectopic heart beats such as premature ventricular contractions (PVCs) contribute to the degradation of image quality (Fig. 13). Multiple studies have demonstrated that the highest image quality of CCTA can be achieved at low heart rates (<65 beats per minute) [101-103]. Adequate patient preparation with medication (e.g. B-blocker) to reduce the heart rate as well as training of the breath-hold commands is mandatory to avoid cardiac and respiratory artifacts. High-attenuation structures, such as calcified plaques or stents may degrade the accuracy of the assessment of stenosis due to beam-hardening artifacts. Several metanalyses demonstrated high-density calcification produces blooming artifacts, which lead to overestimation of the degree of coronary stenosis [104-106]. The specificity of CCTA is reduced in the presence of coronary artery calcium if the Agatston score is >400 [19-37]. The radiation dose associated with CT imaging is a serious concern for both clinicians and manufacturers [22,23]. With increasing application of CCTA in the diagnosis of CAD, the research focus has shifted from the previous emphasis on diagnostic accuracy to the current focus on reduction of radiation dose with acceptable diagnostic images [24,25]. Tremendous progress has been made to reduce the radiation dose by using many of the technologies and strategies however; much effort is still necessary to ensure that CCTA is safely performed in imaging patients with suspected coronary artery disease.

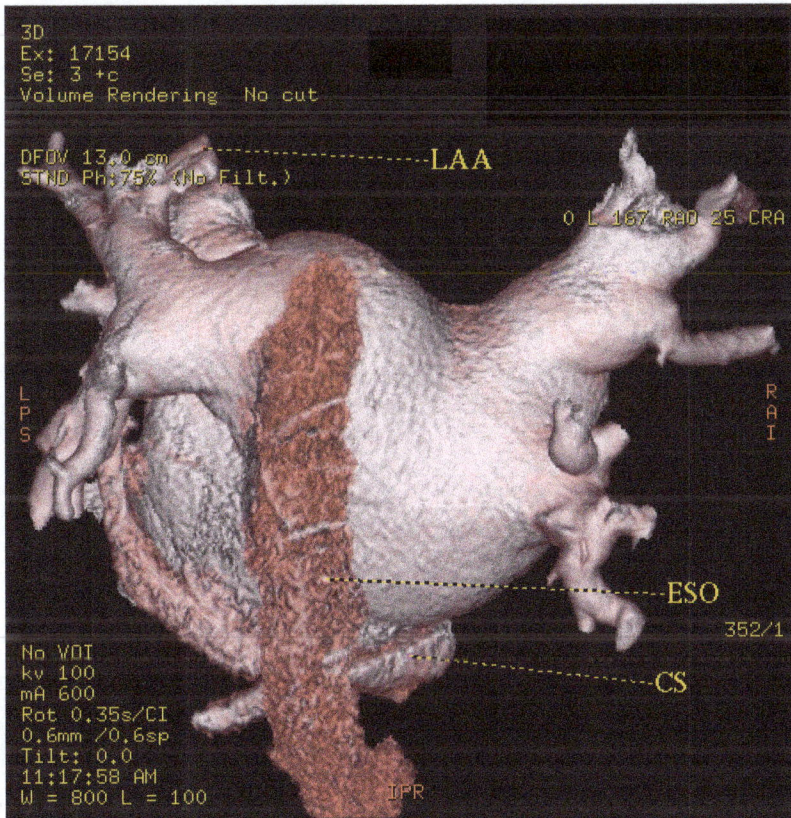

Fig. 12. D reconstructions demonstrating the relationship of coronary sinus (CS) and esophagus (ESO) to the posterior left atrium and left lower pulmonary vein

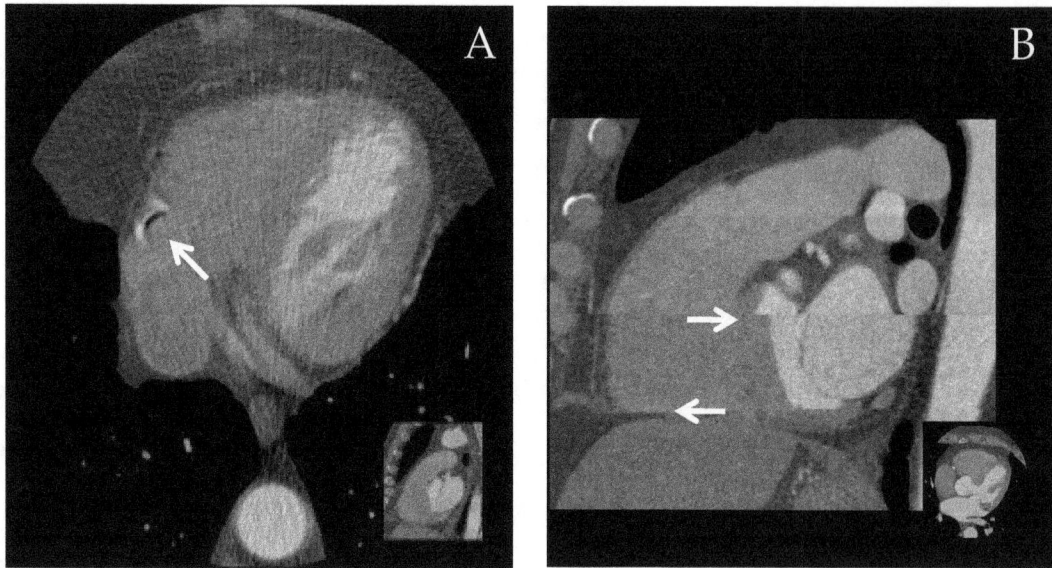

Fig. 13. (A) Patient imaged at heart rate of 77 beats per minute. Axial image at level of mid right coronary artery demonstrates typical appearance of motion artifact (arrow). (B) Patient with multiple extra systolic beats during image acquisition. Stair-step artifacts (arrows) are caused by irregular rhythm

7. CONCLUSION

CCT/CCTA is a well-established cardiac diagnostic modality, which can be used, in various cardiovascular conditions. Major advantages of CCT/CCTA include reliability, safety and the fact it provides both anatomical and functional information. The reduction of radiation dose with acceptable diagnostic image quality is the focus of current and future research.

CONSENT

Not applicable.

ETHICAL APPROVAL

Not applicable.

COMPETING INTERESTS

Authors have declared that no competing interests exist.

REFERENCES

1.   Hurlock GS, Higashino H, Mochizuki T. History of cardiac computed tomography: single to 320-detector row multislice computed tomography. The international Journal of Cardiovascular Imaging. 2009;1:3-42(25 Suppl).

2.   Lim MC, Wong TW, Yaneza LO, De Larrazabal C, Lau JK, Boey HK. Non-invasive detection of significant coronary artery disease with multi-section computed tomography angiography in patients with suspected coronary artery disease. Clinical Radiology. 2006;61(2):174-180.

3.   Halon DA, Gaspar T, Adawi S, Rubinshtein R, Schliamser JE, Peled N, Lewis BS. Uses and limitations of 40 slice multi-detector row spiral computed tomography for diagnosing coronary lesions in unselected patients referred for routine invasive coronary angiography. Cardiology. 2007;108(3):200-209.

4.   Watkins MW, Hesse B, Green CE, Greenberg NL, Manning M, Chaudhry E, Dauerman HL, Garcia MJ. Detection of coronary artery stenosis using 40-channel computed tomography with multi-segment reconstruction. The American Journal of Cardiology. 2007;99(2):175-181.

5.   Grosse C, Globits S, Hergan K. Forty-slice spiral computed tomography of the coronary arteries: assessment of image quality and diagnostic accuracy in a non-selected patient population. Acta Radiologica. 2007;48(1):36-44.

6. Ropers D, Rixe J, Anders K, Kuttner A, Baum U, Bautz W, Daniel WG, Achenbach S. Usefulness of multidetector row spiral computed tomography with 64- x 0.6-mm collimation and 330-ms rotation for the noninvasive detection of significant coronary artery stenoses. The American Journal of Cardiology. 2006;97(3):343-348.

7. Fine JJ, Hopkins CB, Ruff N, Newton FC. Comparison of accuracy of 64-slice cardiovascular computed tomography with coronary angiography in patients with suspected coronary artery disease. The American Journal of Cardiology. 2006;97(2):173-174.

8. Nikolaou K, Knez A, Rist C, Wintersperger BJ, Leber A, Johnson T, Reiser MF, Becker CR. Accuracy of 64-MDCT in the diagnosis of ischemic heart disease. AJR American Journal of Roentgenology. 2006;187(1):111-117.

9. Schlosser T, Mohrs OK, Magedanz A, Nowak B, Voigtlander T, Barkhausen J, Schmermund A. Noninvasive coronary angiography using 64-detector-row computed tomography in patients with a low to moderate pretest probability of significant coronary artery disease. Acta Radiologica. 2007;48(3):300-307.

10. Muhlenbruch G, Seyfarth T, Soo CS, Pregalathan N, Mahnken AH. Diagnostic value of 64-slice multi-detector row cardiac CTA in symptomatic patients. European Radiology. 2007;17(3):603-609.

11. Meijboom WB, Mollet NR, Van Mieghem CA, Weustink AC, Pugliese F, van Pelt N, Cademartiri F, Vourvouri E, de Jaegere P, Krestin GP et al., 64-Slice CT coronary angiography in patients with non-ST elevation acute coronary syndrome heart. 2007;93(11):1386-1392.

12. Herzog C, Zwerner PL, Doll JR, Nielsen CD, Nguyen SA, Savino G, Vogl TJ, Costello P, Schoepf UJ. Significant coronary artery stenosis: comparison on per-patient and per-vessel or per-segment basis at 64-section CT angiography. Radiology. 2007;244(1):112-120.

13. Ehara M, Surmely JF, Kawai M, Katoh O, Matsubara T, Terashima M, Tsuchikane E, Kinoshita Y, Suzuki T, Ito T et al., Diagnostic accuracy of 64-slice computed tomography for detecting angiographically significant coronary artery stenosis in an unselected consecutive patient population: comparison with conventional invasive angiography. Circulation Journal: official

Journal of The Japanese Circulation Society. 2006;70(5):564-571.

14. Hausleiter J, Meyer T, Hadamitzky M, Zankl M, Gerein P, Dorrler K, Kastrati A, Martinoff S, Schomig A: non-invasive coronary computed tomographic angiography for patients with suspected coronary artery disease: the Coronary Angiography by Computed Tomography with the Use of a Submillimeter resolution (CACTUS) trial. European Heart Journal. 2007;28(24):3034-3041.

15. Shabestari AA, Abdi S, Akhlaghpoor S, Azadi M, Baharjoo H, Pajouh MD, Emami Z, Esfahani F, Firouzi I, Hashemian M et al. Diagnostic performance of 64-channel multislice computed tomography in assessment of significant coronary artery disease in symptomatic subjects. The American Journal Of Cardiology. 2007;99(12):1656-1661.

16. Scheffel H, Alkadhi H, Plass A, Vachenauer R, Desbiolles L, Gaemperli O, Schepis T, Frauenfelder T, Schertler T, Husmann L et al. Accuracy of dual-source CT coronary angiography: First experience in a high pre-test probability population without heart rate control. European Radiology. 2006;16(12):2739-2747.

17. Heuschmid M, Burgstahler C, Reimann A, Brodoefel H, Mysal I, Haeberle E, Tsiflikas I, Claussen CD, Kopp AF. Schroeder S: Usefulness of noninvasive cardiac imaging using dual-source computed tomography in an unselected population with high prevalence of coronary artery disease. The American Journal Of Cardiology. 2007;100(4):587-592.

18. Ropers U, Ropers D, Pflederer T, Anders K, Kuettner A, Stilianakis NI, Komatsu S, Kalender W, Bautz W, Daniel WG et al. Influence of heart rate on the diagnostic accuracy of dual-source computed tomography coronary angiography. Journal Of The American College Of Cardiology. 2007;50(25):2393-2398.

19. Leber AW, Johnson T, Becker A, von Ziegler F, Tittus J, Nikolaou K, Reiser M, Steinbeck G, Becker CR, Knez A. Diagnostic accuracy of dual-source multi-slice CT-coronary angiography in patients with an intermediate pretest likelihood for coronary artery disease. European Heart Journal. 2007;28(19):2354-2360.

20. Weustink AC, Meijboom WB, Mollet NR, Otsuka M, Pugliese F, van Mieghem C, Malago R, van Pelt N, Dijkshoorn ML,

Cademartiri F, et al. Reliable high-speed coronary computed tomography in symptomatic patients. Journal of The American College of Cardiology. 2007;50(8):786-794.

21. Alkadhi H, Scheffel H, Desbiolles L, Gaemperli O, Stolzmann P, Plass A, Goerres GW, Luescher TF, Genoni M, Marincek B et al. Dual-source computed tomography coronary angiography: influence of obesity, calcium load, and heart rate on diagnostic accuracy. European Heart Journal. 2008;29(6):766-776.

22. Brenner DJ, Hall EJ. Computed tomography--an increasing source of radiation exposure. The New England Journal of Medicine. 2007;357(22):2277-2284.

23. Hausleiter J, Meyer T, Hermann F, Hadamitzky M, Krebs M, Gerber TC, McCollough C, Martinoff S, Kastrati A, Schomig A et al. Estimated radiation dose associated with cardiac CT angiography. Journal of the American Medical Association. 2009;301(5):500-507.

24. Paul JF, Abada HT. Strategies for reduction of radiation dose in cardiac multislice CT. European Radiology. 2007;17(8):2028-2037.

25. Sun Z, Ng KH. Multislice CT angiography in cardiac imaging. Part III: radiation risk and dose reduction. Singapore Medical Journal. 2010;51(5):374-380.

26. Blankenhorn DH, Stern D. Calcification of the coronary arteries. The American Journal of Roentgenology, Radium Therapy, and Nuclear Medicine. 1959;81(5):772-777.

27. Frink RJ, Achor RW, Brown AL, Jr., Kincaid OW, Brandenburg RO. Significance of calcification of the coronary arteries. The American Journal of Cardiology. 1970;26(3):241-247.

28. Wexler L, Brundage B, Crouse J, Detrano R, Fuster V, Maddahi J, Rumberger J, Stanford W, White R, Taubert K. Coronary artery calcification: pathophysiology, epidemiology, imaging methods, and clinical implications. A statement for health professionals from the American Heart Association. Writing Group. Circulation. 1996;94(5):1175-1192.

29. Agatston AS, Janowitz WR, Hildner FJ, Zusmer NR, Viamonte M, Jr Detrano R. Quantification of coronary artery calcium using ultrafast computed tomography.

Journal of the American College of Cardiology 1990;15(4):827-832.

30. Simons DB, Schwartz RS, Edwards WD, Sheedy PF, Breen JF, Rumberger JA. Noninvasive definition of anatomic coronary artery disease by ultrafast computed tomographic scanning: a quantitative pathologic comparison study. Journal of The American College Of Cardiology. 1992;20(5):1118-1126.

31. Detrano R, Tang W, Kang X, Mahaisavariya P, McCrae M, Garner D, Peng SK, Measham C, Molloi S, Gutfinger D et al. Accurate coronary calcium phosphate mass measurements from electron beam computed tomograms. American Journal of Cardiac Imaging. 1995;9(3):167-173.

32. Mautner GC, Mautner SL, Froehlich J, Feuerstein IM, Proschan MA, Roberts WC, Doppman JL: Coronary artery calcification: assessment with electron beam CT and histomorphometric correlation. Radiology. 1994;192(3):619-623.

33. Budoff MJ, Georgiou D, Brody A, Agatston AS, Kennedy J, Wolfkiel C, Stanford W, Shields P, Lewis RJ, Janowitz WR et al. Ultrafast computed tomography as a diagnostic modality in the detection of coronary artery disease: a multicenter study. Circulation. 1996;93(5):898-904.

34. Guerci AD, Spadaro LA, Popma JJ, Goodman KJ, Brundage BH, Budoff M, Lerner G, Vizza RF: Relation of coronary calcium score by electron beam computed tomography to arteriographic findings in asymptomatic and symptomatic adults. The American Journal of Cardiology. 1997;79(2):128-133.

35. Raggi P, Callister TQ, Cooil B, He ZX, Lippolis NJ, Russo DJ, Zelinger A, Mahmarian JJ: Identification of patients at increased risk of first unheralded acute myocardial infarction by electron-beam computed tomography. Circulation. 2000;101(8):850-855.

36. Ghostine S, Caussin C, Daoud B, Habis M, Perrier E, Pesenti-Rossi D, Sigal-Cinqualbre A, Angel CY, Lancelin B, Capderou A et al. Non-invasive detection of coronary artery disease in patients with left bundle branch block using 64-slice computed tomography. Journal of the American College of Cardiology. 2006;48(10):1929-1934.

37. Budoff MJ, Dowe D, Jollis JG, Gitter M, Sutherland J, Halamert E, Scherer M,

Bellinger R, Martin A, Benton R et al. Diagnostic performance of 64-multidetector row coronary computed tomographic angiography for evaluation of coronary artery stenosis in individuals without known coronary artery disease: results from the prospective multicenter ACCURACY (Assessment by Coronary Computed Tomographic Angiography of Individuals Undergoing Invasive Coronary Angiography) trial. Journal of the American College of Cardiology. 2008;52(21):1724-1732.

38. Vanhoenacker PK, Heijenbrok-Kal MH, Van Heste R, Decramer I, Van Hoe LR, Wijns W, Hunink MG: Diagnostic performance of multidetector CT angiography for assessment of coronary artery disease: meta-analysis. Radiology. 2007;244(2):419-428.

39. Meijboom WB, van Mieghem CA, Mollet NR, Pugliese F, Weustink AC, van Pelt N, Cademartiri F, Nieman K, Boersma E, de Jaegere P et al. 64-slice computed tomography coronary angiography in patients with high, intermediate, or low pretest probability of significant coronary artery disease. Journal of the American College of Cardiology. 2007;50(15):1469-1475.

40. Gilard M, Le Gal G, Cornily JC, Vinsonneau U, Joret C, Pennec PY, Mansourati J, Boschat J. Midterm prognosis of patients with suspected coronary artery disease and normal multislice computed tomographic findings: a prospective management outcome study. Archives of internal medicine. 2007; 167(15):1686-1689.

41. Lesser JR, Flygenring B, Knickelbine T, Hara H, Henry J, Kalil A, Pelak K, Lindberg J, Pelzel J, Schwartz RS. Clinical utility of coronary CT angiography: coronary stenosis detection and prognosis in ambulatory patients. Catheterization and Cardiovascular Interventions : official Journal of the Society for Cardiac Angiography & Interventions. 2007;69(1):64-72.

42. Hadamitzky M, Freissmuth B, Meyer T, Hein F, Kastrati A, Martinoff S, Schomig A, Hausleiter J. Prognostic value of coronary computed tomographic angiography for prediction of cardiac events in patients with suspected coronary artery disease. Jacc Cardiovascular Imaging. 2009;2(4):404-411.

43. Hendel RC, Patel MR, Kramer CM, Poon M, Hendel RC, Carr JC, Gerstad NA, Gillam LD, Hodgson JM, Kim RJ et al. ACCF/ACR/SCCT/SCMR/ASNC/NASCI/SCAI/SIR 2006 appropriateness criteria for cardiac computed tomography and cardiac magnetic resonance imaging: a report of the American College of Cardiology Foundation Quality Strategic Directions Committee Appropriateness Criteria Working Group, American College of Radiology, Society of Cardiovascular Computed Tomography, Society for Cardiovascular Magnetic Resonance, American Society of Nuclear Cardiology, North American Society for Cardiac Imaging, Society for Cardiovascular Angiography and Interventions, and Society of Interventional Radiology. Journal of the American College of Cardiology. 2006;48(7):1475-1497.

44. Hoffmann U, Nagurney JT, Moselewski F, Pena A, Ferencik M, Chae CU, Cury RC, Butler J, Abbara S, Brown DF et al. Coronary multidetector computed tomography in the assessment of patients with acute chest pain. Circulation. 2006; 114(21):2251-2260.

45. Gallagher MJ, Ross MA, Raff GL, Goldstein JA, O'Neill WW, O'Neil B. The diagnostic accuracy of 64-slice computed tomography coronary angiography compared with stress nuclear imaging in emergency department low-risk chest pain patients. Annals of Emergency Medicine. 2007;49(2):125-136.

46. Goldstein JA, Gallagher MJ, O'Neill WW, Ross MA, O'Neil BJ, Raff GL. A randomized controlled trial of multi-slice coronary computed tomography for evaluation of acute chest pain. Journal of the American College of Cardiology. 2007;49(8):863-871.

47. Coles DR, Wilde P, Oberhoff M, Rogers CA, Karsch KR, Baumbach A. Multislice computed tomography coronary angiography in patients admitted with a suspected acute coronary syndrome. The International Journal of Cardiovascular Imaging. 2007;23(5):603-614.

48. Hoffmann U, Bamberg F, Chae CU, Nichols JH, Rogers IS, Seneviratne SK, Truong QA, Cury RC, Abbara S, Shapiro MD et al. Coronary computed tomography angiography for early triage of patients with acute chest pain: the ROMICAT (Rule Out Myocardial Infarction using Computer

Assisted Tomography) trial. Journal of the American College of Cardiology. 2009;53(18):1642-1650.

49. Greenberg MA, Fish BG, Spindola-Franco H. Congenital anomalies of the coronary arteries. Classification and significance. Radiologic Clinics of North America. 1989;27(6):1127-1146.

50. Ropers D, Moshage W, Daniel WG, Jessl J, Gottwik M, Achenbach S. Visualization of coronary artery anomalies and their anatomic course by contrast-enhanced electron beam tomography and three-dimensional reconstruction. The American Journal of Cardiology. 2001;87(2):193-197.

51. Deibler AR, Kuzo RS, Vohringer M, Page EE, Safford RE, Patron JN, Lane GE, Morin RL, Gerber TC. Imaging of congenital coronary anomalies with multislice computed tomography. Mayo Clinic Proceedings Mayo Clinic. 2004;79(8):1017-1023.

52. Datta J, White CS, Gilkeson RC, Meyer CA, Kansal S, Jani ML, Arildsen RC, Read K. Anomalous coronary arteries in adults: depiction at multi-detector row CT angiography. Radiology. 2005;235(3):812-818.

53. Schmid M, Achenbach S, Ludwig J, Baum U, Anders K, Pohle K, Daniel WG, Ropers D. Visualization of coronary artery anomalies by contrast-enhanced multi-detector row spiral computed tomography. International journal of cardiology. 2006;111(3):430-435.

54. Kim SY, Seo JB, Do KH, Heo JN, Lee JS, Song JW, Choe YH, Kim TH, Yong HS, Choi SI et al. Coronary artery anomalies: classification and ECG-gated multi-detector row CT findings with angiographic correlation. Radiographics : AReview Publication of the Radiological Society of North America, Inc. 2006;26(2):317-333; discussion 333-314.

55. Duran C, Kantarci M, Durur Subasi I, Gulbaran M, Sevimli S, Bayram E, Eren S, Karaman A, Fil F, Okur A. Remarkable anatomic anomalies of coronary arteries and their clinical importance: a multidetector computed tomography angiographic study. Journal of Computer Assisted Tomography.2006;30(6):939-948.

56. Kini S, Bis KG, Weaver L. Normal and variant coronary arterial and venous anatomy on high-resolution CT angiography. Ajr American Journal Of Roentgenology. 2007;188(6):1665-1674.

57. Greenland P, LaBree L, Azen SP, Doherty TM, Detrano RC. Coronary artery calcium score combined with Framingham score for risk prediction in asymptomatic individuals. Jama : The Journal of the American Medical Association. 2004;291(2):210-215.

58. Arad Y, Goodman KJ, Roth M, Newstein D, Guerci AD. Coronary calcification, coronary disease risk factors, C-reactive protein, and atherosclerotic cardiovascular disease events: the St. Francis Heart Study. Journal of the American College of Cardiology. 2005;46(1):158-165.

59. Sarwar A, Shaw LJ, Shapiro MD, Blankstein R, Hoffmann U, Cury RC, Abbara S, Brady TJ, Budoff MJ, Blumenthal RS et al. Diagnostic and prognostic value of absence of coronary artery calcification. JACC Cardiovascular Imaging. 2009;2(6):675-688.

60. Ostrom MP, Gopal A, Ahmadi N, Nasir K, Yang E, Kakadiaris I, Flores F, Mao SS, Budoff MJ. Mortality incidence and the severity of coronary atherosclerosis assessed by computed tomography angiography. Journal of the American College of Cardiology. 2008;52(16):1335-1343.

61. van Werkhoven JM, Gaemperli O, Schuijf JD, Jukema JW, Kroft LJ, Leschka S, Alkadhi H, Valenta I, Pundziute G, de Roos A et al. Multislice computed tomography coronary angiography for risk stratification in patients with an intermediate pretest likelihood. Heart. 2009;95(19):1607-1611.

62. Chow BJ, Wells GA, Chen L, Yam Y, Galiwango P, Abraham A, Sheth T, Dennie C, Beanlands RS, Ruddy TD. Prognostic value of 64-slice cardiac computed tomography severity of coronary artery disease, coronary atherosclerosis, and left ventricular ejection fraction. Journal of the American College of Cardiology. 2010;55(10):1017-1028.

63. Hamon M, Lepage O, Malagutti P, Riddell JW, Morello R, Agostini D, Hamon M. Diagnostic performance of 16- and 64-section spiral CT for coronary artery bypass graft assessment: meta-analysis. Radiology. 2008;247(3):679-686.

64. Malagutti P, Nieman K, Meijboom WB, van Mieghem CA, Pugliese F, Cademartiri F, Mollet NR, Boersma E, de Jaegere PP, de Feyter PJ. Use of 64-slice CT in symptomatic patients after coronary bypass surgery: evaluation of grafts and

coronary arteries. European Heart Journal. 2007;28(15):1879-1885.

65. Pache G, Saueressig U, Frydrychowicz A, Foell D, Ghanem N, Kotter E, Geibel-Zehender A, Bode C, Langer M, Bley T. Initial experience with 64-slice cardiac CT: non-invasive visualization of coronary artery bypass grafts. European Heart Journal. 2006;27(8):976-980.

66. Dikkers R, Willems TP, Tio RA, Anthonio RL, Zijlstra F, Oudkerk M. The benefit of 64-MDCT prior to invasive coronary angiography in symptomatic post-CABG patients. The International Journal Of Cardiovascular Imaging. 2007;23(3):369-377.

67. Ropers D, Pohle FK, Kuettner A, Pflederer T, Anders K, Daniel WG, Bautz W, Baum U, Achenbach S. Diagnostic accuracy of noninvasive coronary angiography in patients after bypass surgery using 64-slice spiral computed tomography with 330-ms gantry rotation. Circulation. 2006;114(22):2334-2341; quiz 2334.

68. Meyer TS, Martinoff S, Hadamitzky M, Will A, Kastrati A, Schomig A, Hausleiter J. Improved noninvasive assessment of coronary artery bypass grafts with 64-slice computed tomographic angiography in an unselected patient population. Journal of the American College of Cardiology. 2007;49(9):946-950.

69. Jabara R, Chronos N, Klein L, Eisenberg S, Allen R, Bradford S, Frohwein S. Comparison of multidetector 64-slice computed tomographic angiography to coronary angiography to assess the patency of coronary artery bypass grafts. The American Journal of Cardiology. 2007;99(11):1529-1534.

70. Feuchtner GM, Schachner T, Bonatti J, Friedrich GJ, Soegner P, Klauser A, zur Nedden D. Diagnostic performance of 64-slice computed tomography in evaluation of coronary artery bypass grafts. AJR American Journal of Roentgenology.2007;189(3):574-580.

71. Nazeri I, Shahabi P, Tehrai M, Sharif-Kashani B, Nazeri A. Assessment of patients after coronary artery bypass grafting using 64-slice computed tomography. The American Journal of Cardiology. 2009;103(5):667-673.

72. Maintz D, Juergens KU, Wichter T, Grude M, Heindel W, Fischbach R. Imaging of coronary artery stents using multislice computed tomography: in vitro evaluation. European Radiology. 2003;13(4):830-835.

73. Kumbhani DJ, Ingelmo CP, Schoenhagen P, Curtin RJ, Flamm SD, Desai MY. Meta-analysis of diagnostic efficacy of 64-slice computed tomography in the evaluation of coronary in-stent restenosis. The American Journal of Cardiology. 2009;103(12):1675-1681.

74. Sun Z, Davidson R, Lin CH. Multi-detector row CT angiography in the assessment of coronary in-stent restenosis: a systematic review. European Journal of Radiology. 2009;69(3):489-495.

75. Schlosser T, Scheuermann T, Ulzheimer S, Mohrs OK, Kuhling M, Albrecht PE, Voigtlander T, Barkhausen J, Schmermund A. In vitro evaluation of coronary stents and in-stent stenosis using a dynamic cardiac phantom and a 64-detector row CT scanner. Clinical Research in Cardiology : official Journal of the German Cardiac Society. 2007;96(12):883-890.

76. Annuar BR, Liew CK, Chin SP, Ong TK, Seyfarth MT, Chan WL, Fong YY, Ang CK, Lin N, Liew HB et al. Assessment of global and regional left ventricular function using 64-slice multislice computed tomography and 2D echocardiography: a comparison with cardiac magnetic resonance. European Journal of Radiology. 2008;65(1):112-119.

77. Halliburton SS, Petersilka M, Schvartzman PR, Obuchowski N, White RD. Evaluation of left ventricular dysfunction using multiphasic reconstructions of coronary multi-slice computed tomography data in patients with chronic ischemic heart disease: validation against cine magnetic resonance imaging. The International Journal of Cardiovascular Imaging. 2003;19(1):73-83.

78. Schmermund A, Rensing BJ, Sheedy PF, Rumberger JA. Reproducibility of right and left ventricular volume measurements by electron-beam CT in patients with congestive heart failure. International Journal of Cardiac Imaging. 1998;14(3):201-209.

79. Lang RM, Bierig M, Devereux RB, Flachskampf FA, Foster E, Pellikka PA, Picard MH, Roman MJ, Seward J, Shanewise JS et al. Recommendations for chamber quantification: a report from the American Society of Echocardiography's Guidelines and Standards Committee and the Chamber Quantification Writing Group,

developed in conjunction with the European Association of Echocardiography, a branch of the European Society of Cardiology. Journal of the American Society of Echocardiography : official publication of the American Society of Echocardiography. 2005;18(12):1440-1463.

80. Rumberger JA, Behrenbeck T, Breen JR, Reed JE, Gersh BJ. Nonparallel changes in global left ventricular chamber volume and muscle mass during the first year after transmural myocardial infarction in humans. Journal of the American College of Cardiology. 1993;21(3):673-682.

81. Hirose K, Reed JE, Rumberger JA. Serial changes in left and right ventricular systolic and diastolic dynamics during the first year after an index left ventricular Q wave myocardial infarction. Journal of the American College of Cardiology. 1995;25(5):1097-1104.

82. Richardson P, McKenna W, Bristow M, Maisch B, Mautner B, O'Connell J, Olsen E, Thiene G, Goodwin J, Gyarfas I et al. Report of the 1995 World Health Organization/International Society and Federation of Cardiology Task Force on the Definition and Classification of cardiomyopathies. Circulation. 1996;93(5):841-842.

83. Spodick DH: Pericardial disease. Jama : the journal of the American Medical Association. 1997;278(9):704.

84. Oyama N, Oyama N, Komuro K, Nambu T, Manning WJ, Miyasaka K. Computed tomography and magnetic resonance imaging of the pericardium: anatomy and pathology. Magnetic resonance in medical sciences : MRMS : an official journal of Japan Society of Magnetic Resonance in Medicine. 2004;3(3):145-152.

85. Cook SC, Raman SV. Multidetector computed tomography in the adolescent and young adult with congenital heart disease. Journal of Cardiovascular Computed Tomography. 2008;2(1):36-49.

86. Raman SV, Cook SC, McCarthy B, Ferketich AK. Usefulness of multidetector row computed tomography to quantify right ventricular size and function in adults with either tetralogy of Fallot or transposition of the great arteries. The American Journal of Cardiology. 2005;95(5):683-686.

87. Hoffmann A, Engelfriet P, Mulder B. Radiation exposure during follow-up of adults with congenital heart disease. International Journal of Cardiology. 2007;118(2):151-153.

88. Meijboom WB, Mollet NR, Van Mieghem CA, Kluin J, Weustink AC, Pugliese F, Vourvouri E, Cademartiri F, Bogers AJ, Krestin GP et al. Pre-operative computed tomography coronary angiography to detect significant coronary artery disease in patients referred for cardiac valve surgery. Journal of the American College of Cardiology. 2006;48(8):1658-1665.

89. Reant P, Brunot S, Lafitte S, Serri K, Leroux L, Corneloup O, Iriart X, Coste P, Dos Santos P, Roudaut R et al. Predictive value of noninvasive coronary angiography with multidetector computed tomography to detect significant coronary stenosis before valve surgery. The American Journal of Cardiology . 2006;97(10):1506-1510.

90. Russo V, Gostoli V, Lovato L, Montalti M, Marzocchi A, Gavelli G, Branzi A, Di Bartolomeo R, Fattori R. Clinical value of multidetector CT coronary angiography as a preoperative screening test before non-coronary cardiac surgery. Heart. 2007;93(12):1591-1598.

91. Allman KC, Shaw LJ, Hachamovitch R, Udelson JE. Myocardial viability testing and impact of revascularization on prognosis in patients with coronary artery disease and left ventricular dysfunction: a meta-analysis. Journal of the American College of Cardiology. 2002;39(7):1151-1158.

92. Slart RH, Bax JJ, van Veldhuisen DJ, van der Wall EE, Dierckx RA, de Boer J, Jager PL. Prediction of functional recovery after revascularization in patients with coronary artery disease and left ventricular dysfunction by gated FDG-PET. Journal of nuclear cardiology : official publication of the American Society of Nuclear Cardiology. 2006;13(2):210-219.

93. Kim RJ, Wu E, Rafael A, Chen EL, Parker MA, Simonetti O, Klocke FJ, Bonow RO, Judd RM. The use of contrast-enhanced magnetic resonance imaging to identify reversible myocardial dysfunction. The New England Journal of Medicine. 2000;343(20):1445-1453.

94. Lardo AC, Cordeiro MA, Silva C, Amado LC, George RT, Saliaris AP, Schuleri KH, Fernandes VR, Zviman M, Nazarian S et al. Contrast-enhanced multidetector computed tomography viability imaging after myocardial infarction: characterization

of myocyte death, microvascular obstruction, and chronic scar. Circulation. 2006;113(3):394-404.

95. Gerber BL, Belge B, Legros GJ, Lim P, Poncelet A, Pasquet A, Gisellu G, Coche E, Vanoverschelde JL. Characterization of acute and chronic myocardial infarcts by multidetector computed tomography: comparison with contrast-enhanced magnetic resonance. Circulation. 2006;113(6):823-833.

96. Chang HJ, George RT, Schuleri KH, Evers K, Kitagawa K, Lima JA, Lardo AC. Prospective electrocardiogram-gated delayed enhanced multidetector computed tomography accurately quantifies infarct size and reduces radiation exposure. JACC Cardiovascular Imaging. 2009;2(4):412-420.

97. Wu KC, Lima JA. Noninvasive imaging of myocardial viability: current techniques and future developments. Circulation Research. 2003;93(12):1146-1158.

98. George RT, Jerosch-Herold M, Silva C, Kitagawa K, Bluemke DA, Lima JA, Lardo AC. Quantification of myocardial perfusion using dynamic 64-detector computed tomography. Investigative Radiology 2007;42(12):815-822.

99. Shinbane JS. Cardiovascular computed tomographic angiography in patients with atrial fibrillation: challenges of anatomy, physiology, and electrophysiology. Journal of Cardiovascular Computed Tomography. 2008;2(3):181-182.

100. Garcia MJ. Detection of left atrial appendage thrombus by cardiac computed tomography: a word of caution. JACC Cardiovascular Imaging. 2009;2(1):77-79.

101. Giesler T, Baum U, Ropers D, Ulzheimer S, Wenkel E, Mennicke M, Bautz W, Kalender WA, Daniel WG, Achenbach S.

Noninvasive visualization of coronary arteries using contrast-enhanced multidetector CT: influence of heart rate on image quality and stenosis detection. AJR American Journal of Roentgenology. 2002;179(4):911-916.

102. Schroeder S, Kopp AF, Kuettner A, Burgstahler C, Herdeg C, Heuschmid M, Baumbach A, Claussen CD, Karsch KR, Seipel L. Influence of heart rate on vessel visibility in noninvasive coronary angiography using new multislice computed tomography: experience in 94 patients. Clinical Imaging. 2002;26(2):106-111.

103. Raff GL, Gallagher MJ, O'Neill WW, Goldstein JA: Diagnostic accuracy of noninvasive coronary angiography using 64-slice spiral computed tomography. Journal of the American College of Cardiology. 2005;46(3):552-557.

104. Sun Z, Lin C, Davidson R, Dong C, Liao Y. Diagnostic value of 64-slice CT angiography in coronary artery disease: a systematic review. European Journal of Radiology. 2008; 67(1):78-84.

105. Abdulla J, Abildstrom SZ, Gotzsche O, Christensen E, Kober L, Torp-Pedersen C. 64-multislice detector computed tomography coronary angiography as potential alternative to conventional coronary angiography: a systematic review and meta-analysis. European Heart Journal. 2007;28(24):3042-3050.

106. Mowatt G, Cook JA, Hillis GS, Walker S, Fraser C, Jia X, Waugh N. 64-Slice computed tomography angiography in the diagnosis and assessment of coronary artery disease: systematic review and meta-analysis. Heart. 2008;94(11):1386-1393.

16

Thrombosis of Extra-cardiac Fontan, an Institutional Experience

Mohammed Al-Biltagi[1*], Amjad Al-Kouatli[2], Jameel Al-Ata[3], Ahmad Jamjoom[4] and Heba Abouzeid[5]

[1]*Department of Pediatric, Faculty of Medicine, Tanta University, Egypt.*
[2]*Department of Cardiology, King Faisal Specialist Hospital and Research Center, Jeddah, Saudi Arabia.*
[3]*Department of Cardiology, King Abdulaziz University Hospital, Jeddah, Saudi Arabia.*
[4]*Department of Cardiovascular, Cardiothoracic Surgery Section, King Faisal Specialist Hospital and Research Center, Jeddah, Saudi Arabia.*
[5]*Department of Pediatrics and Cardiovascular, Pediatric Cardiology Section, King Faisal Specialist Hospital and Research Center – Jeddah, Saudi Arabia and Faculty of Medicine, Zagazig University, Egypt.*

Authors' contributions

This work was carried out in collaboration between all authors. Author HA managed the cases, collected the data and wrote the first draft of the manuscript. Authors AA-K and JA-A managed the cases, did the cardiac catheterization and managed the literature searches, author MA-B managed the literature searches, and wrote the final draft of the study and author AJ revised the article and did the surgical part. All authors read and approved the final manuscript.

<u>Editor(s):</u>
(1) Francesco Pelliccia, Department of Heart and Great Vessels, University La Sapienza, Rome, Italy.
<u>Reviewers:</u>
(1) A. Papazafiropoulou, Department of Internal Medicine and Diabetes Center, Tzaneio General Hospital of Piraeus, Tzaneio.
(2) Dmitry Napalkov, Department of Internal Medicine, Moscow First State Medical University, Moscow, Russia.
(3) Pietro Scicchitano, Hospital "F. Perinei" della Murgia – Altamura, Bari, Italy.
(4) Alexander Berezin, Internal Medicine, Medical University, Zaporozhye, Ukraine.

ABSTRACT

Background: Thromboembolism can complicate Fontan surgery. There are few well designed studies in the literature to determine the epidemiology of thrombosis after Fontan.
Methods: We report the experience of King Faisal Specialist Hospital & Research Center- Jeddah, Kingdom of Saudi Arabia; regarding thrombosis of extra-cardiac Fontan pathways in 3 of our

---

*Corresponding author: E-mail: mbelrem@hotmail.com

patients; two patients were post- Fontan operation and one patient was post- Kawashima procedure & hepatic vein incorporation.
Results: The first and second patients developed thrombosis of Fontan pathways at one month & one year postoperatively respectively. In both patients, stenting of the extra-cardiac contegra re-established the patency of Fontan circuit and saved the risks of redo-surgeries. In the third patient, conduit occlusion was diagnosed 5 months postoperatively. Several attempts of cardiac catheterizations failed to penetrate the thrombosed conduit. Surgical re-intervention was inevitable.
Conclusions: The threshold for diagnostic and interventional cardiac catheterization should be lowered in post Fontan operation. Chronic oral anticoagulation may not prevent development of thrombosis despite therapeutic international normalized ratio (INR).

Keywords: Children; fontan; kawashima; thrombosis.

CORE TIP

Fontan surgery can be complicated with thromboembolism. We report the experience of King Faisal Specialist Hospital & Research Center- Jeddah, Kingdom of Saudi Arabia regarding thrombosis of extra-cardiac Fontan pathways in 3 patients; two patients were post-Fontan operation and one patient was post-Kawashima procedure & hepatic vein incorporation. The threshold for diagnostic and interventional cardiac catheterization should be lowered in post Fontan operation. Chronic oral anticoagulation may not prevent development of thrombosis despite therapeutic international normalized ratio (INR).

1. INTRODUCTION

The introduction of the Fontan operation dramatically improved the management of children with a functional single ventricle [1]. Hemodynamic fluctuations and thromboembolic complications are significant areas of concern during the postoperative care and follow up of patients with Fontan operation. Thromboembolic events may occur both in early and late periods after the Fontan procedure at a frequency higher than any other cardiac surgery in children other than prosthetic valve replacement and contribute to the failure of Fontan physiology. Occurrence of these thromboembolic events is not only because of hypercoagulable states but also due to the interaction of different factors including low flow states, stasis in the venous pathways, right-to-left shunts, blind cul-de-sacs, prosthetic material, and atrial arrhythmias [2,3]. The incidence of thrombosis after Fontan surgery has not been determined by prospective trials despite that some cross sectional surveys using transesophageal echocardiography found that the prevalence of thromboembolism following Fontan surgery ranges between 17% and 33%

[4]. The current article reported 3 cases with thromboembolic complications after Fontan and Kawashima procedures.

2. PATIENTS AND METHODS

We reported our own experience of Fontan circuit blockade in 3 patients. The medical records, laboratory data, serial echocardiograms and angiograms of the patients were reviewed by two separate investigators.

2.1 Patient 1

An 8 year old female child presented with the diagnosis of double outlet right ventricle, subpulmonic ventricular septal defect, pulmonary and sub-pulmonary stenosis, d-malposed great arteries and a tiny patent ductus arteriosus. The right ventricle was bipartite with no trabecular portion. The tricuspid valve annulus was overriding the ventricular septum with chordal attachment to the crest.

A bidirectional Glenn shunt, pulmonary artery banding, atrial septectomy & patent ductus arteriosus ligation were performed at the age of 5 months. Till the time of her Glenn surgery, the patient had sinus rhythm then episodes of junctional rhythm & junctional tachycardia were reported and became more frequent later on. After her Glenn shunt, the patient was kept on aspirin.

An extra-cardiac Fontan operation was done at the age of 4.5 years using a contegra size 20 mm to connect the inferior vena cava to the pulmonary arteries confluence. In the intensive care unit, the patient had a history of early post-operative hemothorax, sluggish inferior vena cava flow and low urine output. Cardiac catheterization elucidated stenosis at the junction of the inferior vena cava to contegra, sluggish inferior vena cava flow, a mean pressure of 16 mmHg at Fontan circuit, patent Glenn shunt & a right ventricular end diastolic pressure of 10-12 mm Hg. At this point no intervention was done as there was no gradient across the Fontan stenosis. The patient was managed to be extubated & discharged home in a stable condition. After Fontan operation, warfarin was added for a target PT- INR of 2-3.

Two weeks later, she presented with persistent vomiting & abdominal pain. Chest x-ray showed significant pleural effusion. Echocardiography showed mild pericardial effusion, dilated inferior vena cava and distal hepatic vein (Figs. 1 and 2) and patent Fontan connections with reduced flow velocity. The INR for the patient was within the therapeutic range over the last 6 months before the event.

She had significant hepatomegaly not responding to conservative management, therefore, cardiac catheterization was performed revealing thrombotic blockade of the entire Fontan circuit and the left pulmonary artery. Tissue plasminogen activator infusion was given at the intensive care unit for 48 hours. Repeat catheterization showed significant declotting of Fontan connections with improved but still

sluggish blood flow. Two 45 mm covered stents were used to stent the Fontan circuit (Fig. 3). After stenting, the liver size and abdominal pain showed some improvement and the echocardiography confirmed the patency of Fontan connections with reduced laminar flow velocity in inferior vena cava and hepatic veins, patent right Glenn shunt, with no superior or inferior vena cava dilatation (Fig. 4). At the time of her discharge, liver size regressed to 3 cm below the right costal margin in mid-clavicular line with better oral feeding tolerance and no more abdominal pain.

2.2 Patient 2

An 8 year old boy was diagnosed to have mesocardia, double inlet left ventricle, L-malposed great arteries, and pulmonary and sub-pulmonary stenosis. He presented to us at the age of 8 months with a remarkable desaturation (Oxygen saturation down to 20%); therefore an urgent Glenn shunt was performed. An extra-cardiac Fontan was done at the age of 3.7 years using a contegra size 14 mm with augmentation of proximal left pulmonary artery by bovine pericardium. Similar to the first patient, aspirin was started after the Glenn and warfarin was added after Fontan procedures.

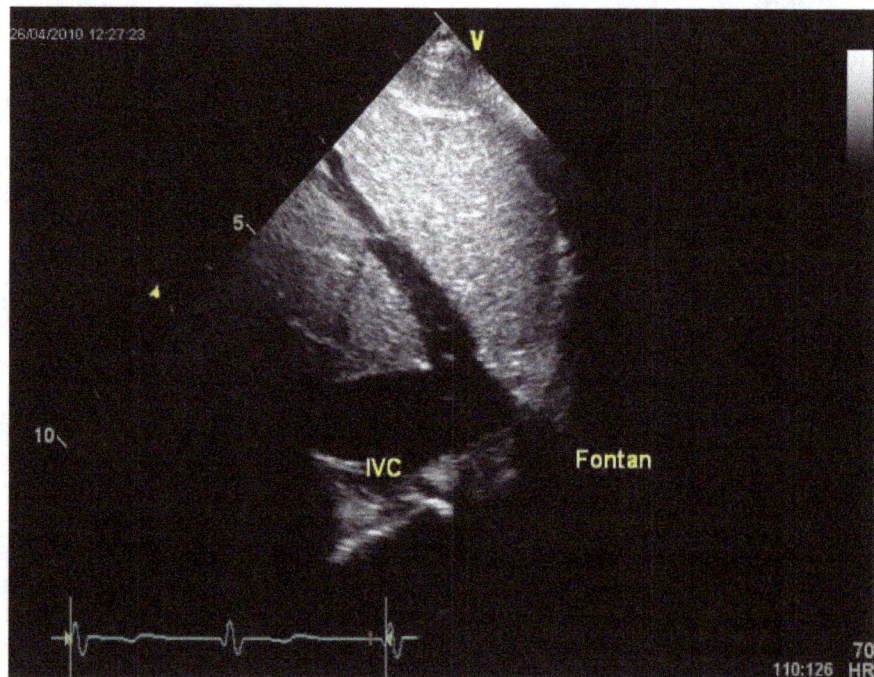

Fig. 1. Two-dimensional image of first patient showing dilated IVC and distal hepatic vein

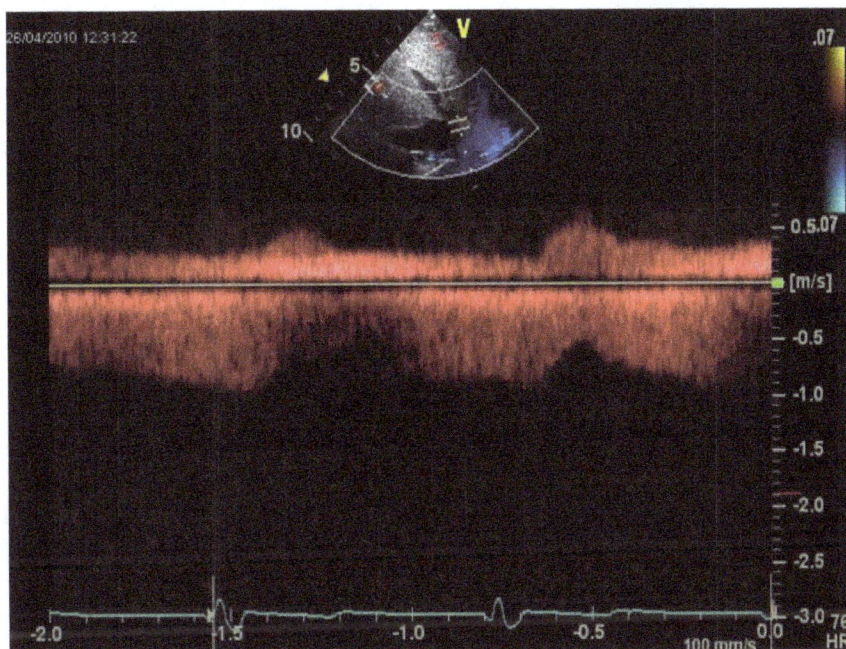

Fig. 2. Pulsed wave Doppler interrogation of IVC in first patient showing preserved respiratory related variation of IVC flow

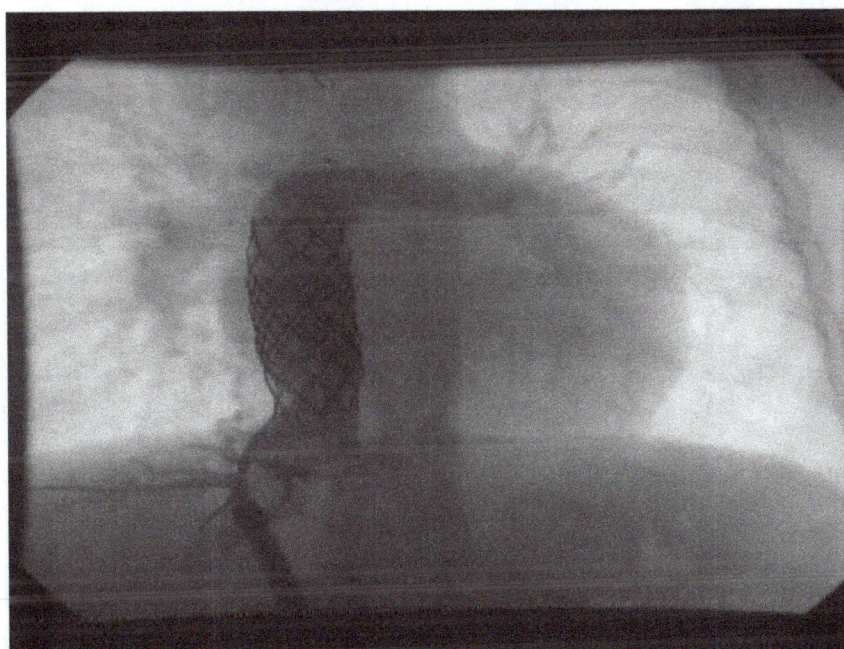

Fig. 3. Stenting of EC fontan contegra in first patient with angiography showing patency of fontan pathways

One year after Fontan operation, during one of the post-operative clinic visits, the family gave a history of an episode of jaundice, dark urine & leg swelling of one week duration and diagnosed as hepatitis at another hospital. On clinical examination, he was found to have an oxygen saturation of 95%, prominent superficial veins over the chest wall with filling from below upwards with an otherwise unremarkable chest examination, grade 1/6 systolic ejection murmur, no hepatomegaly, no lower limb edema, and INR was within the therapeutic range. Echocardiography revealed reduced flow velocity in the inferior vena cava with prominent flow in a hemiazygous vein versus an abnormal venous channel. An urgent cardiac catheterization was arranged to rule out presence of inferior vena caval obstruction and to delineate the venous anatomy. The INR for the patient was within the therapeutic range over the last 6 months before the event.

Cardiac catheterization revealed an inferior vena caval mean pressure of 18 mmHg, and superior vena caval mean pressure of 20 mmHg. Inferior vena caval angiograms showed totally obstructed Fontan contegra with blood clots and aneurysmal dilatation of the contegra. The systemic venous drainage was reaching the pulmonary circulation via dilated azygous & hemiazygous veins and multiple small collateral venous channels. Right internal jugular angiogram showed patent Glenn shunt & good size of right pulmonary artery. The contegra was stented with 2 covered stents 8 x 45 mm and 8 x 39 mm dilated to 15 mm (Fig. 5). After stenting, angiograms revealed stent protrusion into the left pulmonary artery directing the superior vena caval flow to the right pulmonary artery; however, there was a good flow to left pulmonary artery as well. Serial echocardiograms after stenting of the contegra

showed patent Fontan connections (Fig. 6). Shortly after stenting; a lung perfusion scan showed preferential flow to the right lung; 86% compared with 14% for the left lung. Repeat lung perfusion scan 8 months later showed improved left lung perfusion; 71%.

2.3 Patient 3

A 12 year old girl presented shortly after birth with polysplenia, unbalanced atrioventricular septal defect, double outlet right ventricle, and pulmonary stenosis. Her mitral valve was atretic, the ventricles were I-looped, left ventricle was hypoplastic & inferior vena cava was interrupted.

A left bidirectional Kawashima shunt was constructed together with pulmonary arterial banding at the age of 8 months. Three months later; cardiac catheterization revealed multiple large abdomino-pelvic veno-venous malformations. Lung perfusion scan showed no pulmonary arterio-venous malformations.

ECG demonstrated atrial rhythm with sick sinus syndrome at the age of 6 years. Hepatic vein incorporation was performed at the age of 9 years using a fenestrated extra-cardiac Dacron tube size 18 mm to anastomose the hepatic vein confluence to the right pulmonary artery.

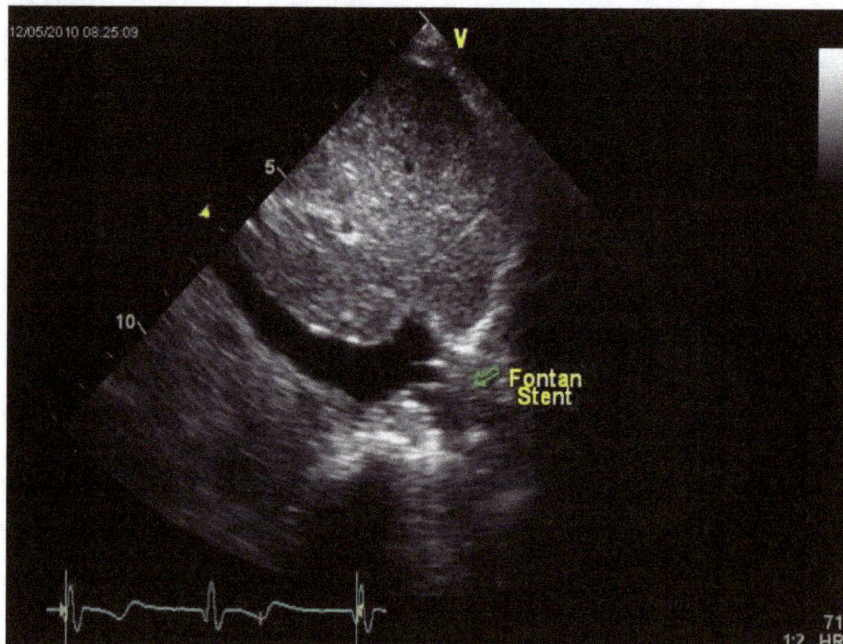

Fig. 4. Two-dimensional image of first patient illustrating the proximal part of Fontan stent with less IVC dilatation compared to Fig. 1

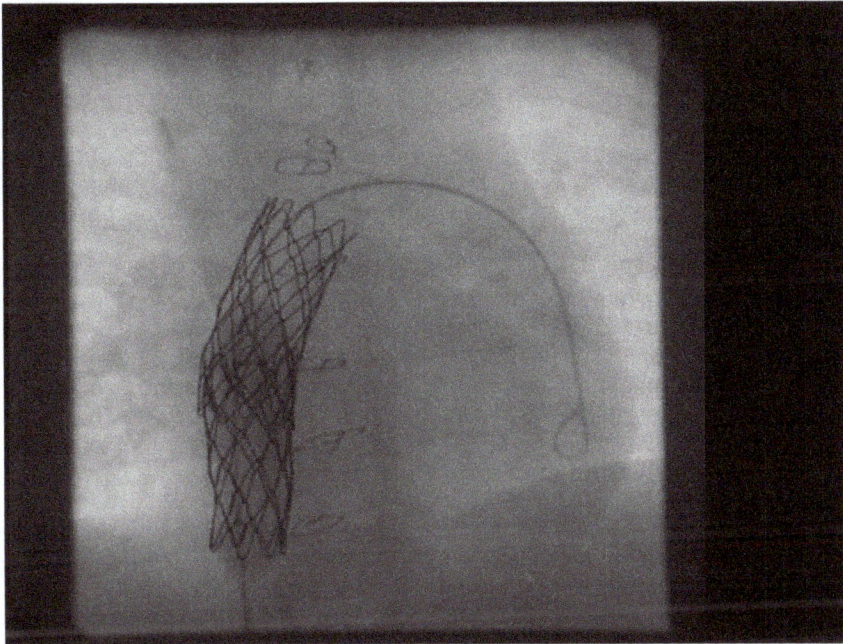

Fig. 5. Stenting of EC fontan contegra in second patient with balloon dilatation of the stent

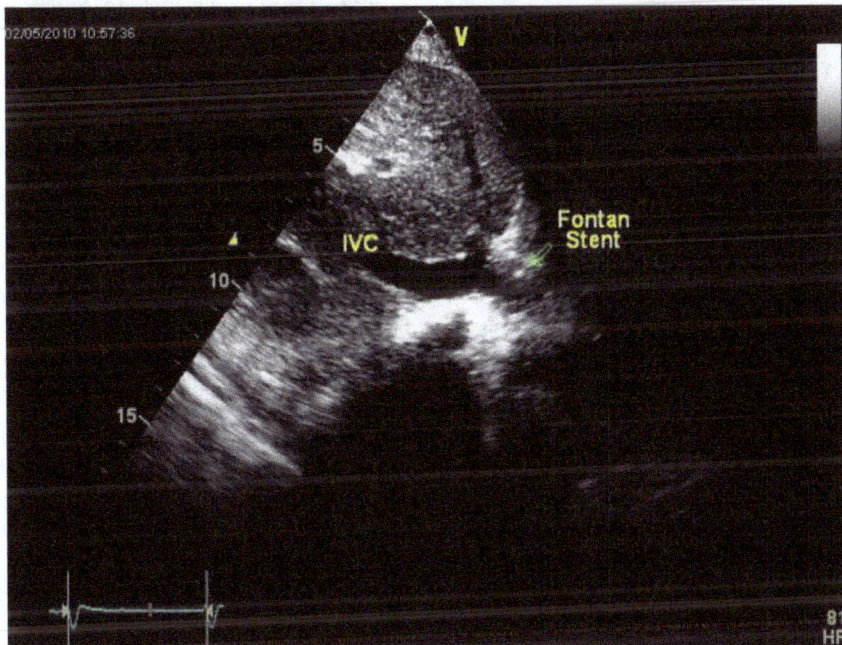

Fig. 6. Two-dimensional echocardiographic image showing the proximal part of Fontan stent in second patient

The main pulmonary artery stump was sutured and closed. A 5 mm fenestration was done between the conduit and the atrium because of the history of recurrent pleural effusion & chylothoraces. A permanent atrial & ventricular pacemaker leads were inserted due to presence of sick sinus syndrome & potential need for pacemaker in future. Postoperative echocardiography confirmed the patency of cavo-pulmonary connections & good ventricular functions. She was discharged home in a stable condition and ECG showing a normal sinus rhythm fluctuating with an adequate junctional rate.

Five months post-hepatic vein incorporation, she had minimal bilateral pitting lower limb edema and mild abdominal distension. Echocardiography revealed thrombosis involving the lower part of the conduit (Fig. 7). She was admitted to hospital with a normal Prothrombin time (PT)-INR as she missed two doses of her warfarin. However, by heparin infusion & resuming warfarin, PT- INR was readjusted to be therapeutic but worsening of thrombosis was detected by MRI. Lower limb edema progressed to be severe with development of ascites & bilateral pleural effusion.

Several catheterization attempts failed to penetrate the hepatic vein thrombosis despite local tissue plasminogen activator infusion into the clot site using the transhepatic & transjugular approaches. Tissue plasminogen activator treatment was complicated with intracranial haemorrhage that was managed conservatively. Surgical intervention was made for hepatic vein thrombectomy and conduit replacement with a Gortex tube size 16 mm. A permanent pacemaker generator was inserted using the old atrioventricular permanent leads.

3. DISCUSSION

The potential advantages of the extra-cardiac Fontan procedure include avoidance of myocardial ischemia (aortic cross-clamping), atrial incision, and intra-atrial suture lines, and the feasibility of early or late fenestration. However, the capacity of this procedure to reduce late atrial arrhythmias and the longevity of the extra-cardiac conduit remain unproven [5-8].

The use of conduits, either intra-cardiac or extra-cardiac, obviates the need of tunneling and has excellent results in patients with normal inferior vena caval drainage. Long-term patency of these conduits continues to be excellent regardless of the material used whether Gore-Tex, homograft tissue, or autologous pericardium [9]. Constructing a competent valve using the xenograft valved conduit (Contegra) in the extra-cardiac Fontan connection may maintain better forward flow into the pulmonary circulation [10]. The importance of hepatic blood flow for prevention or reversal of pulmonary arteriovenous malformation has been reported

[11–14]. Kawashima et al.; reported that pulmonary arteriovenous fistulae develop only rarely in older patients [15]. Arteriovenous fistulae did not develop in any of 14 patients who underwent the Kawashima procedure at age 12 years or older [15,16]. It has been assumed that in older patients, the "putative substance" in hepatic venous blood could be transported to the lung through well-developed systemic-to-pulmonary arterial collaterals [16]. The longevity of the extra-cardiac conduit remains the most controversial aspect of this surgical option. The mechanism of late conduit obstruction is likely longitudinal torsion of the conduit during rapid somatic growth in height. The facility of treating this obstruction by stent placement supports this mechanism [17].

The benefits of prophylactic anticoagulation or antiplatelet therapy for patients undergoing extracardiac conduit (ECC) Fontan procedure still are a matter of debate. Anticoagulant regimens in Fontan patients varied widely with a significant trend for warfarin use in patients with impaired haemodynamics. The options for primary prophylaxis include routine prophylactic anticoagulation with warfarin or antiplatelet agents.

Clearly patients receiving warfarin will have higher probability of bleeding complications compared to those receiving aspirin. Australian data suggests that with a well coordinated pediatric anticoagulation clinic; the annual risk of major bleeding in children on warfarin can be reduced to 0.05% per year. Warfarin requires regular monitoring, that can have a significant impact on family life [18,19]. However, Marrone et al.; evaluated the incidence of thromboembolism among patients undergoing extracardiac (ECC) Fontan procedures who received anticoagulation or antiplatelet therapy. They found that the overall thromboembolism rate was 5.2%. They analyzed the effect of different therapeutic strategies on the occurrence of thromboembolic and bleeding events among those patients. They found that the rate of thromboembolic and bleeding events associated with antiplatelet therapy is similar to that associated with anticoagulation therapy in patient underwent ECC Fontan [20]. A recent study done by Ohuchi et al.; 2015 showed that the haemostatic events occurred in 7% of cases; 45% of these events were haemorrhagic and 55% were thrombo-embolic. They found that low oxygen saturation was the only predictor of early postoperative thrombo-embolic events [21]. Risk factors for thrombotic complications include chronic systemic venous hypertension, protein-losing enteropathy, passive blood flow, atrial arrhythmias, conduit stenosis, coagulation factor abnormalities, and other several patient characteristics [22]. Some reports raise the prospect of warfarin causing reduced bone density in children although further studies are required to confirm this possible effect [23].

A multicenter, randomized clinical trial compared the use of acetylsalicylic acid versus heparin / warfarin targeting international normalized ratio of 2.0 to 3.0 as a primary thromboprophylaxis in children with Fontan procedure in children. The study found no significant difference between the two regimens in the primary thromboprophylaxis in the first 2 years after Fontan surgery. The thrombosis rate was suboptimal for both regimens, suggesting the need for alternative approaches [24]. Low molecular weight heparin (LMWH) demonstrated its safety with cost effectiveness as compared to other heparins [25]. Jacobs, et al.; assessed the impact of aspirin in reducing thromboembolic events after Fontan operation, initiating aspirin therapy from the first post-operative day. On follow up (over forty months), there were no documented thromboembolic events, hemorrhagic events or aspirin-related complications. It was concluded that low dose aspirin can be used safely and effectively in Fontan patients, and more aggressive anticoagulation may be unwarranted [26]. Saheb et al. found that triple antithrombotic therapy was more efficacious in reducing the occurrence of ischemic stroke in patients indicated for chronic oral anticoagulation, compared with double antiplatelet therapy (with aspirin and clopidogrel). However, it significantly increased the major and minor risks of bleeding [27]. Triple therapy with warfarin, aspirin, and a thienopyridine is advised in presence of atrial fibrillation. However, the safety of this regimen appeared suboptimal because of an increased risk of hemorrhagic complications. On the other hand, the combination of oral anticoagulation and an antiplatelet agent is suboptimal in preventing thromboembolic events and stent thrombosis; dual antiplatelet therapy may be considered only when a high hemorrhagic risk and low thromboembolic risk are perceived. Indeed, the need for prolonged multiple-drug antithrombotic therapy increases the bleeding risks when drug eluting stents are used [28]. Till now there are no convincing data that any prophylactic antithrombotic regimen is effective in reducing thromboembolism. Thromboembolic events can occur in patients receiving heparin, aspirin, warfarin, combinations or none of these.

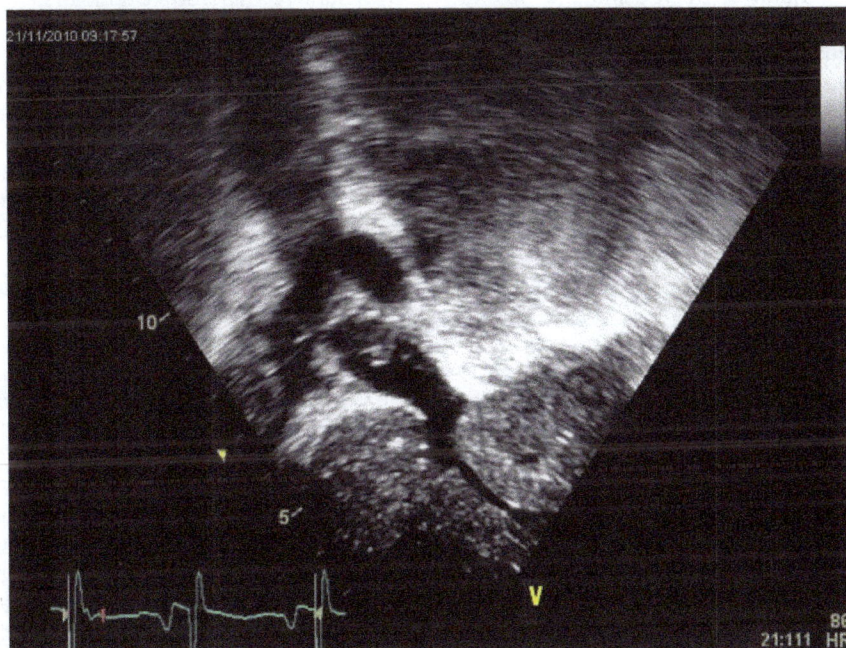

Fig. 7. Subcostal view in the third patient showing thrombosis of hepatic vein. Dilatation of hepatic vein is also noted

4. CONCLUSION AND RECOMMENDA-TION

The issue of anticoagulation therapy after Fontan procedure remains controversial [9,29]. Oral anticoagulation with warfarin did not prevent conduit thrombosis at least in 3 of our patients; hence, it does not seem reasonable to recommend chronic oral anticoagulation in those patients. However, we cannot draw any conclusion on epidemiology of thrombosis after Fontan from this three cases report and further data are needed to confirm this opinion. Perhaps, a smaller diameter conduit should be used in these patients to prevent stagnation of blood predisposing to thrombosis [9]. We emphasize the importance of careful evaluation of post-Fontan patients for thromboembolic events. Clinically suspicious occurrences must be thoroughly investigated. This may include transesophageal echocardiography when there is an alteration from baseline hemodynamics. The threshold for diagnostic and interventional cardiac catheterization should be lowered post-Fontan even in absence of echocardiographic evidence of inferior vena caval obstruction or lack of significant pressure gradient across contegral stenosis respectively. In agreement with Igor et al. [30], we do believe that multi-centre randomized trials are still needed to outline the methods of decreasing the adverse outcomes. The current uncertainty around the optimal primary prophylaxis regimes should be addressed to reduce the risk of thrombosis among children undergoing cardiac surgery in the future.

CONSENT

All authors declare that 'written informed consent was obtained from the patients' parents for publication of the case series and the accompanying images.

ETHICAL REVIEW BOARD

Approved publication of the case series.

COMPETING INTERESTS

Authors have declared that no competing interests exist.

REFERENCES

1.   Fontan F, Baudet E. Surgical repair of tricuspid atresia. Thorax. 1971;26(3):240-8. PMID: 5089489

2.   Canter CE. Preventing thrombosis after the Fontan procedure not there yet. J Am Coll Cardiol. 2011;2;58(6):652-3. DOI: 10.1016/j.jacc.2011.01.062. PMID: 2179843.

3.   Jacobs ML, Pourmoghadam KK. Thromboembolism and the role of anticoagulation in the fontan patient. Pediatr Cardiol. 2007;28(6):457-64. DOI: 10.1007/s00246-007-9006-1. PMID: 17762953

4.   Monagle P, Cochrane A, Roberts R, et al. A multicenter, randomized trial comparing heparin / warfarin and acetylsalicylic acid as primary thromboprophylaxis for 2 years after the Fontan procedure in children. J Am Coll Cardiol. 2011Aug2;58(6):645-51. DOI: 10.1016/j.jacc.2011.01.061. PMID: 21798429.

5.   Azakie A, McCrindle BW, Arsdell GV, et al. Extracardiac conduit versus lateral tunnel cavopulmonary connections at a single institution: impact on outcomes. J Thorac Cardiovasc Surg. 2001;122(6):1219-28. DOI: 10.1067/mtc.2001.116947 PMID: 11726899.

6.   Ovroutski S, Dähnert I, Alexi-Meskishvili V, et al. Preliminary analysis of arrhythmias after the fontan operation with extracardiac conduit compared with intra-atrial lateral tunnel. Thorac Cardiovasc Surg. 2001 Dec;49(6):334-7. DOI: DOI: 10.1055/s-2001-19009 PMID: 11745055.

7.   Kumar SP, Rubinstein CS, Simsic JM, et al. Lateral tunnel versus extracardiac conduit Fontan procedure: a concurrent comparison. Ann Thorac Surg. 2003;76(5):1389-96; discussion 1396-7. DOI: 10.1016/S0003-4975(03)01010-5. PMID: 14602257.

8.   Nakano T, Kado H, Ishikawa S, et al. Midterm surgical results of total cavopulmonary connection: clinical advantages of the extracardiac conduit method. J Thorac Cardiovasc Surg. 2004;127(3):730-7. DOI: 10.1016/S0022-5223(03)01184-X. PMID: 15001901.

9.   Konstantinov IE, Puga FJ, Alexi-Meskishvili VV. Thrombosis of intracardiac or extracardiac conduits after modified Fontan operation in patients with azygous continuation of the inferior vena cava. Ann Thorac Surg. 2001;72(5):1641-4. DOI: 10.1016/S0003-4975(01)03146-0 PMID: 11722058.

10. Baslaim G. Bovine valved xenograft (Contegra) conduit in the extracardiac

Fontan procedure: the preliminary experience. J Card Surg. 2008;23(2):146-9. DOI: 10.1111/j.1540-8191.2007.00524.x. PMID: 18304129.

11. Knight WB, Mee RBB. A cure for pulmonary arteriovenous fistulas? Ann Thorac Surg. 1995;59(4):999-1001. DOI: 10.1016/0003-4975(94)00735-P. PMID: 7695433.

12. King RM, Puga FJ, Danielson GK, et al. Extended indications for the modified Fontan procedure in patients with anomalous systemic and pulmonary venous return. In: Doyle EF, Engle MA, Gersony WM, Rashkind WJ, Talner NS, eds. Pediatric cardiology, proceedings of the Second World Congress. New York: Springer-Verlag, 1986;523–6.

13. Marcelletti C, Corno A, Giannico S, et al. Inferior vena cava-pulmonary artery extracardiac conduit: a new form of right heart bypass. J Thorac Cardiovasc Surg. 1990;100(2):228-32. PMID: 2143549.

14. Rosenkranz ER, Murphy DJ. Modified Fontan procedure for left atrial isomerism: alternative technique. Modified Fontan procedure for left atrial isomerism: alternative technique. Pediatr Cardiol 1995;16:201–3. PMID: 7567669.

15. Kawashima Y, Matsuki O, Yagihara T, et al. Total cavopulmonary shunt operation. Semin Thorac Cardiovasc Surg. 1994 Jan;6(1):17-20. PMID: 8167166.

16. Kawashima Y. Cavopulmonary shunt and pulmonary arteriovenous malformations. Ann Thorac Surg. 1997;63(4):930-2. PMID: 9124964.

17. Giannico S, Hammad F, Amodeo A, et al. Clinical outcome of 193 extracardiac Fontan patients: the first 15 years. J Am Coll Cardiol. 2006 May 16;47(10):2065-73. DOI:10.1016/J.JACC.2005.12.065. PMID: 16697327.

18. Newall F, Savoia H, Campbell J, et al. Anticoagulation clinics for children achieve improved warfarin management. Thromb Res. 2004;114(1):5-9. DOI: 10.1016/j.thromres.2004.03.018. PMID: 15262478 .

19. Andrew M, Marzinotto V, Brooker LA, et al. Oral anticoagulation therapy in pediatric patients: a prospective study. Thromb Haemost. 1994;71(3):265-9. PMID: 8029786.

20. Marrone C, Galasso G, Piccolo R, et al. Antiplatelet versus anticoagulation therapy after extracardiac conduit Fontan: a systematic review and meta-analysis. Pediatr Cardiol. 2011;32(1):32-9. DOI: 10.1007/s00246-010-9808-4. PMID: 20967441.

21. Ohuchi H, Yasuda K, Miyazaki A, et al. Prevalence and predictors of haemostatic complications in 412 Fontan patients: their relation to anticoagulation and haemodynamics. Eur J Cardiothorac Surg. 2015;47(3):511-9. DOI: 10.1093/ejcts/ezu145. PMID: 24699205.

22. Firdouse M, Agarwal A, Chan AK, Mondal T. Thrombosis and Thromboembolic Complications in Fontan Patients: A Literature Review. Clin Appl Thromb Hemost. 2014Jan24;20(5):484-492. DOI: 10.1177/1076029613520464 PMID: 24463598.

23. Barnes C, Newall F, Wong P, et al. Reduced bone density in children on long term warfarin therapy. Pediatr Res. 2005 Apr;57(4):578-81. DOI:10.1203/01.PDR.0000155943.07244.04. PMID: 15695604.

24. Monagle P, Cochrane A, Roberts R, et al. A multicenter, randomized trial comparing heparin/warfarin and acetylsalicylic acid as primary thromboprophylaxis for 2 years after the Fontan procedure in children. J Am Coll Cardiol. 2011Aug2;58(6):645-51. DOI: 10.1016/j.jacc.2011.01.061. PMID: 21798429.

25. Ciccone MM, Cortese F, Corbo F, et al. Bemiparin, an effective and safe low molecular weight heparin: a review. Vascul Pharmacol. 2014;62(1):32-7. DOI: 10.1016/j.vph.2014.03.001. Epub 2014 Mar 19. PMID: 24657810

26. Jacobs ML, Pourmoghadam KK, Geary EM, et al. Fontan's operation: is aspirin enough? Is coumadin too much? Ann Thorac Surg. 2002;73(1):64-8. PMID: 11834064.

27. Saheb KJ, Deng BQ, Hu QS, Xie SL, Geng DF, Nie RQ. Triple antithrombotic therapy versus double antiplatelet therapy after percutaneous coronary intervention with stent implantation in patients requiring chronic oral anticoagulation: a meta-analysis. Chin Med J (Engl). 2013;126(13):2536-42. PMID: 23823830.

28. Mila Menozzi, Andrea Rubboli, Antonio Manari, Rossana De Palma, Roberto Grilli. Triple antithrombotic therapy in patients with atrial fibrillation undergoing coronary artery stenting: hovering among bleeding risk, thromboembolic events, and stent

thrombosis. Thromb J. 2012;10:22. Published online 2012 October 18. DOI: 10.1186/1477-9560-10-22. PMCID: PMC3502192.

29. Monagle P, Cochrane A, McCrindle B, et al. Thromboembolic complications after fontan procedures--the role of prophylactic anticoagulation. J Thorac Cardiovasc Surg. 1998;115(3):493-8. PMID: 9535434.

30. Monagle P. Thrombosis in children with BT shunts, glenns and fontans. Prog Pediatr Cardiol. 2005;21:17-21.

17

Chasing Complications of Balloon Mitral Valvotomy

Shivakumar Bhairappa[1], Prakash Sadashivappa Surhonne[1], Shankar Somanna[1], Rohit Chopra[1*] and Cholenhally Nanjappa Manjunath[1]

[1]*Department of Cardiology, Sri Jayadeva Institute of Cardiovascular Sciences and Research, Rajiv Gandhi University of Health Sciences, Jayanagar 9th Block, BG Road, Bangalore 560069, India.*

Authors' contributions

This work was carried out in collaboration amongst all authors. All authors read and approved the final manuscript.

Editor(s):
(1) Shigenori Ito, Division of Cardiology, Nagoya City East Medical Center Nagoya, Japan.
Reviewers:
(1) Francesco Nappi, Department of Cardiac Surgery, Centre Cardiologique du Nord, France.
(2) Anonymous, University of Bari, Italy.
(3) Anonymous, Michigan State University, USA.

ABSTRACT

Percutaneous balloon mitral valvotomy (BMV) done for mitral stenosis (MS) though largely improved nowadays can be followed by multiple and rare procedure related complications. We present an interesting case of a 45 year old male with symptomatic severe mitral stenosis of rheumatic origin. Ultimately, though he underwent a successful BMV it was ridden with multiple rare procedure related complications. Intra procedural perforation of left atrium with hemopericardium and pericardial tamponade occurred in the first attempt at BMV while rupture of BMV balloon, multiple clots in left atrium (LA) after the procedure and a large pericardial effusion occurred in the second albeit successful attempt. To the best of our knowledge this is the first case to report multiple LA clots post BMV.

Keywords: Left atrial clot; left atrial perforation; complications; tamponade.

1. INTRODUCTION

Rheumatic heart disease (RHD) though uncommon in the developed countries continues to be highly prevalent in the developing nations. In the spectrum of rheumatic heart disease the most commonly affected valve is the mitral valve with Balloon Mitral Valvotomy (BMV) being the

---

Corresponding author: E-mail: drrc2306@gmail.com

most commonly done percutaneous procedure for mitral stenosis (MS) [1].

Over the last few decades the skill of the performing cardiologist as well as the techniques employed in BMV have improved vastly, thus greatly reducing the complications associated with it.

Yet no procedure is free of complications. Our case is one such where BMV done for symptomatic severe rheumatic MS was followed by multiple and rare complications.

2. CASE REPORT

A 45 year old Indian male presented with gradually progressive shortness of breath and exertional palpitations of 3 years duration. Over the last 3 years his shortness of breath and palpitations had worsened to NYHA class II. He had no other complaints and had an insignificant past medical and family history.

On examination he was found to have a regular heart rate of 70/min and blood pressure was 100/70 mm of Hg. Cardiac examination revealed a tapping apical impulse in the fifth intercostal space medial to mid clavicular line and on auscultation a loud first heart sound was heard at the apex. There was an opening snap (OS) followed by a long low pitched rumbling mid diastolic murmur with pre-systolic accentuation and a narrow A2- OS interval. Other systemic examination was within normal limits. An electrocardiogram done on arrival showed sinus rhythm with evidence of left atrial enlargement. Transthoracic echocardiogram (TTE) done showed severe valvular MS with valve area of 0.8 cm^2, enlarged left atrium (LA) (4.3 cm in parasternal long axis view), no mitral regurgitation with a Wilkin's score of 7. A diagnosis of RHD with severe MS was established. He was started on beta blockers and diuretics and a few days later he was admitted for BMV.

His pre procedural stay in the hospital was uneventful with routine haematology and biochemistry investigations being in normal range. A transesophageal echocardiogram (TEE) performed a day before the procedure showed no intracardiac thrombus (Fig. 1). While performing the procedure the next day, after interatrial septal puncture, on attempting to cross the mitral valve there occurred iatrogenic left atrial perforation with development of pericardial effusion and cardiac tamponade manifesting

clinically as hypotension. This called for an abandonment of the procedure and immediate pericardiocentesis was done with removal of 150 ml of bright red blood and a pericardial pigtail catheter was left in situ. He remained clinically stable after the pericardiocentesis with serial echocardiograms showing no further increase in pericardial fluid. After 2 days of observation the pigtail catheter was removed. He was closely observed and was discharged after 5 days with 2D echocardiogram showing mild pericardial effusion.

Two weeks later he was readmitted for a second attempt at BMV. TTE done before the procedure revealed mild pericardial effusion posterior to LA in parasternal long axis view (no increase in size compared to last echocardiogram) with no evidence of any clot in LA. He continued to be in sinus rhythm. The next day he was taken up for BMV and intra-procedurally 1500 units of unfractionated heparin (UFH) was administered initially at the time of sheath insertion and a second bolus of 3500 U (70 u/kg) was given after inter-atrial septal puncture. During the procedure, while inflating mitral valvotomy balloon to dilate the mitral valve the balloon failed to dilate proximally secondary to a tear at the proximal end of the inner layer of the balloon. Therefore this balloon was retrieved and the procedure was continued using a new balloon, with this there was a significant decline in left atrial pressure from 22 to 8 mm Hg after single inflation of 22 cubic centimetres of saline. Immediate post-procedural echocardiography done showed an increase in the mitral valve orifice area from 0.8 cm^2 to 1.7 cm^2 accompanied by a significant decline in gradient across the mitral valve with no suggestion of clinically significant iatrogenic mitral regurgitation or any clots in LA. He continued to remain clinically stable after the procedure.

Surprisingly, TTE performed next day showed mobile clots, one on the left atrial side of the interatrial septum and a second clot visualised near left atrial appendage (Figs. 2 and 3). A possibility of endothelial trauma leading to clot formation was considered and the patient was started on UFH and oral anticoagulation with Acenocoumarol. He was discharged after achievement of target prothrombin time (PT).

A week later he continued to remain unremarkable, his coagulation parameters showed a prothrombin time of 30.7 seconds with an international normalized ratio of 2.15. Review

TTE done showed resolution of both the clots. However, he had now developed a large pericardial effusion with no signs of pericardial tamponade (Fig. 4). There was no drop in his haemoglobin levels, total leucocyte and platelet counts were normal and ESR was mildly elevated (39 mm/hr). His other laboratory parameters continued to remain normal.

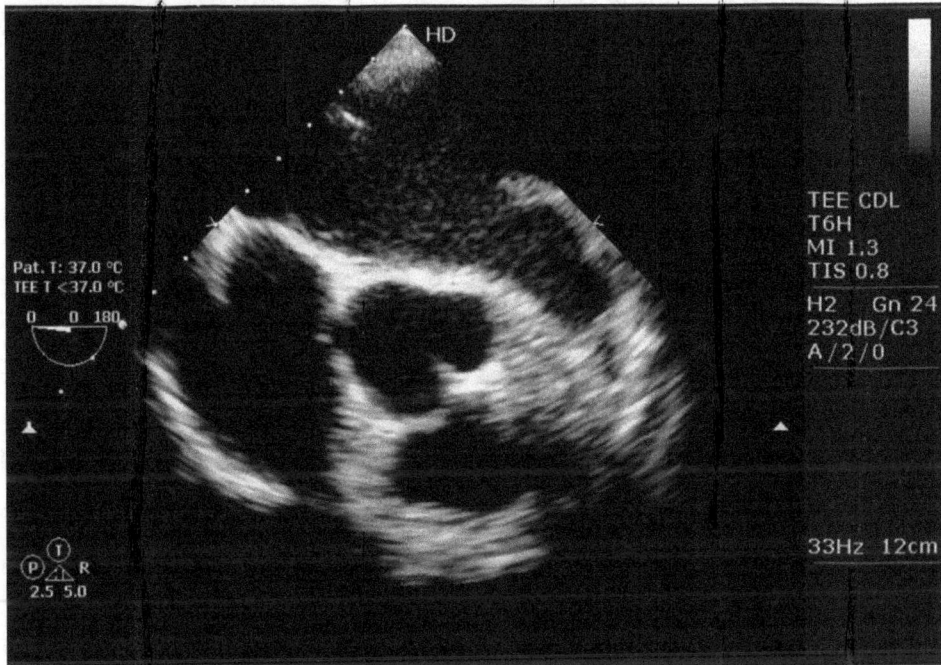

Fig. 1. Transesophageal imaging of the patient at zero degree showing grade I spontaneous ECHO contrast in LA with no clot in left atrium/atrial appendage

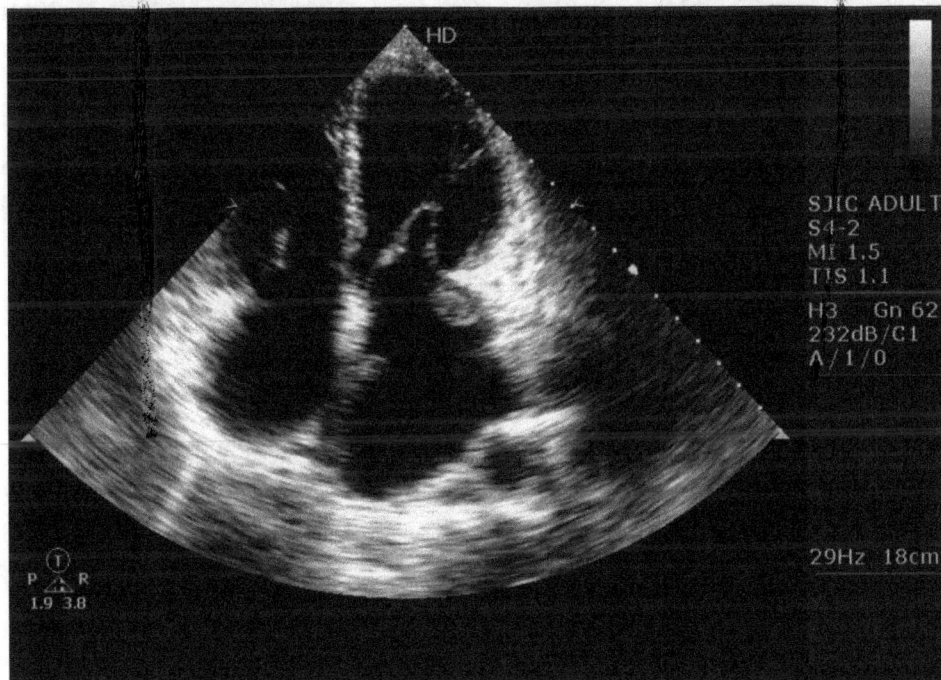

Fig. 2. Apical four chamber view showing clots, one on interatrial septum towards LA and second near left atrial appendage

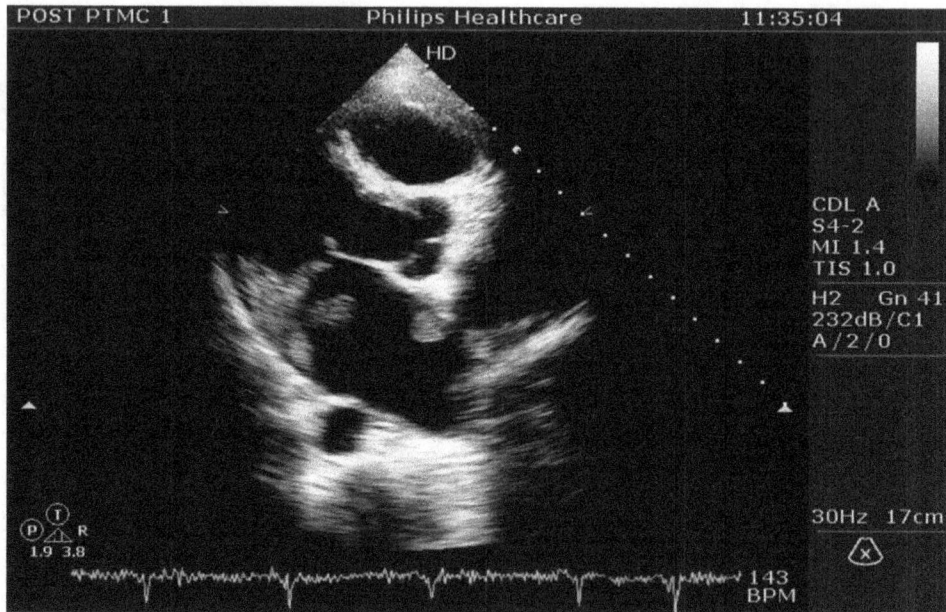

Fig. 3. Parasternal long axis view showing two distinct clots in left atrium

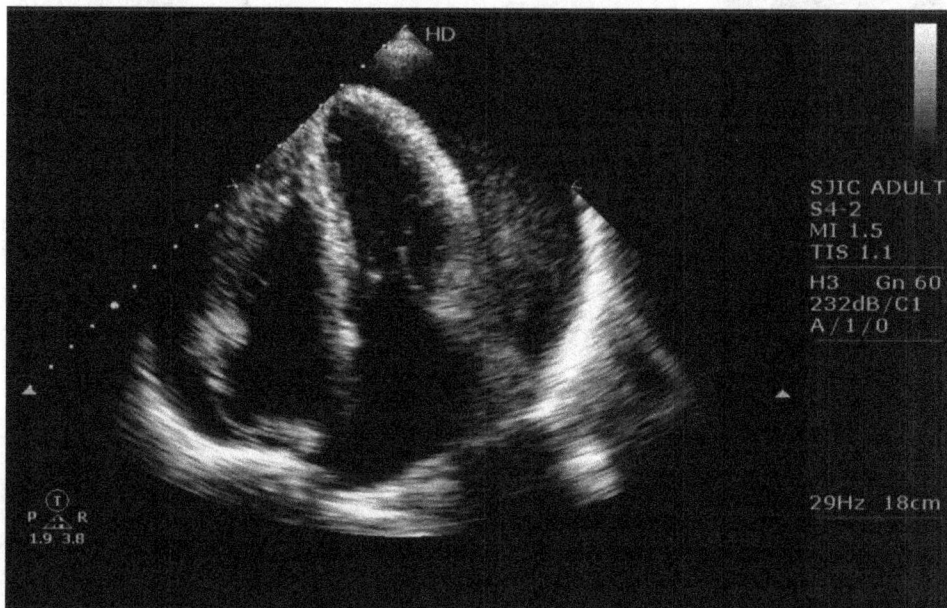

Fig. 4. Large pericardial effusion seen in apical four chamber view

In view of the large pericardial effusion he was readmitted, fresh frozen plasma was administered and Acenocoumarol was withheld. Pericardiocentesis was not considered as he was clinically stable with no hemodynamic compromise. Serial TTE done showed a decrease in pericardial effusion and hence a decision to discharge him was taken after one week of close observation. He was discharged on beta blockers and Acenocoumarol was stopped. A month later he continued to be in good health and TTE performed showed mild pericardial effusion with no clot.

3. DISCUSSION

RHD continues to remain a major cardiac problem with a prevalence rate of 4.54/1000 persons in India [2]. With the advent of BMV, management options have dramatically improved. BMV has shown equal or better success rates and comparable restenosis rates in comparison to surgical mitral commissurotomy [3,4].

Most of the complications of BMV have been noted to occur during the procedure i.e., while performing interatrial septal puncture, manipulating BMV balloon in the LA or while inflating the balloon during commissurotomy [5]. Hemopericardium is the most common serious complication with an incidence of up to 2% [6]. Mortality with hemopericardium is rare with prompt recognition and immediate pericardial drainage either by pericardiocentesis or surgical pericardiotomy. In our case LA rupture was recognized and managed early with pericardiocentesis.

Rupture of valvotomy balloons has been described and is more common with used balloons [7,8]. Clot at interatrial septum following BMV is an extremely rare occurrence with very few case reports having been described in literature [9,10]. To the best of our knowledge, our case is the first case to describe formation of clot at multiple sites in LA namely at the LA side of interatrial septum and near LA appendage, possibly due to endothelial injury sustained while manipulating the hardware in LA. In our case patient developed multiple clots in LA despite anticoagulating the patient during the procedure. As the procedure time was short (around 20 minutes) activated clotting time (ACT) was not monitored.

The development of pericardial effusion 10 days after the procedure could be due to an incompletely healed LA rent which could have led to the development of a gradually increasing pericardial effusion after starting the patient on anticoagulation.

4. CONCLUSION

Left atrial perforation during BMV is a potentially lethal complication. Proper technique of septal puncture and gentle manipulation of hardware in LA can prevent this complication. Patients developing LA perforation should be followed up closely and repeat attempt, after failed initial procedure, should be undertaken only after allowing the rent in LA to heal adequately. Intracardiac clot formation after the procedure, although rare, may still occur despite

anticoagulating with heparin during the procedure. From our experience we suggest that ACT should always be checked and maintained adequately in all patients undergoing BMV.

CONSENT

It is not applicable.

ETHICAL APPROVAL

It is not applicable.

ACKNOWLEDGMENTS

This case has not been presented in any journal or scientific meeting. There were no external funding sources for this case reporting.

COMPETING INTERESTS

Authors have declared that no competing interests exist.

REFERENCES

1. WHO study group, Rheumatic fever and rheumatic heart disease. WHO technical report series No. 764. Geneva: World health organization; 1988.

2. Ahemad MZ JP, Narayanan SN. Rheumatic chorea in children: A study of prevalence of clinical and echocardiographic valvular involvement. Indian Heart J. 1999;51:694.

3. Turi ZG, Reyes VP, Raju BS, Raju AR, Kumar DN, Rajagopal P, Sathyanarayana PV, Rao DP, Srinath K, Peters P. Percutaneous balloon versus surgical closed commissurotomy for mitral stenosis: A prospective, randomized trial. Circulation. 1991;83:1179 –1185.

4. Arora R, Nair M, Kalra GS, Nigam M, Khalilullah M. Immediate and long-term results of balloon and surgical closed mitral valvotomy: A randomized comparative study. Am Heart J. 1993;125:1091-1094.

5. Nobuyoshi M, Hamasaki N, Kimura T, Nosaka H, Yokoi H, Yasumoto H, Horiuchi H, Nakashima H, Shindo T, Mori T. Indications, complications, and short-term clinical outcome of percutaneous transvenous mitral commissurotomy. Circulation. 1989;80:782-792.

6. Martinez-rios MA, Tovar S, Luna J, Eid-Lidt G. Percutaneous mitral commissurotomy. Cardiol Rev. 1999;7:108-116.

7.   Schilling JR, Francis CM, Shaw TRD, Norell MS. Inoue balloon rupture during dilatation of calcified mitral valves. Br Heart. 1995;72:390.

8.   Singla V, Patra S, Patil S, Ramalingam R. Accura balloon rupture during percutaneous trans-septal mitral commissurotomy: A rare and potentially fatal complication. BMJ Case Reports; 2013.
DOI:10.1136/bcr-2013-009819.

9.   Raman VG, Ramachandran P, Kansal N. An unusual complication of cardiac catheterisation during BMV. BMJ Case Rep 2011; 2011.

10.   Yuksel IO, Kucukseymen S, Cagirci G, Arslan S. A case of percutaneous mitral balloon valvuloplasty complicated by pericardial effusion and thrombus formation on the interatrial septum. Turk Kardiyol Dern Ars. 2014;42(8):747-50 (in Turkish).

18

Primary Percutaneous Coronary Intervention in a Patient with Acute Inferior Myocardial Infarction and Agenesis of Right Coronary Artery. "In Search of a Coronary Ostium"

Gabriele Giacomo Schiattarella[1], Fabio Magliulo[1], Vito Di Palma[1], Giovanni Esposito[1] and Plinio Cirillo[1*]

[1]*Department of Advanced Biomedical Sciences, School of Medicine, University of Naples Federico II, Naples, Italy.*

Authors' contributions

This paper was carried out in collaboration between all authors. Authors GGS, FM and PC perform the case and wrote the manuscript. Authors VDP and GE approve the manuscript. All authors read and approved the final manuscript.

Editor(s):
(1) Gen-Min Lin, Division of Cardiology, Hualien-Armed Forces General Hospital, National Defense Medical Center, Taiwan.
Reviewers:
(1) Vasily I. Kaleda, Department of Adult Cardiac Surgery, Ochapowski Regional Hospital #1, Krasnodar, Russia.
(2) Aşkın Ender Topal, Cardiovascular Surgery, Dicle University, Medicine Faculty, Turkey.
(3) Searefttin Demir, General cardiology, Interventional Cardiology, Heart Failure, Heart Disease at Pregnancy, Adana State Hospital, Turkey.

ABSTRACT

Coronary arteries with anomalous origin from the aorta may represent a trouble for interventional cardiologist, in particular in setting of acute coronary syndromes. Research of coronary ostium may cause crucial delay in reperfusion with important consequences for myocardial salvage. We described a case of inferior ST-elevation myocardial infarction (STEMI) complicated by bradyarrythmia and hypotension, and treated with primary percutaneous coronary intervention (PCI) in a patient with agenesis of right coronary ostium. The patient had only a single left coronary artery occluded at the distal portion before a bifurcation with a huge branch that encompassed the theoretical territories of right coronary artery.

*Corresponding author: E-mail: pcirillo@unina.it

Keywords: Coronary anomalies; percutaneous coronary intervention; ST-elevation myocardial infarction.

1. INTRODUCTION

Coronary arteries with anomalous origin from the aorta or anomalous course may represent a trouble for interventional cardiologists. Percutaneous treatment of significant atherosclerotic stenosis of these arteries may be very challenging. These abnormalities are conventionally defined as variants occurring in less than 1% of the general population [1]. Their clinical presentations are widely variant, ranging from diagnosis after autopsy in young subjects with sudden cardiac death to widely asymptomatic forms [1]. Because these anomalous coronary arteries are usually not associated with other congenital cardiac malformations, patients do not show any clinical manifestations, thus, they are usually found, often incidentally, during coronary angiography. In the present report we describe the case of a patient admitted to our hospital with diagnosis of inferior ST-elevation myocardial infarction (STEMI) complicated by bradyarrythmia and hypotension and treated with primary percutaneous coronary intervention (PCI). The peculiarity was that the patient did not have the right coronary artery (RCA) in the coronary tree.

2. CASE REPORT

A 46-year old man, heavy smoker, with history of arterial hypertension was admitted to our emergency room. He presented with chest pain, nausea, hypotension and diaphoresis since 90 minutes ago. At admission, the electrocardiography (ECG) showed elevation of the ST segment in the inferior leads with concomitant reciprocal depression in lateral leads (Fig. 1). In addition, an ultra-sensitivity cardiac troponin T assay was positive and a fast-track echocardiography displayed ipo-akinesia of the inferior and postero-lateral walls. Accordingly, a diagnosis of inferior wall ST-elevation myocardial infarction (STEMI) was made. The patient received 500 mg of acetylsalicylic acid intravenously and 180 mg of ticagrelor orally and was addressed to the cath-lab to perform primary PCI. In the cath-lab, patient had severe bradycardia and hypotension, thus, on the basis of ECG, we decided to immediately approach right coronary artery (RCA) with a 6 French Judkins right guiding catheter (Medtronic, Inc., Minneapolis, MN, USA) in order to obtain reperfusion as soon as possible. Surprisingly, we

were unable to achieve selective cannulation of RCA ostium by using this guiding catheter, thus, we tried to approach the coronary ostium by using other different guiding catheters including both Judkins and Amplatz coronary catheters, with different curves, but our tries were unsuccessful. The patient was stabilized by intravenous use of Atropine as well as fluid administration, and thus, we moved to evaluate left coronary artery by using a 6 French Judkins diagnostic catheter. The angiography of left coronary artery revealed atherosclerotic disease of left main and left anterior descending (LAD) in absence of significant stenosis. Moreover, the angiography showed the thrombotic occlusion of circumflex at its distal portion, close to the origin of three marginal obtuse branches, with a TIMI 0 flow (Figs. 2 A-B). We judged this occlusion to be the culprit lesion responsible for the STEMI. Thus, we approached and crossed it with 0.014 inch Balance Middle Weight Universal, (BMW - Guidant Corp., Santa Clara, California). Then, we performed manual thrombus aspiration with the Export catheter (Medtronic Inc., Minneapolis, Minnesota) obtaining vessel recanalization. Finally, an everolimus eluting stent Xience Xped (3,5 mm x 33 mm, Abbott® Vascular, Santa Clara, USA) was implanted obtaining a TIMI 3 flow. Surprisingly, the final angiography revealed that circumflex extension encompassed the theoretical territories of RCA till the aorta (Figs. 3 A-B). An angiography of aorta was performed to witness that RCA was absent, confirming the agenesis of RCA ostium in the absence of any other anomalies (type I aortic arch). The patient was discharged six days after hospitalization under optimized drugs therapy, with a complete recovery of myocardial function without regional ipo-akinesia.

3. DISCUSSION

Coronary artery anomalies (CAAs) comprise a large number of very different conditions, with an extreme variability in clinical severity. According to the classification of Angelini and coworkers [2], these coronary anomalies may be reduced to the following categories:

- Anomalies of origin and course.
- Anomalous location of coronary ostium outside normal "coronary" aortic sinuses (eventually also located into left or right ventricle, pulmonary artery, aortic arch,

innominate artery, descending thoracic aorta and other) or anomalous origination of coronary ostium from opposite, facing "coronary".

- Anomalies of intrinsic coronary arterial anatomy (such as congenital ostial stenosis or atresia, absent coronary artery of coronary hypoplasia, anomalous coronary course, coronary crossing, anomalous origination of posterior descending artery, split RCA or LAD, and others).
- Anomalies of coronary termination (inadequate ramifications, fistulas).
- Anomalous collateral vessels.

The incidence of CAAs seems to be extremely variable because it changes according to the different studies dealing with this issue. Specifically, Angelini et al. reported, in a series of 1950 patients subjected to coronary angiography, a global incidence of 5.64% [2], with a significant prevalence of anomalous origin of the RCA from the left sinus (0.92%) and of anomalous origin of the left coronary artery from the right sinus (0.15%). Other anomalies, such as myocardial bridge and split RCA, are not considered coronary anomalies but normal variants, due to their high prevalence (>1%) [2]. In another study, a review of the clinical and necropsy charts showed that 33% of sudden cardiac death of young militaries under training was related to anomalous origin of left coronary artery [3] while in a Israelite study concerning suddenly dead subjects < 40 years, the incidence of CAAs was 0.6% [4]. Anomalous origin and course of coronary artery might be discovered in about 0.29% of subjects undergoing coronary angiography; the most frequent types seem to be anomalous origin of Left Circumflex Artery (LCxA) from RCA/right

sinus of Valsalva (0.169%) while anomalous origin of RCA from Left Anterior Descending (LAD) or LCxA is less frequent, with an estimated prevalence of about 0.03% for pathologies involving RCA or left main/LAD [5]. Similarly, anomalous origin of RCA from LAD and/or LCxA artery has an estimated prevalence of 0.036% [5]. Single coronary artery may be associated with other congenital anomalies, such as transposition of the great vessels, coronary arteriovenous fistula, or bicuspid aortic valve [6]; its prognosis appears usually benign. This kind of coronary anomaly is not usually responsible of coronary hypoperfusion, but a potential increased risk of ischemic heart disease has been reported (till to 15% of prevalence in some studies) [7]. However, it is intuitive that a stenosis of a coronary artery in subjects with a single coronary vessel has a such different clinical meaning than in patients with a normal coronary tree. Thus, coronary abnormality must be always kept in mind specially in those cases in which the coronary ostium is not easy to engage or visualize by direct injection of contrast medium. The suspect of anomalies of the coronary tree has an important role in approaching patients with STEMI, because "the search of the ostium" might be time consuming and finally it leads to delay in the reperfusion time and, consequently, in prognosis. In the present case, after few attempts with several guiding catheters of engaging the right coronary ostium, we suspected a coronary anomaly and decided to perform angiography of the left coronary artery to evaluate and treat an hypothetical culprit lesion of this vessel. In such contexts, injection of contrast medium into the sinus of Valsalva and aortic angiography, preferably in two different projections, can help to individuate any form of CAAs.

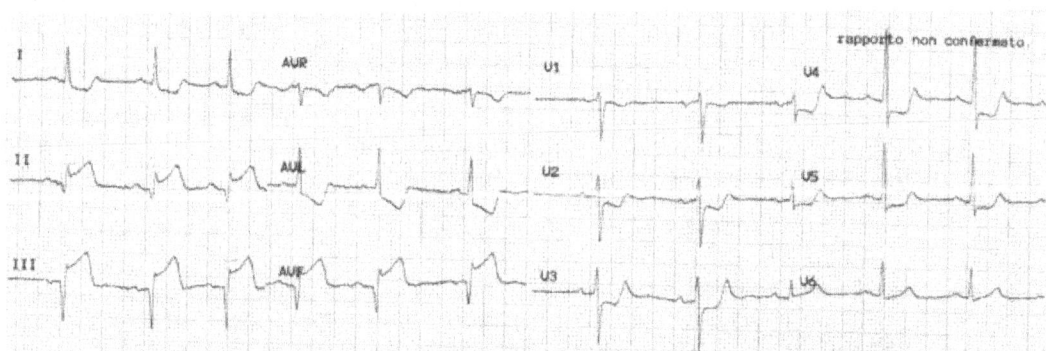

Fig. 1. An ECG revealing significant ST segment elevation in II, III and aVF leads with significant ST segment depression with high R waves in V2-V5 leads

A

B

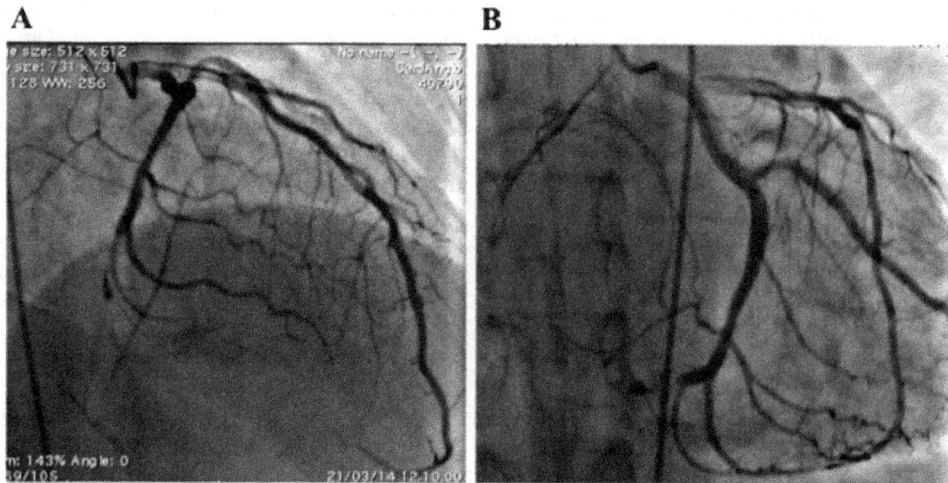

Fig. 2. A coronary angiography revealed a thrombotic occlusion of the distal portion of circumflex branch of left coronary artery visualized in both left anterior oblique projection (A) and anteroposterior caudal projection (B)

A

B

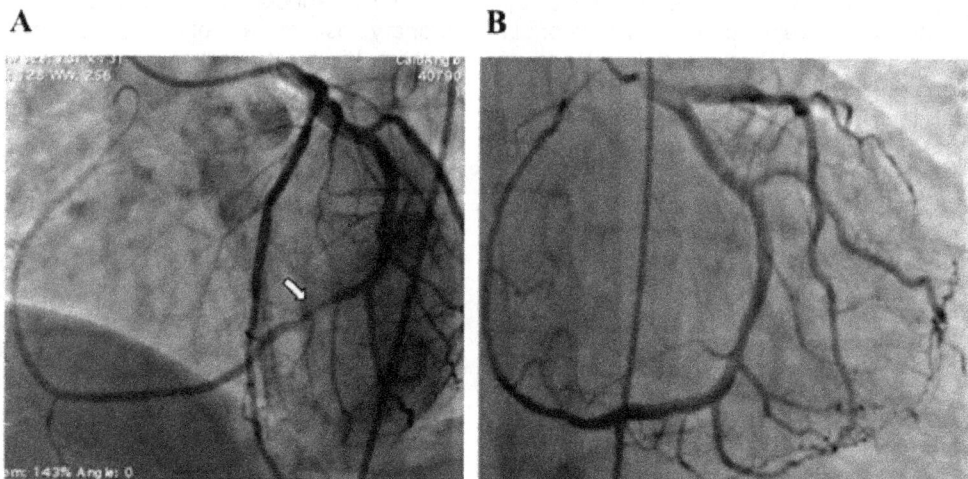

Fig. 3. A. An angiography after manual thrombus aspiration with the Export catheter showed partial vessel recanalization and a critical stenosis of circumflex branch (arrow). B. The final angiography after everolimus-eluting-stent (Xience Xped 3,5 mm in diameter x 33 mm long) implantation showed excellent result without thrombus evidence, TIMI grade 3 and a long patent vessel extending to the theoretical territories of RCA

Few other cases of unexpected RCA agenesis at coronary angiogram have been described in the context of acute coronary syndromes. Turhan and colleagues reported the case of patient evaluated for chest pain and ECG signs of myocardial ischemia. The angiography revealed a RCA arising from distal LCxA, following course, retrogradely, of the normal artery and terminating near sinus of Valsalva [6]. In another report, Papadopoulos et al. presented a case of acute coronary syndrome in which coronary angiography revealed agenesis of RCA ostium

and RCA originating from distal LCxA. [8]. Moreover, Chung et al. described the case of a 77-year-old man subjected to angiographic study for chest pain. Left coronary angiography showed a dominant LCxA, with an aberrant RCA from distal LCxA, which crossed the crux and continued to the right atrioventricular groove, covering the territory of the right coronary artery. After several unsuccessful attempts to engage RCA ostium, aortography confirmed the absence of the RCA ostium, and a subsequent contrast-enhanced 64-slice multi-detector cardiac tomography also confirmed the absence of this vessel showing an extended LCxA supplying RCA territory [9]. Finally, Pourbehi et al described a coronary angiography demonstrated a single coronary artery originating from the left Valsalva sinus. The angiography revealed significant stenosis in the mid-portion of the LAD and in the distal portion of the LCxA, where there was the origin of an aberrant RCA. Angioplasty and stenting of the LAD and LCxA were done with durable resolution of symptoms [10]. In all these cases, patients were at "low risk" for acute coronary syndromes, on the contrary, in the present report we deal with an ST-elevation myocardial infarction with unstable clinical conditions in which the anomalous LCxA was the culprit vessel, causing hemodynamic instability.

4. CONCLUSION

The main lesson to extrapolate from this case and the cited ones is: never forget the eventuality of a CAAs during a coronary angiography exam! The suspicion is often the first way to find them, so interventional cardiologists should always keep their existence in mind.

CONSENT

All authors declare that written informed consent was obtained from the patient for publication of this case report and accompanying images.

ETHICAL APPROVAL

It is not applicable.

COMPETING INTERESTS

Authors have declared that no competing interests exist.

REFERENCES

1. Angelini P, Velasco JA, Flamm S. Coronary anomalies: incidence, pathophysiology, and clinical relevance. Circulation. 2002;105:2449-2454.

2. Angelini P. Coronary artery anomalies: an entity in search of an identity. Circulation. 2007;115:1296-1305.

3. Eckart RE, Scoville SL, Campbell CL, et al. Sudden death in young adults: a 25-year review of autopsies in military recruits. Ann Intern Med. 2004;141:829-834.

4. Drory Y, Turetz Y, Hiss Y, et al. Sudden unexpected death in persons less than 40 years of age. Am J Cardiol. 1991;68:1388-1392.

5. Yuksel S, Meric M, Soylu K, et al. The primary anomalies of coronary artery origin and course: A coronary angiographic analysis of 16,573 patients. Exp Clin Cardiol. 2013;18:121-123.

6. Turhan H, Duru E, Yetkin E, et al. Right coronary artery originating from distal left circumflex: an extremely rare variety of single coronary artery. Int J Cardiol. 2003; 88:309-311.

7. Shirani J, Roberts WC. Solitary coronary ostium in the aorta in the absence of other major congenital cardiovascular anomalies. J Am Coll Cardiol. 1993;21: 137-143.

8. Papadopoulos DP, Moyssakis I, Athanasiou A, et al. Right coronary ostium agenesis with absence of the right coronary artery: a rare case of non-ST elevation coronary syndrome. Clin Anat. 2006;19:345-346.

9. Chung SK, Lee SJ, Park SH, et al. An extremely rare variety of anomalous coronary artery: right coronary artery originating from the distal left circumflex artery. Korean Circ J. 2010;40:465-467.

10. Pourbehi MR, Amini A, Farrokhi S. Single coronary artery with anomalous origin of the right coronary artery from the distal portion of left circumflex artery: a very rare case. J Tehran Heart Cent. 2013;8:161-163.

19

Non-linear Analysis of Heart Rate Variability Improves Differential Diagnosis between Parkinson Disease and Multiple System Atrophy

Donatella Brisinda[1], Francesco Fioravanti[1], Emilia Iantorno[1], Anna Rita Sorbo[1], Angela Venuti[1], Claudia Cataldi[1], Kristian Efremov[1] and Riccardo Fenici[1*]

[1]Clinical Physiology-Biomagnetism Center, Catholic University of Sacred Heart, Rome, Italy.

Authors' contributions

This work was carried out in collaboration between all authors. Authors DB and RF designed the study, wrote the protocol. Authors DB and EI managed the literature searches, performed patient's recordings and compiled clinical database. Authors EI, CC, FF, KE and AV performed signal analyses and statistical evaluation of the results of the study. Author DB wrote the first draft of the manuscript. Author RF edited the final version of the manuscript. All authors read and approved the final manuscript.

Editor(s):
(1) Anonymous.
Reviewers:
(1) Patricia Siques, Institute of Health Studies, Universidad Arturo Prat, Chile.
(2) Anonymous, Safarik's Universitz, Slovakia.

ABSTRACT

Aims: Parkinson's disease (PD) and multiple system atrophy (MSA) are neurodegenerative disorders characterized by motor "parkinsonian" symptoms and non-motor symptoms related to autonomic nervous system (ANS) dysfunction. The latter can be quantified with the analysis of Heart Rate Variability (HRVa) and of its complexity. In this study nonlinear (NL) HRV complexity parameters were calculated to assess their predictive accuracy as markers of "disease" useful for early differentiation between PD and MSA in parkinsonian syndromes of uncertain diagnosis.
Study Design: Observational study.
Place and Duration of Study: Clinical Physiology-Biomagnetism Center, Policlinico A. Gemelli, Rome Italy. Patients enrolled from January 2010 to October 2013.
Methodology: 51 patients [25 with "certain" diagnosis of PD, 9 with a "highly probable" diagnosis of MSA and 17 with parkinsonian syndromes of uncertain neurological definition (6 with "undefined

Corresponding author: E-mail: feniciri@rm.unicatt.it

parkinsonism" and 11 with "suspected MSA")] and 40 age-matched healthy control subjects were studied. Short-term NL HRVa was performed during daily activity and during REM/NREM sleep from 24 h ECG recordings. Discriminant analysis (DA) was used to identify which NL HRV parameters (or their combination) were efficient to differentiate between PD and MSA in cases of uncertain diagnosis.

Results: Compared with healthy controls, most NL HRV parameters were significantly altered in patients ($p<0.05$), during both active and passive awakeness and during sleep. Most evident HRV abnormalities were found during active awakeness in MSA. DA of recurrence plot parameters provided the best predictive accuracy (76.5%) for the classification of parkinsonian patients with uncertain diagnosis.

Conclusion: NL HRVa is efficient in differentiating MSA from PD and may improve earlier diagnosis in patients with parkinsonian symptoms of uncertain nature, useful to address second level diagnostic steps and to guide more individualized drug treatment.

Keywords: Autonomic nervous system; Parkinson disease; multiple system atrophy; non linear HRV analysis; discriminant analysis.

1. INTRODUCTION

Parkinson's disease (PD) and multiple system atrophy (MSA) are neurodegenerative disorders belonging to the family of alpha-synucleinopaties [1], characterized by symptoms of "parkinsonism", such as bradykinesia, tremor at rest, muscle rigidity, postural instability, ataxia, which can occur in different combinations and gravity.

PD is the most common movement disorders and affects about 1% of people over the age of sixty. In most cases the etiology is unknown (idiopathic form), but are described both familiar [1] and genetically determined forms [2]. MSA is a sporadic neurodegenerative disease of unknown etiology that predominantly affects males between fifty and sixty years, with a prevalence of 4.6 cases per 100,000 people [1,3]. Both diseases are characterized by the combination of motor and non-motor symptoms. Among the latter, undoubtedly the dysfunction of the autonomic nervous system (ANS) is one of the main determinants of the altered quality of life of patients [4-8].

In PD autonomic dysfunction may precede even many years the typical motor signs, may be evident already in the first phase or dominate throughout the entire course of the disease [5,9].

The dominance of autonomic symptoms (orthostatic hypotension, urinary dysfunction, impaired intestinal motility, body temperature dysregulation) is a hallmark of MSA, in variable combination with typical signs of "parkinsonism", cerebellar ataxia and/or pyramidal signs [3]. Although it is known that ANS dysfunction is a consequence of the degenerative phenomena occurring in both central nervous system and in peripheral ganglia [10-14], the mechanisms responsible for motor and non-motor symptoms are somehow different and not fully understood [15-17]. Along the last 30 years the diagnosis of ANS derangement, relevant for prognostic judgment and therapeutic decisions, has been one of the major challenges for neurologists dealing with "parkinsonism" of uncertain nature. For this reason, several methods, including the Ewing Protocol [3,18,19], thermoregulation assessment [20], myocardial scintigraphy with iodine-123 meta-Iodobenzylguanidine (123I MIBG) [21] and Heart Rate Variability (HRV) analysis [8,10,14,22-25], have been proposed to attempt quantification of ANS derangement and to provide early differentiation between PD and MSA [26-29].

In most recent studies, time-domain (TD) and frequency-domain (FD) HRV parameters were efficient to assess cardiovascular dysautonomia in parkinsonian syndromes [23-25]. In particular, TD parameters were sensitive for the assessment of early stage of the PD whereas alteration of FD parameters was associated with the disease's duration [24,25].

It was also shown that HRVa in combination with the Ewing protocol provides a better assessment of cardiovascular dysautonomia in parkinsonian syndromes, useful to differentiate PD from MSA [23].

Although recent literature has shown that the Discriminant analysis (DA) of nonlinear (NL) HRV parameters can be more efficient that linear HRV parameters to investigate certain ANS conditions [30,31], their diagnostic accuracy to distinguish parkinsonian syndromes of uncertain origin has been little investigated [32,33]. These nonlinear techniques are expected to provide additional information about the nonlinearity and complexity of autonomic cardiovascular control which cannot be reflected by linear HRV analysis. The goal is not that NL HRV techniques would replace the linear analysis, but they have to be considered as an addition, yielding information about a specific aspect of scaling behavior, complexity or chaos in the underlying system [34].

The aim of this study was to evaluate the predictive accuracy of NL HRV parameters to identify markers of dysautonomia sensitive to differentiate PD from MSA in early stage of parkinsonian syndromes of uncertain diagnosis.

2. MATERIALS AND METHODS

2.1 Patients Population

51 consecutive ambulatory patients (35 males and 16 females) (mean age 63±10 years) presenting with parkinsonian symptoms (Table 1) and 40 age-matched healthy subjects (20 males and 20 females), as case control, were included in the study.

Preliminarily patients were clinically classified according to standardized diagnostic criteria [17,27,28]. 25 patients (49%) had a "certain" diagnosis of PD, 9 (18%) a "highly probable" diagnosis of MSA (7 MSA-p, 2 MSA-c). 17 patients (33%) had an uncertain neurological definition, (6 "undefined parkinsonism" and 11 "suspected MSA") (Table 1). 62,8% of patients were under pharmacological treatment with a mean LED (Levodopa dose equivalent) of 495.35, not significantly different in PD (485.6) from MSA (497.2), (p = 0.95), which was not discontinued the day of Holter recording. Patients treated with medications that could interfere with the sympatho-vagal balance (e.g. β -blockers, calcium channel blockers and vasodilators), were excluded.

After careful clinical history, physical examination and ECG recording in basal conditions, to verify the possible presence of spontaneous arrhythmias, twenty-four hours 12-lead Holter ECG was recorded (*H-Scribe -Mortara-Rangoni Instruments*).

Since factors, such as circadian rhythm, body position, activity level prior to recording, medication, verbalization, and breathing condition may influence the HRV, special precautions were taken to maintain similar condition in all patients, such as starting Holter session approximately at the same time of day (usually in the mid-late morning, after a light breakfast). Moreover all patients were instructed to perform some moderate physical activity at least twice during daytime before and after lunch, and to note accurately the timing of resting in bed, sleep, and eventual awakeness intervals during the night.

The study was approved by the local ethics committee and was performed in accordance with the ethical standards of the 1964 declaration of Helsinki. All patients gave informed consent to all clinical examinations and to the possible anonym inclusion of their data in scientific reports.

2.2 Heart Rate Variability Analysis

Quantitative HRV analysis was performed according to the European Society of Cardiology and the North American Society of Pacing and Electrophysiology guidelines [22] as follows. First raw ECG data were extracted from the Holter recordings with a custom software routine and edited to manually remove technical artifacts and/or physiological artifacts. The fraction of total RR intervals labeled as normal-to-normal (NN) intervals was used as a measure of data reliability, with the purpose to exclude records with a ratio less than a 95% threshold. Then a further editing was performed by visual analysis of the tachogram and of corresponding ECG, with manual correction of possible residual artifacts. Finally, HRV parameters were calculated in the TD, FD and with NL methods [30-41], using the Kubios HRV software (version 2.1) [42]. The "Smoothness Priors regularization" (lambda value: 500) was used to remove "non-stationary" low-frequency components [43].

The following methods were chosen for Non Linear Heart Rate Variability analysis (NL HRVa):

2.2.1 Poincare' plot

The Poincare' plot is a common graphical representation of the correlation between successive RR intervals, which analysis consists in fitting an ellipse oriented according to the line-of-identity and computing the standard deviation of the points perpendicular to and along the line-of-identity referred as *sd1* and *sd2*, respectively (*sd1* describes short-term variability; *sd2* describes long-term variability; *sd1/sd2 ratio* that is a measure of the interaction between short-term and long- term variability) [30,35,36]. In a study investigating correlation amongst TD, FD and NL HRV parameters SD1 was highly correlated to RMSSD (r=0.99) (thus parasympathetic modulation) and SD2 to SDNN (r=0.95) [44].

Table 1. Demographic of the 51 investigated patients

Disease	Age	Therapy	UPDRS III: 0-68	HOEN & YAHR
MSA-c	65	no	30	3
MSA-c	67	no	n.a.	n.a.
MSA-c	69	no	55	5
MSA-p	45	Carbidopa, Levodopa/Benserazide	47	5
MSA-p	63	Levodopa/Carbidopa, Pramipexole	41	3
MSA-p	63	no	38	4
MSA-p	64	Levodopa/Carbidopa	62	5
MSA-p	69	Levodopa/Carbidopa, Ropirinol	n.a.	n.a.
MSA-p	77	Levodopa/Carbidopa	41	4
MSA-p	77	Levodopa/Carbidopa	n.a.	n.a.
PD	38	no	27	2
PD	48	Levodopa/carbidopa, Selegiline	41	n.a.
PD	51	Rasagiline	n.a.	n.a.
PD	53	Levodopa/Benserazide, Selegiline	13	2
PD	56	Rasagiline	25	2
PD	57	Rasagiline, Mevelodopa/Carbidopa, Ropirinol	16	2
PD	58	Rasagiline	9	1
PD	60	Rasagilina, Mevelodopa/Carbidopa, Ropirinol	26	2
PD	61	no	26	2
PD	62	Levodopa/benserazide, Ropirinol, Selegiline	n.a.	n.a.
PD	62	Rasagiline	26	2
PD	63	Levodopa/Carbidopa, Ropirinol	22	2
PD	65	Ropirinol	20	2
PD	65	Levodopa/Carbidopa, Entecapone	17	2
PD	65	Pramipexole, Levodopa/Carbidopa, Selegiline	n.a.	n.a.
PD	69	Levodopa/Carbidopa	32	2.5
PD	70	no	22	2
PD	71	Levodopa/Benserazide	33	2
PD	72	Levodopa/Benserazide, Ropirinolo	n.a.	n.a.
PD	72	Levodopa/Benserazide	18	2
PD	76	Levodopa/carbidopa, Ropirinol	31	3
PD	77	Levodopa/Benserazide	20	2
PD	77	Levodopa/Benserazide	n.d.	n.d.
PD	85	no	19	2
susp MSA-c	41	no	n.a.	n.a.
susp MSA-c	51	no	n.a.	n.a.
susp MSA-c	57	no	n.a.	n.a.
susp MSA-c	63	no	n.a.	n.a.
susp MSA-c	64	no	n.a.	n.a.
susp MSA-c	66	no	15	n.a.
susp MSA-c	69	no	n.a.	n.a.
susp MSA-p	57	Pramipexole, Carbidopa, Rasagiline	n.a.	n.a.
susp MSA-p	65	Levodopa/Benserazide	n.a.	n.a.
susp MSA-p	66	Levodopa/Benserazide	30	4
susp MSA-p	67	no	n.a.	n.a.
Und park	43	Pramipexole, Selegiline	n.a.	n.a.
Und park	57	Rotigotine	24	2
Und park	67	no	n.a.	n.a.
Und park	68	Selegiline	n.a.	n.a.
Und park	71	no	n.a.	n.a.
Und park	74	no	n.a.	n.a.

PD: Parkinson Disease, MSA-c: Multiple System Atrophy- cerebellar type; MSA-p: Multiple System Atrophy- Parkinsonian type; und: Undefined; susp: Suspected; n.a: Not available

2.2.2 Recurrence plot

The Recurrence plot analyzes the complexity of a given time series [30,37] divided in several parameters [mean line length (*lmean*), max line length (*lmax*), recurrence rate (*rec*), determinism (*det*), Shannon Entropy (*shanen*)].

2.2.3 Entropy

a) Approximate entropy (*apen*) is a measurement of the irregularity or complexity of the signal [30,38,39], b) Sample entropy (*sampen*) similar to *apen* [39,40], measures regularity or randomness of heart rate variations. Higher values indicate greater irregularity and are commonly a feature of health. Sample entropy decreases by moving from supine to orthostatic posture, thus with an increase of sympathetic modulation [45].

2.2.4 Detrended fluctuation analysis

Detrended fluctuation analysis (DFA), quantifies the fractal correlation properties of physiological signals [41,42]. DFA detects self-similarity and its variables are *dfα1* (short term scaling component: 4-11 beats) and *dfα2* (intermediate term scaling component: >11 beats). An α value of 0.5 suggests that the signal is truly random (white-noise) with larger values suggesting less noise. In previous studies, it was shown that DFA values rise with vagal blockade and decrease with sympathetic blockade [46,47].

2.2.5 The correlation dimension

The correlation dimension (*d2*) another way to measure the complexity of a time series. It gives information on the minimum number of dynamic variables needed to model the underlying system [30].

Quantitative HRV analysis was carried out from 5-minutes (Standard Short-Term, SST) time intervals selected during daytime, at rest (passive awakeness), during moderate physical activity (active awakeness) and during physiological sleep, identifying whenever possible NREM and REM stages. Given their short duration and transient variations, only 1-minute time-segments were used for HRV analysis during REM phases. For comparison and to evaluate the effect of shorter segment duration on quantitative assessment of NL

parameters, HRV was also calculated from 2-minutes and 1-minute time-segments within the 5-minutes intervals during awakeness and NREM sleep.

The criteria chosen to validate the selection of the time-segments used for HRV calculation within each explored condition were: 1) the highest possible "stationarity" of the RR signal (defined as the absence of arrhythmias and of any kind of artifacts at visual analysis of corresponding ECG recordings) and 2) the best coherence among spectral output obtained with the Fast Fourier Transform (FFT) and autoregressive (AR) methods.

2.3 Statistical Analysis

All statistical calculations were performed with SPSS software, version 13.0 (*SPSS Inc., Chicago, Illinois*) [48]. Results are expressed as mean value ± standard deviation (SD). The significance between different groups was assessed by the chi-square test for discrete variables and by unpaired Student t-test for continuous variables. A probability level of $P<.05$ was chosen as the least significant difference. Factors differentiating between PD and MSA were tested by univariate and multivariate analyses. Independent variables for entry into the multivariate analysis were selected according to their weight on univariate testing (p values and shorter 95% confidence intervals) [49].

Discriminant Analysis (performed also with *Addinsoft XLSTAT, Version 2013.4.07*) was used to evaluate if HRV parameters were adequate to provide a separation between PD and MSA patients. DA search for linear combinations of the input features that can provide an adequate separation between the investigated subjects, in this study [31]. The discriminant functions used by linear DA are built up as a linear combination of the variables that seek to maximize the differences between the investigated groups. The classification accuracy of the method is defined as the ability to discriminate between the investigated groups.

The formula (F1, see section 3.2) obtained with DA of HRV data of patients with "certain PD" and "highly probable MSA" [31], was applied to classify the subpopulation of patients with parkinsonian symptoms of uncertain diagnosis.

3. RESULTS

3.1 Comparison between Patients (PD + MSA) and Controls

Independently from the length of the time segments explored, the majority of NL HRV parameters were significantly altered in patients as compared with healthy controls, especially during active awakeness. Several parameters were also altered during passive awakeness and during NREM sleep. Only sd1, sd2, dfa2 and d2 were abnormal during REM sleep (Table 2).

DA applied to NL HRV parameters had high predictive accuracy (above 80%) in differentiating patients (PD+MSA) from healthy controls in all conditions, reaching 91.3% with parameters calculated during the REM sleep (Table 3).

3.2 Comparison between PD and MSA Patients

When confronting patients with "certain" PD and "high probable" MSA, only recurrence plot parameters calculated during active awakeness and dfa2 during passive awakeness were significantly different (Table 4).

At DA (Table 5), the classification accuracy of single parameters ranged between 58,8 and 73.5%. The best accuracy (76.5%) was obtained with a combination of parameters *rplmean*, *rpadet* and *rpshen*, in formula (F1):

F1= -0.61 × rplmean + 0.15 x rpadet + 6.51 × rpshen - 27.53

In which: -0.61, 0.15, and 6.51 are the coefficients derived from the discriminant function of the DA for each parameter, while -27.53 is the constant derived from the same function.

When the formula F1 (if <0, the patient was classified as MSA, otherwise as PD) was applied to reclassify the seventeen patients with an uncertain clinical diagnosis, nine of them were classified as PD and six as MSA, only 2 remain unclassified.

Out of them, when comparing the HRV results with the definitive neurological diagnosis during the outcome during follow-up, five of the six

patients with initial diagnosis of "undefined parkinsonism" were confirmed correctly classified as PD and one as MSA. Out of the eleven patients initially considered "suspected MSA", in five of the six patients classified as MSA on the basis of HRV criteria the diagnosis was confirmed by the clinical evolution during the follow-up. In the remaining six patients with shorter follow-up a definitive diagnosis is still uncertain.

4. DISCUSSION

The evaluation of autonomic dysfunction from heart rate pattern has proven useful for the stratification of risk associated with numerous diseases [50] including heart failure, hypertension, ischemic heart disease, diabetes, sepsis and neurological diseases linked to brain damage, especially patients with parkinsonism syndromes, to attempt early differentiation between PD and MSA and to define prognosis [3,18-20,22,23,26].

In spite of the increasing number of clinical studies, univocal criteria for the use of HRV a as a diagnostic tool in parkinsonian syndromes are still lacking [6,8,51,52]. This may be due to differences study protocols and/or experimental conditions not taking uniformly into account variables related to physiological variation of sympatho/vagal modulation due to circadian rhythm, physical activity, different phase of sleep etc.

Furthermore, quantitative HRV analysis can be affected by eventual non-stationarity of physiological conditions even during standard short-term analysis. Moreover, linear HRV analysis (in the TD and FD) may not be adequate to highlight the complexity of the autonomic cardiovascular modulation even in physiological conditions [42,43].

In this view, the use of methods based on NL mathematical models and on chaos theory (*Poincaré plot analysis, Recurrence Plot analysis, Correlation Dimension, Entropy*, etc.) which have proven efficient in improving the predictive value of HRVa in several other diseases [31,53,54], could be more efficient than linear HRV analysis also in the study of parkinsonian dysautomia.

Table 2. Comparison between NL HRV of 51 patients (PD + MSA) and 40 healthy controls

A

| | Passive awakeness (2 min) | | | | | | Active awakeness (2 min) | | | | | |
| | Controls | | PD+MSA | | P | | Controls | | PD+MSA | | P |
	Mean	SD	Mean	SD			Mean	SD	Mean	SD	
sd1/sd2	0.47	± 0.16	0.67	± 0.25	<.05		0.45	± 0.17	0.66	± 0.26	<.05
sd1	16.96	± 10.49	10.56	± 8.26	<.05		17.52	± 10.06	8.99	± 7.63	<.05
sd2	37.53	± 20.64	18.25	± 16.09	<.05		40.94	± 20.76	15.73	± 13.38	<.05
rplmean	9.24	± 2.51	8.24	± 4.77	n.s.		9.62	± 3.15	8.03	± 3.84	<.05
rplmax	91.70	± 48.03	52.18	± 35.14	<.05		85.60	± 42.44	55.57	± 32.63	<.05
rprec	27.43	± 7.65	23.68	± 14.64	n.s.		29.06	± 8.33	24.20	± 12.87	<.05
rpadet	97.03	± 2.03	94.93	± 2.84	<.05		97.39	± 1.88	95.20	± 2.93	<.05
rpshen	2.89	± 0.30	2.64	± 0.43	<.05		2.90	± 0.33	2.66	± 0.36	<.05
dfa1	1.28	± 0.27	0.99	± 0.30	<.05		1.31	± 0.27	1.02	± 0.33	<.05
dfa2	0.38	± 0.14	0.44	± 0.14	n.s.		0.38	± 0.13	0.45	± 0.14	<.05
apen	0.82	± 0.10	0.78	± 0.10	n.s.		0.83	± 0.09	0.84	± 0.11	n.s.
sampen	1.63	± 0.34	1.75	± 0.40	n.s.		1.66	± 0.37	1.58	± 0.30	n.s.
d2	1.20	± 1.41	0.25	± 0.67	<.05		1.30	± 1.31	0.15	± 0.52	<.05

B

| | NREM sleep (2 min) | | | | | | REM sleep (1 min) | | | | | |
| | Controls | | PD+MSA | | P | | Controls | | PD+MSA | | P |
	Mean	SD	Mean	SD			Mean	SD	Mean	SD	
sd1/sd2	0.85	± 0.25	0.89	± 0.29	n.s.		0.5	± 0.2	0.5	± 0.2	n.s.
sd1	28.75	± 17.57	14.25	± 9.54	n.s.		27.6	± 17.9	13.1	± 7.9	<.05
sd2	33.24	± 15.89	17.27	± 12.19	n.s.		55.5	± 26.7	27.1	± 16.6	<.05
rplmean	8.42	± 2.89	7.29	± 2.43	<.05		9.9	± 5.6	8.1	± 2.7	n.s.
rplmax	41.85	± 15.83	35.47	± 15.17	n.s.		43.9	± 12.9	41.3	± 18.4	n.s.
rprec	19.49	± 4.07	16.22	± 4.19	<.05		30.2	± 13.2	25.7	± 11.1	n.s.
rpadet	95.85	± 1.62	94.17	± 3.11	<.05		97.3	± 2.1	96.0	± 2.7	n.s.
rpshen	2.69	± 0.27	2.53	± 0.28	<.05		2.6	± 0.3	2.5	± 0.3	n.s.
dfa1	0.69	± 0.27	0.69	± 0.25	n.s.		1.2	± 0.2	1.3	± 0.3	n.s.
dfa2	0.20	± 0.11	0.29	± 0.11	<.05		0.4	± 0.2	0.5	± 0.2	<.05
apen	0.66	± 0.09	0.71	± 0.09	<.05		0.5	± 0.1	0.5	± 0.1	n.s.
sampen	1.84	± 0.32	1.87	± 0.41	n.s.		1.4	± 0.4	1.6	± 0.4	n.s.
d2	1.72	± 1.48	0.40	± 0.95	<.05		1.5	± 0.9	0.6	± 0.9	<.05

Table 3. Predictive accuracy of NL parameters in differentiating patients from healthy controls

Condition	Sensitivity	Specificity	Predictive accuracy
Passive awakeness	77.8%	89.7%	84.9%
Active awakeness	66.7%	89.5%	81.4%
REM sleep	91.3%	91.3%	91.3%

Table 4. Comparison between NL HRV parameters of patients with certain PD and highly probable MSA diagnosis

	Passive awakeness (2 min)					Active awakeness (2 min)					NREM sleep (2 min)				
	certain PD		highly probable MSA		P	certain PD		highly probable MSA		P	certain PD		highly probable MSA		P
	Mean	SD	Mean	SD		Mean	SD	Mean	SD		Mean	SD	Mean	SD	
sd1/sd2	0.6	± 0.2	0.7	± 0.2	n.s.	0.6	± 0.2	0.8	± 0.3	n.s.	0.9	± 0.2	1.0	± 0.4	n.s.
sd1	10.7	± 7.3	9.2	± 7.5	n.s.	8.4	± 3.6	7.4	± 4.5	n.s.	14.8	± 9.1	11.0	± 8.4	n.s.
sd2	18.4	± 12.9	14.1	± 10.8	n.s.	15.6	± 9.5	10.9	± 8.4	n.s.	17.9	± 10.4	10.9	± 6.2	n.s.
rplmean	7.8	± 2.4	8.2	± 3.7	n.s.	8.0	± 2.3	6.0	± 1.4	< .05	7.3	± 1.5	7.3	± 3.1	n.s.
rplmax	57.7	± 35.6	44.9	± 32.1	n.s.	57.4	± 30.2	34.6	± 18.7	< .05	34.4	± 9.5	35.4	± 18.3	n.s.
rprec	23.6	± 10.1	23.8	± 12.6	n.s.	23.7	± 8.5	16.6	± 6.9	< .05	16.9	± 3.9	15.1	± 3.9	n.s.
rpadet	95.3	± 2.8	94.8	± 2.7	n.s.	95.8	± 2.2	93.0	± 2.4	< .05	94.6	± 3.4	94.0	± 2.9	n.s.
rpshen	2.6	± 0.3	2.7	± 0.4	n.s.	2.7	± 0.3	2.4	± 0.2	n.s.	2.6	± 0.2	2.5	± 0.4	n.s.
dfa1	1.0	± 0.3	1.0	± 0.2	n.s.	1.1	± 0.3	0.9	± 0.4	n.s.	0.7	± 0.2	0.6	± 0.3	n.s.
dfa2	0.4	± 0.1	0.6	± 0.2	< .05	0.5	± 0.1	0.4	± 0.1	n.s.	0.3	± 0.1	0.3	± 0.1	n.s.
apen	0.8	± 0.1	0.8	± 0.1	n.s.	0.8	± 0.1	0.9	± 0.1	n.s.	0.7	± 0.1	0.7	± 0.1	n.s.
sampen	1.7	± 0.3	1.8	± 0.4	n.s.	1.6	± 0.3	1.6	± 0.2	n.s.	1.9	± 0.5	1.7	± 0.3	n.s.
d2	0.3	± 0.7	0.2	± 0.6	n.s.	0.1	± 0.4	0.0	± 0.0	n.s.	0.5	± 1.1	0.1	± 0.3	n.s.

PD: Parkinson Disease, MSA: Multiple System Atrophy

Table 5. Performance of the classification rules (PD vs MSA) based on single NL HRV parameter and combination of parameters

	Classified as PD if			Sens	Spec	PPV	NPV	PA
dfa2	passive awakeness	<	0.440	80.00%	55.56%	83.33%	50.00%	73.53%
rprec	active awakeness	>	18.744	60.87%	75.00%	87.50%	40.00%	64.52%
rplmean	active awakeness	>	7.471	48.00%	88.89%	92.31%	38.10%	58.82%
rpadet	active awakeness	>	95.039	76.00%	66.67%	86.36%	50.00%	73.53%
rpshen	active awakeness	>	2.622	72.00%	77.78%	90.00%	50.00%	73.53%
F1	active awakeness	>	0	80.00%	66.67%	86.96%	54.55%	76.47%

F1 = −0.61 × rplmean + 0.15 × rpadet + 6.51 × rpshen − 27.53

PD: Parkinson Disease, MSA: Multiple System Atrophy, Sens: Sensitivity, Spec: Specificity, PPV: Positive Predictive Value; NPV: Negative Predictive Value

The present study focused on the application of NL HRVa from short-term time segments of different lengths (5-2-1 min), taking into account also different phases of daily activity (both passive and active awakeness) and of sleep (NREM and REM), to attempt a more comprehensive quantification of different degrees of cardiovascular autonomic dysfunction detected in patients with "parkinsonian" movement disorders, but due to illness with very different prognosis and outcome.

In a first phase of the study we compared HRV parameters of patients (PD + MSA) with those of age-matched control group. As expected, the majority of NL HRV parameters were significantly abnormal in parkinsonian patients ($P<.05$) compared to healthy subjects, during both active and passive awakeness as well as during NREM sleep, thus confirming the well-known altered autonomic control of RR variability and complexity (Table 2) [23-25,32,33]. Such decreased value of complexity measures reflects a change towards more stable and periodic behavior of the heart rate in patients, which may be associated with "decoupling of multimodal integrated networks and deactivation of control-loops within the cardiovascular system" [31].

However the real clinical challenge is to provide the neurologist with additional tools improving non-invasive early differentiation between PD and MSA, especially in patients with uncertain clinical patterns.

Whereas previous studies questioned the value of comprehensive autonomic nervous system testing for risk assessment of patients with parkinsonism [50-52], in the present study NL HRV parameters were significantly more altered in MSA compared to PD, especially during active awakeness. This result indicate a greater impairment of sympathetic autonomic response during daily activity, which could be responsible for the increased prevalence and severity of orthostatic hypotension in MSA compared to PD.

The performance of the classification rules based on DA of NL parameters distinguished between the two diseases with accuracy provided by single NL parameters ranging between 58.8% and 73.5%.

Since clinical experience with the analysis of HRV complexity and regularity in parkinsonian patients is still limited, it is difficult at the moment to speculate about their physiological meaning in

different abnormal conditions and about possible reasons why only few NL parameters were significant in differentiating between MSA and PD in this study. However it may be interesting to note that the combination of NL parameters *rplmean*, *rpadet*, *rpshen*, in the formula F1 (Table 5), improved the predictive accuracy of evolution in MSA to a 76.5%, which may be a reasonably good additional information to attempt an early differentiation between parkinsonian syndromes with different prognosis. In fact, by applying F1 to attempt a better classification of the seventeen patients with a uncertain diagnosis, more than half of them were properly classified as demonstrated by the evolution of the clinical picture during the follow-up.

4.1 Limitations of the Study

A first obvious limitation of the study is certainly the limited number of enrolled patients, especially patients with highly probable MSA, but we must consider that the disease is very disabling and often limits the "patient's compliance" to participate to clinical studies.

Second, for accurate evaluation of ANS balance, one should study patients either before the beginning of pharmacological treatment or after an appropriate period of drug washout. Unfortunately, this is often impossible, particularly in cases with severe motor impairment and/or marked dysautonomia, since, in the absence of therapy, the patients could not be evaluated in terms of mobility and of daily life activities.

Finally, as there are now sensitive second-level diagnostic tools that allow very accurate and precise diagnosis of alpha-synucleinopatie diseases, such as *Datscan* and brain *Pet* [55,56] as well as myocardial scintigraphy with meta-iodobenzylguanidine [21] for studying cardiac sympathetic innervation, the lack of these data in some of our patients with uncertain diagnosis is still limiting the evaluation of the results of this paper.

On the other hand HRVa is a non-invasive tool, that requires only a good quality electrocardiographic recording which is applicable to most patients, even in uncomfortable clinical conditions. Thus it may be an optimal first level additional tool for a better early diagnostic classification at very low cost and with no need to expose the patient to ionizing radiation.

5. CONCLUSION

NL HRVa might be a simple and quick method to improve the quantization of the degree of derangement of cardiovascular autonomic modulation in patients with parkinsonian neurodegenerative syndromes associated with signs of dysautonomia [3,23]. Furthermore the assessment of the degree of ANS impairment is certainly more pronounced in MSA compared to PD and this element seems better highlighted by investigating the complexity of HRV with NL methods which seem to have a greater stability, probably because less affected by non-stationarity conditions [29-35].

In this study NL analysis provided satisfactory differentiation between patients with a "certain or highly probable" diagnosis of PD or MSA with a good (76.5) predictive accuracy. The classification rules could be useful for an earlier definition of prognostic evolution toward one or other type of disease in patients with parkinsonian symptoms of uncertain nature, to address second level assessment and to guide the choice of early and more individualized drug treatment.

ACKNOLEDGMENTS

The authors are grateful to the colleagues Prof. Anna Rita Bentivoglio and Dr. Carla Piano for constructive discussion and for referring some of the patients included in this study.

COMPETING INTERESTS

Authors have declared that no competing interests exist.

REFERENCES

1. Samii A, Nutt JG, Ransom BR. Parkinson's disease. The Lancet. 2004;363(9423):1783-93.
2. Trinh J, Farrer M. Advances in the genetics of Parkinson disease. Nat Rev Neurol. 2013;9(8):445-54. DOI:10.1038/nrneurol.2013.132. Epub 2013 Jul 16.
3. Albanese A, Colosimo C, Bentivoglio AR, Fenici R, Melillo G, Tonali P. Multiple system atrophy presenting as parkinsonism: Clinical features and diagnostic criteria. J Neurol Neurosurg Psychiatry. 1995;59:144-151.
4. Quinn N. Multiple system atrophy: The nature of the beast. J Neurol Neurosurg Psychiatry. 1989;52:78-89.
5. Ziemssen T, Reichmann H. Cardiovascular autonomic dysfunction in Parkinson's disease. J Neurol Sci. 2010;289:74-80.
6. Jain S. Multi-organ autonomic dysfunction in Parkinson disease. Parkinsonism Relat Disord. 2011;17(2):77-83.
7. Chaudhuri KR, Healy DG, Schapira AH. Non-motor symptoms of Parkinson's disease: Diagnosis and management. The Lancet Neurol. 2006;5:235-45.
8. Valappil RA, Black JE, Broderick MJ, Carrillo O, Frenette E, Sullivan SS, et al. Exploring the electrocardiogram as a potential tool to screen for premotor Parkinson's disease. Mov. Disord. 2010;25 (14):2296-2303.
9. Antonini A, Barone P, Marconi R, Morgante L, Zappulla S, Pontieri FE, et al. The progression of non-motor symptoms in Parkinson's disease and their contribution to motor disability and quality of life. J Neurol. 2012;259(12):2621-31. DOI:10.1007/s00415-012-6557-8. Epub 2012 Jun
10. Goldestein DS. Dysautonomia in Parkinson's disease: Neurocardiological abnormalities. The Lancet Neurol. 2003;2 (11):669-76.
11. Goldestein DS. Neuroscience and heart-brain medicine: The year in review. Cleve Clin J Med. 2010;77(3):S34-S39.
12. Walter BL. Cardiovascular autonomic dysfunction in patients with movement disorders. Cleve Clin J Med. 2008;25(2):S54-S58.
13. Holmberg B, Kallio M, Johnels B, Elam M. Cardiovascular reflex testing contributes to clinical evaluation and differential diagnosis of Parkinsonian syndromes. Mov Disord. 2001;16(2):217-25.
14. Barbic F, Perego F, Canesi M, Gianni M, Biagiotti S, Costantino G, et al. Early abnormalities of vascular and cardiac autonomic control in Parkinson's disease without orthostatic hypotension. Hypertension. 2007;49(1):120-26.
15. Aerts MB, Synhaeve NE, Mirelman A, Bloem BR, Giladi N, Hausdorff JM. Is heart rate variability related to gait impairment in patients with Parkinson's disease? A pilot study. Parkinsonism Relat Disord. 2009;15:712-15.
16. Spiegel J, Hellwing D, Farmakis G, Jost WH, Samnick S, Fassbender K, et al.

Myocardial sympathetic degeneration correlates with clinical phenotype of Parkinson's disease. Mov Disord. 2007; 22(7):1004-08.

17. Köllensperger M, Geser F, Ndayisaba JP, Boesch S, Seppi K, Ostergaard K, et al. Presentation, diagnosis, and management of multiple system atrophy in Europe: Final analysis of the European multiple system atrophy registry. Mov Disord. 2010; 25(15):2604-12.

18. Ewing DJ. Cardiovascular reflex and autonomic neuropathy. Clin Sci Mol Med. 1978;55:321-27.

19. Kimpinski K, Iodice V, Burton DD, Camilleri M, Mullan BP, Lipp A, et al. The role of autonomic testing in the differentiation of Parkinson's disease from multiple system atrophy. J Neurol Sci. 2012;317(1-2):92-6.

20. Weimer LH. Autonomic testing: Common techniques and clinical applications. Neurologist. 2010;16(4):215-22.

21. Kikuchi A, Baba T, Hasegawa T, Sugeno N, Konno M, Takeda A. Differentiating Parkinson's disease from multiple system atrophy by [123I] meta-iodobenzylguanidine myocardial scintigraphy and olfactory test. Parkinsonism Relat Disord. 2011;17(9): 698-700.

22. Task force of the European Society of Cardiology and the North American Society of pacing and Electrophysiology. Heart rate variability. Standards measurement, physiological interpretation, and clinical use. Eur Heart J. 1996;17:354-81.

23. Brisinda D, Sorbo AR, Di Giacopo R, Venuti A, Bentivoglio AR, et al. Cardiovascular Autonomic Nervous System Evaluation in Parkinson Disease and Multisystem Atrophy. J Neurol Sci. 2014;336(1-2):197-202.
DOI: 10.1016/j.jns.2013.10.039. Epub 2013 Nov 6.

24. Maetzler W, Karam M, Berger MF, Heger T, Maetzler C, Ruediger H, et al. Time- and frequency-domain parameters of heart rate variability and sympathetic skin response in Parkinson's disease. J Neural Transm; 2014. [Epub ahead of print]

25. Harnod D, Wen SH, Chen SY, Harnod T. The association of heart rate variability with parkinsonian motor symptom duration. Yonsei Med J. 2014;55(5):1297-302.

26. O'Sullivan SS, Massey LA, Williams DR, Silveira-Moriyama L, Kempster PA, Holton JL, et al. Clinical outcomes of progressive supranuclear palsy and multiple system atrophy. Brain. 2008;131:1362–72.

27. Lipp A, Sandroni P, Ahlskog JE, Fealey RD, Kimpinski K, Iodice V, et al. Prospective differentiation of multiple system atrophy from Parkinson's disease, with and without autonomic failure. Arch Neurol. 2009;66(6):742–50.

28. Litvan I, Bhatia KP, Burn DJ, Goetz CG, Lang AE, McKeith I, et al. Movement Disorders Society Scientific Issues Committee report: SIC Task Force appraisal of clinical diagnostic criteria for Parkinsonian disorders. Mov Disord. 2003; 18(5):467-86.

29. Jankovic J. Parkinson's disease: Clinical features and diagnosis. J. Neurol. Neurosurg. Psychiatr. 2008;79(4):368–76.

30. Chua KC, Chandran V, Acharya UR, Min LC. Computer-based analysis of cardiac state using entropies, recurrence plots and Poincare geometry. J Med Eng Technol UK. 2008;32(4):263-72.
DOI: 10.1080/03091900600863794.

31. Melillo P, Bracale M, Pecchia L. Nonlinear Heart Rate Variability features for real-life stress detection. Case study: Students under stress due to university examination. Biomed Eng Online. 2011;10:96.
DOI: 10.1186/1475-925X-10-96.

32. Kallio M, Suominen K, Bianchi AM, Mäkikallio T, Haapaniemi T, Astafiev S, et al. Comparison of heart rate variability analysis methods in patients with Parkinson's disease. Med Biol Eng Comput. 2002;40(4):408-14.

33. Pursiainen V, Haapaniemi TH, Korpelainen JT, Huikuri HV, Sotaniemi KA, Myllylä VV. Circadian heart rate variability in Parkinson's disease. J Neurol. 2002;249 (11):1535-40.

34. Vandeput S. Heart Rate Variability: Linear and nonlinear analysis with applications in human physiology. Dissertation. Arenberg Doctoral School of Science, Engineering & Technology Faculty of Engineering Department of Electrical Engineering Katholieke Universities Leuwen. 2010;10.

35. Brennan M, Palaniswami M, Kamen P. Do existing measures of Poincare plot geometry reflecect nonlinear features of heart rate variability. IEEE Trans Biomed Eng. 2001;48(11):1342-1347.

36. Kamen PW, Krum H, Tonkin AM. Poincare plot of heart rate variability allows quantitative display of parasympathetic

nervous activity. Clin Sci. 1996;91:201–208.

37. Eckmann JP, Kamphorst SO, Ruelle D. Recurrence plots of dynamical systems. Europhys Lett. 1987;4:973–977.

38. Pincus SM, Viscarello RR. Approximate entropy: A regularity measure for heart rate analysis. Obstet Gynecol. 1992;79:249–55.

39. Richman JA, Moorman JR. Physiological time-series analysis using approximate entropy and sample entropy. Am J Physiol. 2000;278:H2039-H2049.

40. Cysarz D, Bettermann H, van Leeuwen P. Entropies of short binary sequences in heart period dynamics. Am J Physiol Heart Circ Physiol. 2000;278:H2163–H2172.

41. Yeh JR, Peng CK, Lo MT, Yeh CH, Chen SC, Wang CY, et al. Investigating the interaction between heart rate variability and sleep EEG using nonlinear algorithms. J Neurosci Methods. 2013;219(2):233-9. DOI: 10.1016/j.jneumeth.2013.08.008. Epub 2013 Aug 18.

42. Tarvainen MP, Niskanen JP, Lipponen JA, Ranta-Aho PO, Karjalainen PA. Kubios HRV--heart rate variability analysis software. Comput Methods Programs Biomed. 2014;113(1):210-20.

43. Tarvainen MP, Ranta-aho PO, Karjalainen PA. An advanced detrending method with application to HRV analysis. IEEE Transactions on Biomedical Engineering. 2002;49:172–175.

44. Hoshi R, Pastre C, Vanderlei L, Godoy M. Poincare plot indexed of heart rate variability: Relationships with other nonlinear variables. Auton Neurosci 2013; 177:271-274.

45. Porta A, Gnecchi-Ruscone T, Tobaldini E, Guzzetti S, Furlan R, Montano N. Progressive decrease of heart period variability entropy-based complexity during graded head-up tilt. J Appl Physiol. 2007;103:1143-1149.

46. Castiglioni P, Parati G, di Rienzo M, Carabalona R, Cividjian A, Quintin L. Scale exponents of blood pressure and heart rate during autonomic blockade as assessed by detrended fluctuation analysis. J Physiol 2011;589:355-369.

47. Millar P, Cotie L, Amand T, McCartney N, Ditor D. Effects of autonomic blockade on nonlinear heart rate dynamics. Clin Auton Res. 2010;20:241-247.

48. SPSS Inc. Released 2004. SPSS Statistics for Windows, Version 13.0. Chicago: SPSS Inc.

49. Larsen RJ, Marx ML. An introduction to mathematical statistics and its application. Pearson Education. Boston, Mass, USA; 2012.

50. Günther A, Witte OW, Hoyer D. Autonomic dysfunction and risk stratification assessed from heart rate pattern. Open Neurol J. 2010;4:39-49.

51. Riley DE, Chelimsky TC. Autonomic nervous system testing may not distinguish multiple system atrophy from Parkinson's disease. J Neurol Neurosurg Psychiatry. 2003;74(1):56-60.

52. Reimann M, Schmidt C, Herting B, Prieur S, Junghanns S, Schweitzer K, et al. Comprehensive autonomic assessment does not differentiate between Parkinson's disease, multiple system atrophy and progressive supranuclear palsy. J Neural Transm. 2010;117(1):69-76.

53. Voss A, Schroeder R, Vallverdú M, Schulz S, Cygankiewicz I, Vázquez R, et al. Short-term vs long-term heart rate variability in ischemic cardiomyopathy risk stratification. Front Physiol. 2013;4:364.

54. Tobaldini E, Nobili L, Strada S, Casali KR, Braghiroli A, Montano N. Heart rate variability in normal and pathological sleep. Front Physiol. 2013;4:294.

55. Brooks DJ. Imaging approaches to Parkinson disease. J Nucl Med. 2010;51 (4):596–609.

56. Di Giuda D, Camardese G, Bentivoglio AR, Cocciolillo F, Guidubaldi A, Pucci L, et al. Dopaminergic dysfunction and psychiatric symptoms in movement disorders: A 123i-FP-CIT SPECT study. Eur J Nucl Med Mol Imaging. 2012;39(12):1937-48.

20

What's New and What Gaps in 2013 European Guidelines for the Management of Arterial Hypertension: A Reappraisal

Pietro Scicchitano[1], Michele Gesualdo[1], Santa Carbonara[1], Pasquale Palmiero[2],
Pietro Nazzaro[3], Annapaola Zito[1], Gabriella Ricci[1], Luisa de Gennaro[4],
Pasquale Caldarola[4], Francesca Cortese[1] and Marco Matteo Ciccone[1*]

[1]*Department of Emergency and Organ Transplantation (DETO), Cardiovascular Diseases Section, University of Bari, Piazza G. Cesare 11–70124, Bari, Italy.*
[2]*Department of Cardiology, Local Health Service-Brindisi, Italy.*
[3]*Department of Basic Medical Sciences, Neurosciences and Sense Organs, Division of Neurology-Stroke Unit, Hypertension, University of Bari, Bari, Italy.*
[4]*Department of Cardiovascular Disease, "San Paolo" Hospital, Bari, Italy.*

Authors' contributions

This work was carried out in collaboration between all authors. Authors MMC, PS, MG, PP, PC and PN designed the study and wrote the first draft of the manuscript, contributed in answering the comments of the reviewers. Authors SC, AZ, GR, LDG and FC managed the literature searches and revised the draft of the paper. All authors read and approved the final manuscript.

<u>Editor(s):</u>
(1) Anonymous.
<u>Reviewers:</u>
(1) Anonymous, King George's Medical University, India.
(2) Xing Li, Division of Biomedical Statistics and Informatics and Department of Health Sciences Research, Mayo Clinic College of Medicine, USA.

ABSTRACT

Arterial hypertension is the most common cardiovascular risk factor causing over 9 million deaths worldwide. Its treatment is crucial in preventing adverse outcomes, in reducing morbidity and mortality and related socio-economic impact of cardiovascular diseases. The European Society of Cardiology and the European Society of Hypertension recently published the new guidelines for the management of hypertension in order to provide physicians diagnostic and therapeutic tools and indications for improving health outcomes. Despite the new advances proposed by the authors,

---

Corresponding author: E-mail: marcomatteo.ciccone@uniba.it

gaps in evidences still persist. The aim of our paper is to give an overview about the new aspects proposed in the arterial hypertension management and the dark side of the knowledge still persisting about such a matter.

Keywords: Arterial hypertension; hypertension management; gaps in evidence; guidelines.

1. INTRODUCTION

Hypertension is a well-known risk factor for cardiovascular disease (CVD) [1]. Increased values of arterial pressure lead to organ damages and clinical adverse events such as ischemic heart disease, stroke, heart and kidney failure. Due to its asymptomatic features, hypertension is considered as a "silent killer" responsible for about nine million deaths each year all over the world [1].

The European Society of Hypertension (ESH) and the European Society of Cardiology (ESC) recently developed an update of the Guidelines on the Management of Hypertension [2] to be followed by cardiologists, family practitioners, nephrologists, internists and endocrinologists. These new guidelines were determined from a drafting panel composed by eminent scientists and academics from European Society of Hypertension and European Society of Cardiology in order to give a frank overview and methods in the general management of hypertensive condition.

These new guidelines point out new advances as compared to previous position papers [3,4], although many gaps still persist in the general management of hypertensive patients.

The 2013 manuscript [2] tries to summarize the specific recommendations in order to fast the consultation processes. This is a novelty for guidelines presentation which is linked to the high level of evidence reached for each point of the recommendations. Only 29% of the recommendations presents level of evidence C (i.e. derived from a consensus of opinions of experts and/or small studies, retrospective studies or registries) and this is due to an increased availability of data from randomized clinical trials. This increases the value of the document and suggests that treatments based on evidence medicine are now available in the general management of arterial hypertension [5]. Despite such positive aspects, the presence of several gaps still persists and deserves much more attention from the international scientific community.

The aim of this paper is to give an overview about both advances and gaps in the general management of arterial hypertension, in relation to the new ESC/ESH guidelines (see also Table 1).

2. CARDIOVASCULAR RISK PROFILE ASSESSMENT

The introduction section focused on the cardiovascular risk profile assessment of patients suffering from arterial hypertension, pointing out the definitions of the terms adopted in order to make a uniform evaluation of such patients all over the European nations whoever may be the physician involved [2].

Although the proposed definitions are equal to those written in the previous guidelines [4,5], some novelties can be outlined.

The first one is represented by the introduction of the SCORE (Systematic Coronary Risk Evaluation) risk charts in order to assess cardiovascular risk, in line with the ESC guidelines on CVD prevention [6] and dyslipidemia management [7]. This model expresses the estimated 10-year risk of cardiovascular mortality by including parameters such as age, gender, smoking status, total cholesterol and systolic blood pressure [8].

Nevertheless, SCORE "underscores" the estimation of the global cardiovascular risk of the patients because it did not consider additional risk-modifying factors such as sedentary lifestyle, obesity, impaired metabolism of carbohydrates, high serum levels of triglycerides or low concentrations of high-density lipoprotein cholesterol, a family history of cardiovascular disease at early age (before 55 years for men and 65 years for women). Furthermore, asymptomatic organ damage can be considered as a potential, new risk-modifier: the presence of left ventricular hypertrophy, carotid intima-media thickening ($\geq$0.9 mm) or atherosclerotic plaques, carotid/femoral pulse wave velocity (PWV), which utility was emphasized lowering the normal values from >12 m/s (ESC-ESH 2007) to actual >10 m/s [3] and urine albumin/creatinine ratio $\geq$90th percentile predict cardiovascular mortality independently of SCORE model [9-11].

Table 1. New advances and still persisting gaps in guidelines for the management of arterial hypertension

What's new?

- Unique systolic blood pressure target:
- Less than 140 mmHg for all healthy subjects (140-150 mmHg for patients older than 80 years if their mental and physical heath allow it).
- Diastolic blood pressure target:
- <90 mmHg, with the exception of diabetic patients whose target is <85 mmHg.
- Adjunct value of Home and Ambulatory blood pressure monitoring in accurate risk assessment.
- Reduction in salt intake to 5-6g/day to reduce blood pressure.
- Individualized approach to drug therapy based on global cardiovascular risk and comorbidities of patient.
- No treatment for subjects with high normal blood pressure.
- Catheter-based renal denervation seems to be a promising approach for resistant hypertension.

What gaps?

- In the global risk-assessment algorithm, elderly people per se should be considered a category at moderate to high cardiovascular risk.
- Emerging cardiovascular risk factors should be considered in total risk stratification
- Home blood pressure monitoring could cause discomfort or concern in some patients

Aware of such limitations of the SCORE charts, the 2013 ESC guidelines [2] proposed a second chart for the assessment of the cardiovascular risk which includes the evaluation of asymptomatic cardiovascular diseases expressions as able to further increase the patients' risk profile. Despite this implementation, the new guidelines did not provide any indication about the predictive value of each chart nor the incremental value of each organ damage markers in the context of hypertensive patient risk stratification. This generates confusion above all among general practitioners who, unaware of the main and specialized tools and parameters showed by guidelines, remain unable to advice patients for the best tool to study and evaluate their disease state.

One more novelty of 2013 ESC-ESH guidelines is that no mention is for patients showing normal pressure but risk factors or even organ damages. In contrast to the previous 2007 recommendations, the authors did not consider lifestyle changes or at least drug therapy when considering patients at normal pressure values. This seems quite unusual in relation to the great weight that 2013 ESC-ESH paper gives to organ damages and cardiovascular risk factors when considering a hypertensive patient.

Furthermore, while patients with three risk factors were previously compared to those with established organ damage, chronic kidney disease or diabetes, the current guidelines, strangely separate these categories by

considering the former at favorable prognosis than the latter.

3. METHODS FOR BLOOD PRESSURE ASSESSMENT

The 2013 ESC/ESH guidelines pointed out the new approach to methods for blood pressure assessment in relation to the continental nationwide laws. In particular, they pointed out the out-of-order use of mercury sphygmomanometer due to its dangerousness although the use of the semiautomatic instrument deserves a tight attention in daily and home monitoring of blood pressure. No other great variations in the methodology for the blood pressure monitoring and measurement can be outlined from standard international guidelines.

In opposition to previous recommendations, the 2013 ESC guidelines emphasized "out of office" blood pressure (BP) monitoring in form of home blood pressure monitoring (HBPM) and ambulatory blood pressure monitoring (ABPM), by favoring the former rather than the latter, in agreement with recent evidences showing that blood pressure values detected with these two methods predict organ damage and risk of cardiovascular outcomes better than BP assessed in the office (office pressure measurement) [12-14]. Although office pressure measurement, i.e. the blood pressure evaluation in the medical environment, represents the gold standard for the diagnosis of arterial hypertension, the guidelines underline the complementary role of HBPM and ABPM in the general assessment of BP. This is the reason why the 2013 paper contains more accurate definitions about the cut-off values for diagnosis of the office, home and ambulatory blood pressure measurements, paying more attention to technical procedures or their evaluations.

Furthermore, 2013 guidelines offer a sort of simplification of ABPM interpretation which makes the guidelines more useful and practical than previous one. The paper considered as main prognostic factor the mean BP value recorded over 24 hours (cut-off values $\geq$130 mmHg for systolic and/or $\geq$80 mmHg for diastolic blood pressure). This is really important because enhances the relevance of the masked hypertension outlined by 24 h BP monitoring and defined as normal BP at the office measurement with increased BP levels at ABPM or HBPM. This condition is considered equivalent to sustained hypertension in term of predictor of major cardiovascular events [15]. Although the ESC 2013 guidelines did not advise to perform ABPM in all subjects with normal blood pressure values and other cardiovascular risk factors, the relevance of ABPM is particularly sustained.

4. ORGAN DAMAGE ASSESSMENT

The section devoted to organ damage assessment repeats the directions of previous guidelines, in relation to the effectiveness and low cost of the available techniques used for early detection of vascular injuries (i.e. PWV and ankle-brachial index). More importance has now been assigned to the role of magnetic resonance imaging (MRI) for cerebral microbleeds evaluation (observed in 5% of individuals) and for the study of silent brain lesions in hypertensive patients. Although the guidelines do not recommend the routine use of MRI due to lack of data [16], they promote the management of more trials evaluating the predictive value of MRI in hypertensive patients. Furthermore, retinopathy grades III and IV are actually considered to be more predictive of cardiovascular mortality than mild lesions of fundus oculi.

5. TARGET BLOOD PRESSURE VALUES

The 2013 guidelines simplify the goals for antihypertensive treatment: in opposition to the 2007 version which indicated different blood pressure targets in relation to age, gender and co-morbidities. Not only the actual guidelines did not consider anymore the cardiovascular risk in normotensives but, focusing more on high blood pressure values, the new document only recommends a systolic BP target <140 mmHg as the best target to be reached in hypertensive patients. This cut-off is strongly recommended (Class I) for patients with low-to-moderate cardiovascular risk and with diabetes [2], while it shows a class IIa recommendation for patients with history of stroke and transient ischemic attack, coronary artery disease and chronic kidney disease [2]. In patients older than 80 years the systolic BP target should be maintained between 140-150 mmHg if their mental and physical health allow it. According to the diastolic blood pressure, it is recommended a target value <90 mmHg, with the exception of patients with diabetes mellitus whose target should be <85 mmHg [2].

6. METABOLIC ASSESSMENT

The metabolic syndrome is not recognized anymore as independent risk factor but all its components are considered as single factors. There is no mention in the current guidelines about the metabolic syndrome as a whole. The authors of the new guidelines considered only the single features of metabolic syndrome in the general assessment of the patient suffering from hypertension. This is a point of criticism when considering the new guidelines: the metabolic syndrome gathers features and conditions that increase too much the cardiovascular risk profile of hypertensive patients. Thus, much more attention should be paid to the patient suffering from metabolic syndrome.

7. THERAPEUTIC APPROACH

The section dealing with the treatment strategies presents the major novelties of this document, mainly arising from randomized controlled trials performed in recent years, but also from the need to reform the previous organization. First of all, pharmacological treatment should be based on patient's overall risk, determined by clinic blood pressure values and other cardiovascular risk factors, such as subclinical organ damage, diabetes mellitus, symptomatic cardiovascular disease or chronic kidney disease [2], outlining not to give (Class IIIA) any drugs in case of high normal blood pressure (systolic values between 130 and 139 mmHg) but recommending to encourage life style changes.

According to pharmacological treatment, the new guidelines substantially reconfirm the 5 major classes of antihypertensive drugs (thiazide diuretics, beta-blockers, calcium channel blockers, angiotensin-converting enzyme [ACE] inhibitors, angiotensin II receptor blockers, [ARBs]) for the initiation and maintenance of treatment, either as monotherapy or in association (Class IA) [2]. Nevertheless, for the first time the paper contraindicated the combination therapy between ACE inhibitors and ARBs in relation to the results of ongoing Telmisartan Alone and in combination with Ramipril Global Endpoint Trial (ONTARGET) [17].

Furthermore, the 2013 version updated the recommendations about the starting of combined therapy in high cardiovascular risk patients or with high blood pressure values (Class IIb) in relation to the findings coming from three large-scale clinical trials published after 2007 (Avoiding Cardiovascular events through combination therapy in Patients Living with Systolic Hypertension [ACCOMPLISH], Action in Diabetes and Vascular disease: Preterax and diamicron Controlled Evaluation [ADVANCE] and (ONTARGET). The current hypertension guidelines dedicate a whole subsection to aliskiren, the first selective inhibitor of plasma renin activity. This drug, alone or in combination, reduces systolic and diastolic BP in all age hypertensive patients [18], increases its effectiveness in association with a thiazide diuretic, a renin-angiotensin system blocker on a different site [19] or a calcium channel blocker [20] and finally improves asymptomatic organ damage indices [21]. Despite the large initial expectations, this drug was not included in the recommendations of new guidelines due to the poor results coming from literature [22,23]. The altitude study, for example, randomized diabetic patients to receive aliskiren in addition to an ace inhibitor or an ARB. it was discontinued due to the onset of renal complications, hyperkalemia and hypotension [22]. In subjects with reduced left ventricular ejection fraction, aliskiren did not reduce cardiovascular mortality or readmission rate at 6 months, nor showed any clinical benefit within one year [23].

8. DRUG-RESISTANT HYPERTENSION

Unlike the previous version, the 2013 ESC guidelines on arterial hypertension management amply dealt with the problem of resistant hypertension, defined as blood pressure that remains high despite treatment with at least three antihypertensive agents at the maximum tolerated dose [2]. Its diagnosis requires a careful assessment of blood pressure values through ABPM and an evaluation of patient's compliance to drug therapy, after a prudent exclusion of all the causes which can sustain high blood pressure. The true resistant hypertension is a relevant public health problem due to its role in increasing the risk of developing complications such as myocardial infarction, stroke, heart or kidney failure, death regardless of age, gender and/or other associated diseases [24-26]. Therefore, high costs for the national health system are related to resistant hypertension. The current guidelines underlined that resistant hypertensive patients should be evaluated by an appropriate and thoroughly trained team in order to optimize anti-hypertensive drugs administration or consider minimally invasive treatments [2].

The non-pharmacological approaches to resistant hypertension are another novelty in 2013 guidelines. Although the paper outlined the lack of large cohort studies and long-term efficacy, safety, morbidity and mortality data, non-pharmacological, invasive approaches to hypertension is considered the future of hypertensive patients' treatment. Implantable device stimulating the carotid baroreceptors can be an optimal treatment option with few side effects [27,28], as well as renal artery sympathetic denervation by radiofrequency [29-31]. The ESH believes that, although the conclusion of Simplicity HTN-3 depicts the renal denervation as an ineffective technique [32], more trials are needed in order to better validate these pathophysiological concepts, the efficacy in specific subgroups of patients and the clinical outputs obtained through different devices employed.

9. GAPS

The 2013 guidelines confirm a therapeutic approach to hypertensive patients according to total cardiovascular risk highlighting the need for a tailored treatment. In elderly patients, the document recommends a systolic BP target between 140-150 mmHg (class IA) in subjects younger than 80 years or <140 mmHg if case of healthy patient (class IIb C); in individuals older than 80 years the systolic BP target still continues to be set at 140-150 mmHg if mental and physical heath allow it (class IB). Thus, in the global risk-assessment algorithm the age is considered as a risk factor when overcome 55 years in men and 65 years in women.

Nevertheless, old adults, especially the frail elderly, should be *per se* considered as a category at moderate to high cardiovascular risk due to their co-morbidities. Older adults often suffer from isolated systolic hypertension which decreases vascular compliance and increases pulse pressure, which are powerful predictor of cardiovascular events even more than the single values of systolic or diastolic blood pressure [33]. Furthermore, the impact of cardiovascular risk factors on vascular outcomes is greater in very elderly subjects and this should be taken into account [34,35]. Other medical conditions such as urinary incontinence, falls and fractures, depression, cognitive dysfunction, functional impairment with lack of moderate or vigorous exercise and delirium can negatively influence the outcome of the elderly patients. For this reason geriatricians use the term "geriatric syndromes" to gather the condition of the elder with his/her co-morbidities [36,37]. The novel targets proposed for hypertensive old persons are really interesting above all because point out that antihypertensive therapy should be carefully tailored in such category of patients in order to avoid a steeper decrease in diastolic pressure which could compromise the blood perfusion of important organs, such as heart and brain. Although such particular attention to elderly people, the 2013 guidelines did not consider the evaluation of their physical and mental performance and, therefore, no indicators were provided for optimization of the treatments in relation to subject's health state while, for the first time, cerebral microvascular lesions are considered as target organ damage.

The new guidelines on hypertension management are particularly endowed with stratification of cardiovascular risk profile of individuals. Nevertheless, they did not consider nontraditional risk factors which contribute to atherosclerosis development and to increase cardiovascular risk. Hyperuricemia is currently recognized as an independent risk factor for cardiovascular disease: Baseline serum uric acid (SUA) levels can effectively predict cardiovascular mortality [38-40]. The association between SUA and increased risk for cardiovascular events/all-cause mortality was demonstrated in untreated subjects with essential hypertension [41]. Elevated plasma levels of homocysteine (HCY is deemed a powerful marker of cardiovascular diseases [42,43]. Elevated HCY plasma values ameliorate risk prediction in subjects considered at "intermediate risk" according to Framingham risk

score [44]. In patient with established coronary artery disease, increased HCY levels are strong predictors of cardiovascular mortality. HCY concentrations are slightly associated with angiographic extent of coronary atherosclerosis and strongly related to history of myocardial infarction, impaired left ventricular ejection fraction and death due to cardiac causes [45]. Moreover, high HCY levels have an important value in predicting re-stenosis and major adverse cardiac events after successful coronary angioplasty [46]. The evaluation of such a molecule is not fully considered in the overall text of the guidelines and this limits the complete evaluation of cardiovascular risk score of hypertensive patients.

Furthermore, the guidelines briefly refer to lipoprotein(a) and C-reactive protein, declaring that risk may be higher than indicated in the charts in patients with increased levels of such compounds [47,48]. Additional assessment of the serum levels of these molecules should be taken into account in order to fully predict cardiovascular events [49].

Our opinion is that guidelines should win the reticence in recommending screening for nontraditional risk factors, in relation to the wide evidences supporting their prognostic power and the amelioration of cardiovascular risk when a reduction in their serum levels is reached [50-53].

Thus, in clinical practice and management of hypertensive patients, the screening of emerging risk factors should be encouraged to complete and enhance the global risk assessment of cardiovascular disease.

By considering the instrumental approach to hypertensive patients, the guidelines support the HBPM approach for a more accurate cardiovascular risk assessment to obtain a careful picture of blood pressure profile, evaluate the efficacy of pressure-lowering therapy and increase the adherence of patients to treatments. Nevertheless, BP presents short-term fluctuations over the 24-hour cycle [54]. At the moment, it is not establish whether antihypertensive treatment should aim at reducing absolute BP values or shall counteract BP variability. Furthermore, the HBPM could cause discomfort or worry to the patients during the performance. Thus, such a monitoring might be lived with concern by patients and this emotional stress might cause increasing blood pressure by itself.

Finally, the cardiovascular risk algorithm is also based on organ damage assessment that requests several laboratory and instrumental examinations. This struggles with long waiting lists in public hospitals and high costs of private healthcare that not allows all patients to bear the fees due to of the great economic difficulties of these times.

10. 2013 ESH/ESC GUIDELINES vs. EIGHTH JOINT NATIONAL COMMITTEE GUIDELINES

The 8th JNC guidelines on hypertension [55] are the expression of general and worldwide guidelines for the management of hypertension and they are the evolution of the previous 7th JNC guidelines [56]. The 2013 ESC/ESH guidelines [2] also differ from the extra-continental one [55] as some points and cut-offs are not equal from each other. One of the major differences that can be pointed out regards the evaluation of the role of age per se in the general management of hypertensive condition. JNC 8th effectively gave a great importance to age by considering it as a fundamental characteristics able to make the physician changed his/her pharmacological or interventional management of the hypertensive patient [55]. While 2013 European guidelines considered "age" as a common cardiovascular risk parameter in the SCORE model for cardiovascular risk stratification, preferring cardiovascular risk stratification as the leading factors for maneuvers in hypertension condition [2], the JNC 8th underlined the need for an "age-based therapy" [55]. Nevertheless, a great positive advantage of the JNC 8 report was the consideration of "race" as a condition able to induce a change in pharmacological treatment of the patients. The black population, in particular, deserved different approaches as compared to non-black one in relation to the different characteristics of their hypertensive state [55]. Such a consideration is not pointed out in the 2013 ESC guidelines and even the SCORE model for cardiovascular risk stratification did not contemplate any remind to race as able to influence the treatment of hypertension. This is a great limitation of the European guidelines above all in relation to the great immigration flows in the continental lands [57]. Nevertheless, despite such a positive aspect, the JNC 8th did not offer a full representation of the cardiovascular risk profile of individuals. In contrast to 2013 ESC/ESH guidelines, the JNC 8th did not provide any reference about a model for cardiovascular risk

evaluation of patients and a different pharmacological strategy for hypertension management in relation to the different total cardiovascular risk profile of the patients.

11. CONCLUSION

In conclusion, the 2013 guidelines on hypertension management offer new diagnostic and therapeutic possibilities on the basis of numerous clinical trials and updates performed during the last years. Many points, however, remain to be clarified such as: Blood pressure values at treatment starts and target BP values in elderly patients; the quantification of the eventual reduction in cardiovascular morbidity and mortality by adopting the new therapeutic approaches for resistant hypertension; the benefits of the drug treatment in subjects at high cardiovascular risk and with high-normal blood pressure. Therefore, we think that new randomized controlled trials will resolve all the issues pointed out in this overview in order to improve the management of that part of hypertensive patients still not on perfect BP control. Furthermore, we think that more attention should be paid to age and patients' frailty: the general practitioners will be able to really help specialists in reaching a full evaluation of all the aspects related to hypertension and finally overcome the gaps in evidence. Practically, a tight collaboration among researchers and medical doctors is the basis for the reduction of the great number of limitations of the current perspective on hypertension, in order to obtain a full control of this cardiovascular risk factor.

CONSENT

It is not applicable.

ETHICAL APPROVAL

It is not applicable.

COMPETING INTERESTS

Authors have declared that no competing interests exist.

REFERENCES

1.   Go AS, Mozaffarian D, Roger VL, Benjamin EJ, Berry JD, Blaha MJ, et al. Heart disease and stroke statistics-2014

update: A report from the American Heart Association. Circulation. 2014;129:e28-e292.

2. Mancia G, Fagard R, Narkiewicz K, Redon J, Zanchetti A, Böhm M, et al. ESH/ESC guidelines for the management of arterial hypertension: The Task Force for the management of arterial hypertension of the European Society of Hypertension (ESH) and of the European Society of Cardiology (ESC). Eur Heart J. 2013;34: 2159-219.

3. Mancia G, De Backer G, Dominiczak A, Cifkova R, Fagard R, Germano G, et al. Guidelines for the management of arterial hypertension: The Task Force for the management of arterial hypertension of the European Society of Hypertension (ESH) and of the European Society of Cardiology (ESC). Eur Heart J. 2007;28:1462-536.

4. Mancia G, Laurent S, Agabiti-Rosei E, Ambrosioni E, Burnier M, Caulfield MJ, et al. Reappraisal of European guidelines on hypertension management: A European Society of Hypertension task force document. J. Hypertens. 2009;27:2121-58.

5. Anguita Sánchez M. Grupo de Trabajo de la SEC sobre la guía de hipertensión arterial ESC/ESH 2013, revisores expertos de la guía de hipertensión arterial ESC/ESH 2013 y Comité de Guías de Práctica Clínica de la SEC. Comments on the ESC/ESH guidelines for the management of arterial hypertension 2013. A report of the Task Force of the Clinical Practice Guidelines Committee of the Spanish Society of Cardiology. Rev Esp Cardiol. 2013;66:842-847.

6. Perk J, De Backer G, Gohlke H, Graham I, Reiner Z, Verschuren M, et al. European Guidelines on cardiovascular disease prevention in clinical practice (version 2012). The Fifth Joint Task Force of the European Society of Cardiology and Other Societies on Cardiovascular Disease Prevention in Clinical Practice (constituted by representatives of nine societies and by invited experts). Eur Heart J. 2012;33:1635-701.

7. Reiner Z, Catapano AL, De Backer G, Graham I, Taskinen MR, Wiklund O, et al. ESC/EAS Guidelines for the management of dyslipidaemias: The Task Force for the management of dyslipidaemias of the European Society of Cardiology (ESC) and the European Atherosclerosis Society (EAS). Eur Heart J. 2011;32:1769-818.

8. Conroy RM, Pyörälä K, Fitzgerald AP, Sans S, Menotti A, De Backer G, et al. Estimation of ten-year risk of fatal cardiovascular disease in Europe: The SCORE project. Eur Heart J. 2003;24:987-1003.

9. Sehestedt T, Jeppesen J, Hansen TW, Wachtell K, Ibsen H, Torp-Pedersen C, Hildebrandt P, Olsen MH. Risk prediction is improved by adding markers of subclinical organ damage to SCORE. Eur Heart J. 2010;31:883-91.

10. Sehestedt T, Jeppesen J, Hansen TW, Rasmussen S, Wachtell K, Ibsen H, Torp-Pedersen C, Olsen MH. Thresholds for pulse wave velocity, urine albumin creatinine ratio and left ventricular mass index using SCORE, Framingham and ESH/ESC risk charts. J Hypertens. 2012; 30:1928-36.

11. Volpe M, Battistoni A, Tocci G, Rosei EA, Catapano AL, Coppo R, et al. Cardiovascular risk assessment beyond Systemic Coronary Risk Estimation: A role for organ damage markers. J. Hypertens. 2012;30:1056-64.

12. Ward AM, Takahashi O, Stevens R, Heneghan C. Home measurement of blood pressure and cardiovascular disease: Systematic review and meta-analysis of prospective Studies. J. Hypertens. 2012; 30:449-56.

13. Fan HQ, Li Y, Thijs L, Hansen TW, Boggia J, Kikuya M, et al. Prognostic value of isolated nocturnal hypertension on ambulatory measurement in 8711 individuals from 10 populations. J Hypertens. 2010;28:2036-45.

14. Gaborieau V, Delarche N, Gosse P. Ambulatory blood pressure monitoring versus self-measurement of blood pressure at home: Correlation with target organ damage. J. Hypertens. 2008;26: 1919-27.

15. Fagard RH, Cornelissen VA. Incidence of cardiovascular events in white-coat, masked and sustained hypertension versus true normotension: A meta-analysis. J. Hypertens. 2007;25:2193-8.

16. Henskens LH, van Oostenbrugge RJ, Kroon AA, Hofman PA, Lodder J, de Leeuw PW. Detection of silent cerebrovascular disease refines risk stratification of hypertensive patients. J Hypertens. 2009;27:846-53.

17. Yusuf S, Teo KK, Pogue J, Dyal L, Copland I, Schumacher H, et al. Telmisartan, ramipril or both in patients at high risk for vascular events. N. Engl J. Med. 2008;358:1547-59.

18. Gradman AH, Schmieder RE, Lins RL, Nussberger J, Chiang Y, Bedigian MP. Aliskiren, a novel orally effective renin inhibitor, provides dose-dependent antihypertensive efficacy and placebo-like tolerability in hypertensive patients. Circulation. 2005;111:1012-8.

19. O'Brien E, Barton J, Nussberger J, Mulcahy D, Jensen C, Dicker P, Stanton A. Aliskiren reduces blood pressure and suppresses plasma renin activity in combination with a thiazide diuretic, an angiotensin-converting enzyme inhibitor or an angiotensin receptor blocker. Hypertension. 2007;49:276-84.

20. Littlejohn TW, 3rd, Trenkwalder P, Hollanders G, Zhao Y, Liao W. Long-term safety, tolerability and efficacy of combination therapy with aliskiren and amlodipine in patients with hypertension. Curr Med Res Opin. 2009;25:951-9.

21. Seed A, Gardner R, McMurray J, Hillier C, Murdoch D, MacFadyen R, et al. Neurohumoral effects of the new orally active renin inhibitor, aliskiren, in chronic heart failure. Eur J. Heart Fail. 2007;9:1120-7.

22. Parving HH, Brenner BM, McMurray JJ, de Zeeuw D, Haffner SM, Solomon SD, et al. Cardiorenal end points in a trial of aliskiren for type 2 diabetes. N Engl J. Med. 2012;367:2204-13.

23. Gheorghiade M, Böhm M, Greene SJ, Fonarow GC, Lewis EF, Zannad F, et al. Effect of aliskiren on postdischarge mortality and heart failure readmissions among patients hospitalized for heart failure: The ASTRONAUT randomized trial. JAMA. 2013;309:1125-35.

24. Myat A, Redwood SR, Qureshi AC, Spertus JA, Williams B. Resistant hypertension. BMJ. 2012;345:e7473.

25. Daugherty SL, Powers JD, Magid DJ, Tavel HM, Masoudi FA, Margolis KL, et al. Incidence and prognosis of resistant hypertension in hypertensive patients. Circulation. 2012;125:1635-42.

26. De la Sierra A, Segura J, Banegas JR, Gorostidi M, de la Cruz JJ, Armario P, et al. Clinical features of 8295 patients with resistant hypertension classified on the basis of ambulatory blood pressure monitoring. Hypertension. 2011;57:898-902.

27. Lovic D, Manolis AJ, Lovic B, Stojanov V, Lovic M, Pittaras A, Jakovljevic B. The pathophysiological basis of carotid baroreceptor stimulation for the treatment of resistant hypertension. Curr Vasc Pharmacol. 2014;12:16-22.

28. Doumas M, Faselis C, Kokkinos P, Anyfanti P, Tsioufis C, Papademetriou V. Carotid baroreceptor stimulation: A promising approach for the management of resistant hypertension and heart failure. Curr Vasc Pharmacol. 2014;12:30-7.

29. Krum H, Schlaich M, Whitbourn R, Sobotka PA, Sadowski J, Bartus K, et al. Catheter-based renal sympathetic denervation for resistant hypertension: A multicentre safety and proof-of-principle cohort study. Lancet. 2009;373:1275-81.

30. Symplicity HTN-2 Investigators, Esler MD, Krum H, Sobotka PA, Schlaich MP, Schmieder RE, Böhm M. Renal sympathetic denervation in patients with treatment-resistant hypertension (The Symplicity HTN-2 Trial): A randomised controlled trial. Lancet. 2010;376:1903-9.

31. Witkowski A, Prejbisz A, Florczak E, Kądziela J, Śliwiński P, Bieleń P, et al. Effects of renal sympathetic denervation on blood pressure, sleep apnea course and glycemic control in patients with resistant hypertension and sleep apnea. Hypertension. 2011;58:559-65.

32. Bhatt DL, Kandzari DE, O'Neill WW, D'Agostino R, Flack JM, Katzen BT, et al. A controlled trial of renal denervation for resistant hypertension. N. Engl J. Med. 2014;370:1393-401.

33. Madhavan S, Ooi WL, Cohen H, Alderman MH. Relation of pulse pressure and blood pressure reduction to the incidence of myocardial infarction. Hypertension. 1994; 23:395-401.

34. Kagiyama S, Matsumura K, Ansai T, Soh I, Takata Y, Awano S, et al. Chronic kidney disease increases cardiovascular mortality in 80-year-old subjects in Japan. Hypertens Res. 2008;31:2053-8.

35. Shastri S, Tighiouart H, Katz R, Rifkin DE, Fried LF, Shlipak MG, et al. Chronic kidney

disease in octogenarians. Clin J. Am Soc Nephrol. 2011;6:1410-7.

36. Fried LP, Kronmal RA, Newman AB, Bild DE, Mittelmark MB, Polak JF, et al. Risk factors for 5-year mortality in older adults: The cardiovascular health study. JAMA. 1998;279:585-92.

37. Inouye SK, Studenski S, Tinetti ME, Kuchel GA. Geriatric syndromes: Clinical, research and policy implications of a core geriatric concept. J. Am Geriatr Soc. 2007; 55:780-91.

38. Strasak AM, Kelleher CC, Brant LJ, Rapp K, Ruttmann E, Concin H, et al. Serum uric acid is an independent predictor for all major forms of cardiovascular death in 28,613 elderly women: A prospective 21-year follow-up study. Int J. Cardiol. 2008; 125:232-9.

39. Huang H, Huang B, Li Y, Huang Y, Li J, Yao H, et al. Uric acid and risk of heart failure: A systematic review and meta-analysis. Eur J. Heart Fail. 2014;16:15-24.

40. Feig DI, Kang DH, Johnson RJ. Uric acid and cardiovascular risk. N. Engl J. Med. 2008;359:1811-21.

41. Verdecchia P, Schillaci G, Reboldi G, Santeusanio F, Porcellati C, Brunetti P. Relation between serum uric acid and risk of cardiovascular disease in essential hypertension. The PIUMA study. Hypertension. 2000;36:1072-8.

42. Clarke R, Daly L, Robinson K, Naughten E, Cahalane S, Fowler B, Graham I. Hyperhomocysteinemia: An independent risk factor for vascular disease. N. Engl J. Med. 1991;324:1149-55.

43. Antoniades C, Antonopoulos AS, Tousoulis D, Marinou K, Stefanadis C. Homocysteine and coronary atherosclerosis: From folate fortification to the recent clinical trials. Eur Heart J. 2009;30:6-15.

44. Veeranna V, Zalawadiya SK, Niraj A, Pradhan J, Ference B, Burack RC, et al. Homocysteine and reclassification of cardiovascular disease risk. J. Am Coll Cardiol. 2011;58:1025-33.

45. Nygård O, Nordrehaug JE, Refsum H, Ueland PM, Farstad M, Vollset SE. Plasma homocysteine levels and mortality in patients with coronary artery disease. N. Engl J. Med. 1997;337:230-6.

46. Schnyder G, Roffi M, Flammer Y, Pin R, Hess OM. Association of plasma homocysteine with restenosis after percutaneous coronary angioplasty. Eur Heart J. 2002;23:726-33.

47. Erqou S, Kaptoge S, Perry PL, Di Angelantonio E, Thompson A, White IR, et al. Lipoprotein (a) concentration and the risk of coronary heart disease, stroke and nonvascular mortality. JAMA. 2009;302: 412-23.

48. Lagrand WK, Visser CA, Hermens WT, Niessen HW, Verheugt FW, Wolbink GJ, Hack CE. C-reactive protein as a cardiovascular risk factor: More than an epiphenomenon? Circulation. 1999;100: 96-102.

49. Kaptoge S, Di Angelantonio E, Pennells L, Wood AM, White IR, Gao P, et al. C-reactive protein, fibrinogen and cardiovascular disease prediction. N. Engl J. Med. 2012;367:1310-20.

50. Nordestgaard BG, Chapman MJ, Ray K, Borén J, Andreotti F, Watts GF, et al. Lipoprotein (a) as a cardiovascular risk factor: Current status. Eur Heart J. 2010; 31:2844-53.

51. Rentoukas E, Tsarouhas K, Tsitsimpikou C, Lazaros G, Deftereos S, Vavetsi S. The prognostic impact of allopurinol in patients with acute myocardial infarction undergoing primary percutaneous coronary intervention. Int J. Cardiol. 2010;145:257-8.

52. Rajendra NS, Ireland S, George J, Belch JJ, Lang CC, Struthers AD. Mechanistic insights into the therapeutic use of high-dose allopurinol in angina pectoris. J. Am Coll Cardiol. 2011;58:820-8.

53. Ridker PM, Danielson E, Fonseca FA, Genest J, Gotto AM. Jr, Kastelein JJ, et al. Rosuvastatin to prevent vascular events in men and women with elevated C-reactive protein. N. Engl J. Med. 2008;359:2195-207.

54. Parati G, Ochoa JE, Lombardi C, Bilo G. Assessment and management of blood-pressure variability. Nat Rev Cardiol. 2013; 10:143-55.

55. James PA, Oparil S, Carter BL, Cushman WC, Dennison-Himmelfarb C, Handler J, et al. Evidence-based guideline for the management of high blood pressure in adults report from the panel members

appointed to the Eighth Joint National Committee (JNC 8). JAMA. 2014;311:507-20.

56. Chobanian AV, Bakris GL, Black HR, Cushman WC, Green LA, Izzo JL. Jr, et al. The seventh report of the Joint National Committee on Prevention, Detection, Evaluation and Treatment of High Blood Pressure: The JNC 7 report. JAMA. 2003; 289:2560-72.

57. Modesti PA, Bianchi S, Borghi C, Cameli M, Capasso G, Ceriello A, et al. Cardiovascular health in migrants: Current status and issues for prevention. A collaborative multidisciplinary task force report. J. Cardiovasc Med (Hagerstown). 2014;15:683-92.

21

Approaching Long Term Cardiac Rhythm Monitoring Using Advanced Arm Worn Sensors and ECG Recovery Techniques

William D. Lynn[1][*], Omar J. Escalona[1] and David J. McEneaney[2]

[1]*University of Ulster, School of Engineering, Engineering Research Institute, Newtownabbey, BT37 0QB, UK.*
[2]*Craigavon Area Hospital, Southern Health and Social Care Trust, Cardiac Unit, SHSCT, Portadown, BT63 5QQ, UK.*

Authors' contributions

This work was carried out in collaboration between all authors. Author WDL designed the study, managed the literature searches and wrote the first draft of the manuscript. Author OJE managed the experimental process. Author DJM wrote the protocols and the ethical approval application. All authors read and approved the final manuscript.

Editor(s):
(1) Francesco Pelliccia, Department of Heart and Great Vessels, University La Sapienza, Rome, Italy.
Reviewers:
(1) Anonymous, Qatar.
(2) Anonymous, Italy.
(3) Anonymous, China.
(4) Anonymous, India.

ABSTRACT

According to recent British Heart Foundation statistics, one in six men and more than one in ten women die from coronary heart disease (CHD) in the UK. This equates to almost 74,000 deaths per annum from CHD alone. More worryingly, every week, 12 apparently fit and healthy young people aged 35 and under, die from undiagnosed cardiac conditions. In both circumstances, monitoring is preformed only when triggered by an event. Unfortunately, this may be too late in the large majority of cases. For instance, there is evidence suggesting that most indiscernible cardiac abnormalities are made detectable by ECG through the act of suddenly standing upright. This infers that the condition would be detectable during the course of everyday ambulatory activity and highlights the need for a long term monitoring device. Current diagnostic equipment consists of the Holter monitor

*Corresponding author: E-mail: Lynn-WD@email.ulster.ac.uk

for extended periods up to 36 hours and the implantable loop recorder (ILR) for monitoring up to 3 years. The diagnostic yield of the ECG monitoring strategy is greatly increased as the monitoring period increases. Therefore, for subjects that exhibit symptoms of cardiac involvement that are transient in nature, the ILR offers the best opportunity for diagnosis. However, the ILR is inserted under the surface of the skin in the upper chest area and requires a surgical procedure, with associated risks, which makes ILR's a costly and inconvenient option in many cases.

The need for a non-invasive long term monitoring device, which is comfortable to wear along the arm and able to provide reliable ECG monitoring, has been addressed by many, in several lines of approach to a solution. This review details the current state of the art and any pending limitations. It then presents key multidisciplinary solutions on the different aspects of the problem, which will still require integration in order to realise such a device.

Keywords: ECG; long term; monitor; arm worn; dysrhythmia.

1. INTRODUCTION

As heart disease remains a prevalent killer of both the old and the young [1], there is a strong case for the development of a long term monitoring technology that is non-invasive and comfortable to wear. Also, with recent research alluding toward an increased detectability of latent cardiac abnormalities once the subject stands from a seated position [2], the desirability and marketability of an arm worn sensor is increasingly realised [3].

The effect of drugs on the heart rhythm is widely noted in the literature. An example being those which are linked with QT elongation or torsade de pointes. Domperidone, for instance has been associated with a small increased risk of serious ventricular dysrhythmia or sudden cardiac death [4,5]. A warning strategy for patients continuously monitored during their course of treatment would significantly de-risk the administration period.

Atrial fibrillation (AF) affects almost 800,000 people in the UK, predominantly over 75 year olds with an affect rate of 10%. AF is uncommon in younger people; however, it may be coincidental with other heart defects such as heart valve problems [6]. Gauging the time a patient spends in paroxysmal atrial fibrillation will determine the treatment plan. Current analysis and recording equipment, such as the Omron HCG801 [7] (Fig. 1 (a)), do not give a good temporal picture because the recording is not continuous. The Holter monitor (Fig. 1 (b)) is a continuous data storage device; however, it is a short term technology, offering recording over time periods of 24hrs to 2 weeks. For longer recording periods, in the region of 28 days, an External Loop Recorder or Event Loop Recorder (ELR) may be selected by the clinician to act as a diagnostic tool. The ELR (Fig. 1 (c)) is available

in two forms - permanently worn (looping memory) or as a post applied recorder (non-looping memory). The permanently worn device may be automatically triggered by a threshold crossing of the patient's heart rate or patient triggered once he has become aware of a dysrhythmia. The post event recorder is not worn continuously and as a result does not store any historical precursor to the dysrhythmic event. The post event recorder depends on the patient's compliance with general operational protocols, the patient remaining sufficiently coherent to operate the event trigger and the maintenance of consciousness during the scope of the dysrhythmia.

Real time monitoring of the cardiac output can be achieved using a fusion of ELR and cellular phone technology in the form of the Mobile Cardiac Output Telemetry recorder (MCOT) [8] (Fig. 1 (d)). MCOT recorders are a recent development and provide the wearer with a 24 hr full, high resolution data recording device. The device can provide the clinician with real time, streamed data over a cellular interface, hence delimiting the storage capacity. The technology may also be configured as a looping, non-looping, event triggered and patient triggered device, capable of delivering a recording directly to the clinician.

The Implantable Loop Recorder (ILR) overcomes patient noncompliance through surgical intervention. A small device, similar in size to a USB memory stick (Fig. 1 (e)), is implanted under the skin on the wall of the upper chest. The ILR is event triggered or can be patient triggered by placing an activator proximally on the chest. The more recent generations of this device are designed to operate in excess of 2 years [9] and have wireless communication capability offering the provision of fast delivery of data for interpretation and subsequent clinical decision.

Thus, depending on the device time application, the available technology can operate in three time-range categories: limited to short term monitoring, up to 1 month, or very long term, in excess of 2 years. Without the risk and cost of the surgically implanted ILR, the middle category is not catered for. It is also notable that a continuous full data recording device is not yet available for periods over 1 month.

Several key factors influence the success of a proposed very long term monitor. Firstly, the comfort of such a monitor is paramount. The

ambulatory patient must be virtually unaware of the monitor's presence to ensure that the urge to tamper with, or completely remove the device prematurely is mitigated. Several authors have suggested comfort sites for wearable electronics [10,11]. Gemperle et al. and Shackel et al. discuss the many factors that contribute to a subject feeling comfortable. Shackel discusses ergonomics of work place design, specifically chair comfort while Gemperle tested the design of wearable forms by studying subjects while they perform activities. Each subject rated the forms perceived comfort to allow the construction of a body position comfort model - shown in Fig. 2.

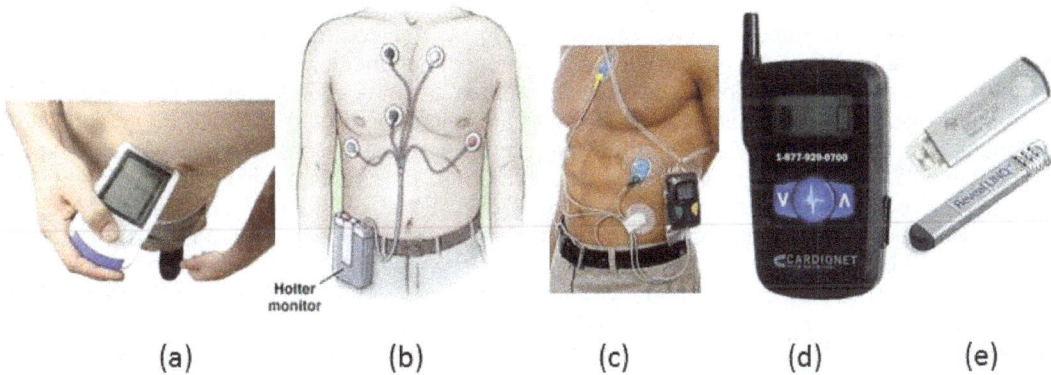

Fig. 1. (a) Omoron HCG801 post applied non-looping recorder; (b) standard short term holter recording device; (c) Event Loop Recorder (ELR); (d) Mobile Cardiac Output Telemetry(MCOT); (e) Implantable Loop Recorder (ILR), standard and wirelessly enabled

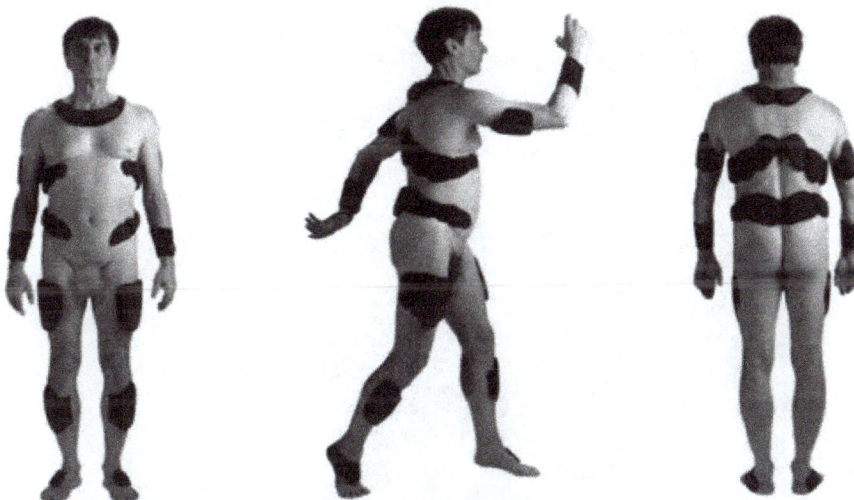

Fig. 2. Body sites for comfortable "wearability" (Gemperle et al.) [4]

Lynn (2013). concluded, by analysis of the data from a clinical study, that a significant reduction in ECG signal occurred on the right arm [12], an opinion supported by Hung-Chi Yang et al [13]. Hence all attempts at a successful arm worn device refer to data collected on the left limb. Yang developed a flexible foil electrode that can be conveniently wrapped around a limb and will facilitate the recording of ECG information – Fig. 3. He successfully extracted QRS information from the upper left arm (bicep region) and elbow position. However, attempts to recover ECG data from the wrist were unsuccessful. Yang has declared that the ECG signal at the wrist is "very weak" and is easily disrupted by electromyographic (EMG) noise. It is also notable that the signal processing used during his study was simplistic, consisting of bandwidth narrowing to remove power line and EMG noise. Yang's chosen noise mitigation technique will have suppressed desired signal information ratio metrically with the noise component, as the frequency domain of the desired signal and the unwanted noise component are overlapped. The electrode design is of interest however. It is also probable that the recordings used in the Yang publication are best case selections and that a dry electrode, of the type described in the experiment, will produce large amounts of electrical noise should the subject move.

1.1 The Noise Issue

As is the case in most areas of measurement, the decisive boundary of detectability of a weak signal is determined by the presence of unwanted, random signals - or noise. Noise obscures the desired signal and poses a major challenge in the recovery of biological signals.

The problem of noise is not limited to weak, low amplitude signals. The measurement accuracy and repeatability of comparatively large amplitude signals can also be affected by the presence of a noise component. When discussing the recovery of cardiac electrical activity, the signals can be described as low amplitude and low energy [14]. This means that the electrical signal produced by the heart is incapable of driving a low impedance load. The conditions described by physicist Georg Ohm, govern and predict the capability and behaviour of all measurement systems [15]. Consider Fig. 4; the component Z_{BM} simulates the body impedance model, if the measurement system is 'ideal' and has an input impedance of infinity, the maximum amplitude will be measured. If the measurement system impedance is equal to Z_{BM}, the measured signal amplitude will appear to be 50% of that measured from the 'ideal' system. The degradation continues as the input impedance of the measurement system decreases. In order to achieve a reasonable signal amplitude, a measurement system design with an input impedance of Z_{BM} or greater is typically chosen. The trade-off being that the high impedance input also allows any noise component to be readily evident in the measured signal.

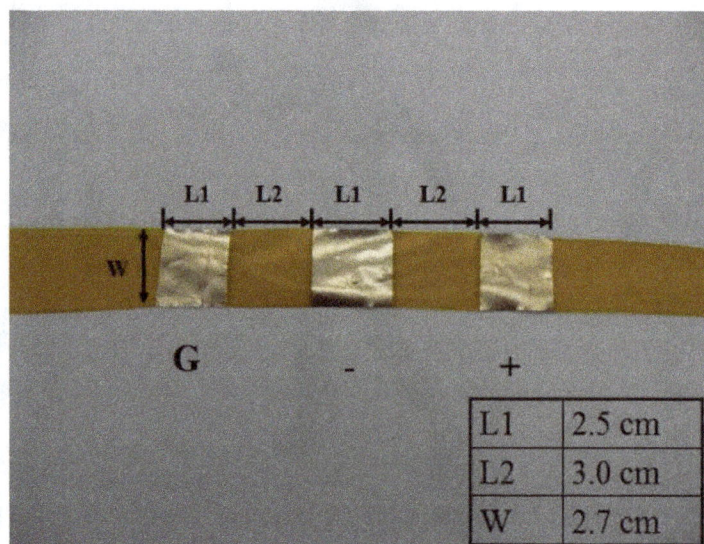

L1	2.5 cm
L2	3.0 cm
W	2.7 cm

Fig. 3. Flexible printed circuit electrode trialled by Yang H et al. 2011. [7]

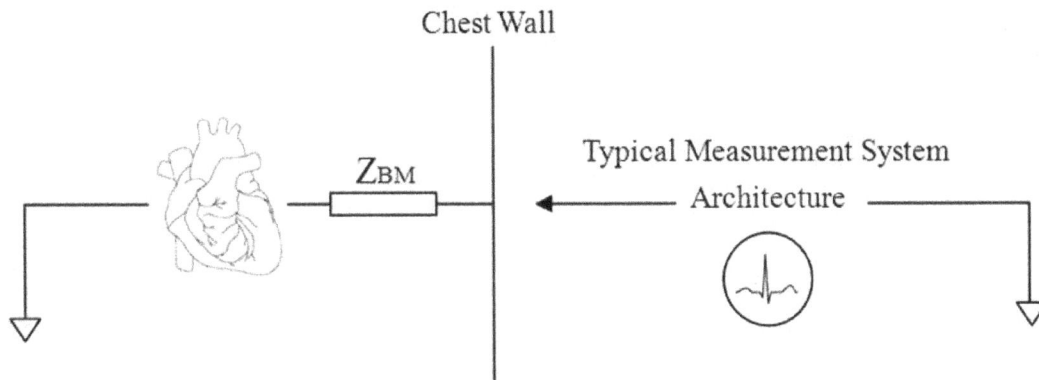

Fig. 4. Illustration showing measurement system interaction with the human body model impedance

Noise falls into two main types - conducted and radiated. Conducted noise is that which is unavoidably present in the final signal. An example of which would be electromyographic disturbances. This type of noise can often be removed by signal averaging or bandwidth narrowing. Radiated noise is that which is propagated through the environment and electromagnetically coupled onto the bioamplifier high impedance input. Radio interference and mains (50Hz/60Hz) interference are examples of this. Radiated noise is often a function of physical layout of the system. Careful positioning of wires, electrodes and power cables can, along with filtering, reduce its affects.

2. POTENTIAL SOLUTIONS

2.1 Signal Denoising Techniques

2.1.1 Signal averaging

Signal averaging (SA) is a reasonably simplistic approach to noise removal from repetitive signals - the ECG, due to its rhythmic nature, is ideal for this approach. The technique requires a fiducial [16] or datum point to be identified. All subsequent repetitions of the signal are temporally aligned and the noise signals are expected to annihilate. The SA technique requires that the noise signals are non-coherent for successful filtering to take place. Power line interference and electromyographic noise sources, through their repetitive nature, often confound this technique.

Temporal misalignment of the fiducial datum has the unwanted effect of integrating the output response, e.g. a pulse stream averaged and processed using an ideal, perfect temporal alignment will reproduce a perfect square pulse as an output. However if the fiducial point is subject to jitter, the output will be a smoothed pulse, ie the high frequency edges will have been lost. This phenomenon was discussed by Escalona et al [16] and William Craelius et al. [17]. Craelius also suggests that a temporal misalignment can add signal components to the filtered signal as well as subtract, producing false triggering of any beat extraction algorithm. A lot can be done to optimise the SA technique and reduce the levels of fiducial point jitter; however, a 'real time' beat to beat comparison is not achievable, therefore a successful clinical implementation of this technique is unlikely.

2.1.2 Empirical mode decomposition

Empirical Mode Decomposition (EMD) was developed by N. E. Huang [18] in 1998. EMD uses an iterative process to decompose a signal into a series of Intrinsic Mode Functions (IMF's) subject to the following conditions.

1) In the whole data set the number of extreme and the number of zero crossings must be either equal or differ by, at most, one.
2) At any time the mean value of the envelope of the local maxima and the envelope of the local minima must equal zero.

The IMF's represent the oscillatory modes embedded in the signal x(t). Each IMF is actually a zero mean monocomponent AM-FM signal of the form $x(t)=a(t)\cos\Phi(t)$. As most naturally occurring signals contain more than one oscillatory mode they cannot be classed as IMF's. The EMD process is designed to sift through the signal, breaking it down further with each pass, exposing the intrinsic oscillatory modes. The sifting process is defined by Zhao Zhidong et al. [19] as follows:-

Find the local extrema and join the upper Xup(t) and lower envelopes Xlow(t) using a smooth cubic spline.

Subtract the mean of the two envelopes m1(t) = ((Xup(t) + Xlow(t))/2) to get their difference h1(t) = x(t)-m1(t).

Repeat steps 1 and 2 until the signal h1(t) meets the criteria set out for an IMF - define as c1(t). The first IMF contains the highest frequency component of x(t). The residual r1(t) is given by r1(t)= x(t)-c1(t).

Repeat steps 1,2 and 3 using r1(t) until all IMF's have been extracted and rn(t) becomes monotonic.

Simply, EMD decomposes a non-stationary signal into narrow band components with decreasing frequency. The original signal is defined as the summation of the IMF's + rn(t) , therefore filtering is achieved by excluding the IMF containing the unwanted information prior to reconstruction by summation.

A comparison of SA and EMD was presented by Lynn et al [20] and showed a promising, low latency method of rhythm artefact extraction from recordings recovered from the upper left arm.

2.1.3 Ensemble empirical mode decomposition

A major disadvantage of the classical EMD method is the mode-mixing effect. This becomes evident when pulsed high frequency components are mixed with a lower frequency constant wave. Again the ECG is an example of this type of signal, where the QRS complex is subject to base line drift caused by EMG or 50Hz mains. Mode mixing is said to occur when the IMF is not monotonic. This can be overcome by the use of the Ensemble Empirical Mode Decomposition (EEMD).

The EEMD technique [21] overcomes the mode mixing problem by mixing white noise to the residual (rn(t)) before each resubmission to the

IMF extraction algorithm. This has the effect of increasing the frequency of the splinic envelope and hence eliminating the aliasing effect which causes mode mixing.

2.1.4 Wavelet analysis

An alternative to EMD is the wavelet transform. A method referred to as wavelet transform thresholding is discussed by Alfaouri and Daqroug [22]. The thresholding method is similar to the EMD and EEMD technique, in that it uses the Discrete Wavelet Transform (DWT) to decompose the original into its wavelet series, then it passes the series through a threshold, which removes the coefficients below a certain value, before taking the inverse DWT. The mother wavelet suggested by Alfaouri et al is Daubechies DB4. However, a paper on a similar topic by Singh et al. [23] suggest using DB8. Singh provides evidence based proof for using DB8 and suggests that it produces least root mean square errors (RMSE) and also preserves the peaks of the ECG signal. Alfaouri's work is directed at preserving the lower frequency aspects of the complex, the P wave and T wave.

The work carried out by Alfaouri and Singh is directed at denoising and recovery of the ECG complex. Each work has a different agenda but has proved the DWT to be useful in extracting a detailed signal from noise. The technique compares the mother wavelet of choice in both time and scale across the data set and calculates a best fit with the data. This technique can also be used as a syntactic method of QRS detection, as described by M. Bahoura et al. [24]. Bahoura's technique is an alternative to non-syntactic methods such as the Pan-Tomkins [25] method. Non-syntactic techniques tend to suffer from two problems.

1) It has been found that the bandwidth of the QRS may alter between patients and in some cases the same patient at different times.
2) The bandwidth of the noise and the QRS overlap making filtering difficult. As mentioned earlier, this is especially problematic when mains noise at 50 or 60 Hz is involved. Bahoura's [24] proposed DWT technique is aimed at P and T wave extraction and has been tested on the MIT arrhythmia database. It was suggested that this tool could be used in the post processing of Holter recordings when assessing possible beat arrhythmias.

3. LOW NOISE SIGNAL ACQUISITION

In order to record the ECG signal from remote regions of the body such as the forearm, wrist or thigh, an innovative, low noise signal recovery method will be required to support any signal processing technique. Failure to recover the desired signal is irreversible; no amount of post processing will facilitate extraction.

A wrist worn device that will extract and monitor a clinical quality heart rate and or rhythm is described in US patent 4938228 [26], wrist worn heart rate monitor by William H. Righter et al. Righter, describes several of the essential features required by a wrist worn monitor in his patent.

1) The necessity for the device to be worn on an arm or leg, for example, rather than the chest area.
2) The requirement for the device to utilise a dry electrode arrangement for long term skin contact is highlighted
3) It is suggested that, in order to extract an adequate biometric signal, the acquisition should be in a differential mode.

The Righter patent, although describing an ideal embodiment of the wrist worn clinical ECG monitor, disappoints by underachieving and details claims based around a monitor that requires the application of an oppositely polarised body part, ie the finger of the opposite hand. This creates a significantly large potential across the differential inputs, in the order of 1-2 mV, while the 'true' wrist measured ECG is in the microvolts scale. Righter does not seem to mention the failing of this approach and continues to describe techniques to validate the detection of a QRS complex. His technique is based around maximum coherence matching of the real-time sampled data with a reference waveform. This technique requires that the data to be acted on is sufficiently filtered and free from noise [27].

Any design for a wrist worn monitor that is capable of continuous monitoring of an ECG signal will require analogue signal recovery to be carefully considered. For instance, typical clinical ECG recording equipment is a 'single-ended' recovery system, i.e. each channel is referred to a common point electrode, sometimes referred to as the CMS terminal. This means that the recovered signals are highly susceptible to common mode offset from the electrode potential and to environmental noise. The system also suffers greatly from crosstalk due to the both conducted and radiated noise. In a standard ECG, recording is not noticeably affected. However, when extracting a very low level ECG signal, about one thousand times smaller, from a similar noise environment, then crosstalk can becomes a major issue. A fully differential recovery would provide a solution to handle the effect of crosstalk.

3.1 Biopotential Amplifiers Solutions

Many texts describe the use of differential biopotential amplifiers. Nagel, J. H. [28] and Webster, J.G. [29] discuss the basic requirements of a biopotential amplifier and suggest that the minimum criteria are –

The physiological process should not be influenced by the measurement process.
The measured signal should be high fidelity
The amplifier stage should offer high noise rejection

The 'standard' amplifier type used to acquire biological signals is the differential or instrumentation amplifier. This is referenced in the majority of the literature surrounding the topic of instrumentation for biopotential acquisition. There are many variations on the topology from the standard differential conduction amplifiers to non-contact, high impedance amplifiers [30]. Wayne J. Smith et al describe a method of ECG recovery using an innovative, non-contact biopotential electrode. Their technique utilises an OPA129 FET op-amp from Burr-Brown in, what is essentially an open loop gain, differential input. A small portion of negative feedback has been applied to the non-inverting input via a 500 GΩ resistor to prevent the amplifier from saturating. Smith states that the circuit is a charge amplifier with an overall gain of 2 when the capacitively coupled electrode is about 5 mm from the body. Smith has quoted noise figures for his design in the order of 70uV/√Hz to 9.4uV/√Hz dependent of frequency. He has suggested an improvement may be made to the system noise figure by changing to an op-amp with a lower bias current and suggests the INA116 device.

Smith's method requires that the measurement system be referenced to the body by means of a contact electrode, therefore is not ideal for a wrist or arm located monitor. However, under some circumstances the technique may be adaptable to be of use.

Thomas J. Sullivan et al. [31] has developed an integrated sensor specifically for the purpose of EEG and ECG recovery in non-contact mode. Sullivan has used the INA116 device as suggested by Smith [31]. He has highlighted the areas where wet and dry contact electrodes can prove to be unreliable if used for long periods. It is also worth noting that both contact technologies are susceptible to variation in performance due to the wide range of skin types seen in application. This variation is evident across the relatively small sample size recorded in Lynn et al. (2013) clinical study [12], conducted at the Craigavon Area Hospital cardiac research facility.

Sullivan has solved the referencing issue experienced by Smith by using an annular design electrode topology – Fig. 5. The central copper of the electrode layout is a capacitive sense element, as reported by Smith. The guarded output of the INA116 device is used to drive a guard ring that surrounds the central positive electrode. It is also used to drive a shielding layer that is displaced directly behind the capacitive electrode and overlapping the guard ring. The input current is extremely small, 3fA, but if left uncontrolled will eventually drive the INA116 into saturation. Smith combats this phenomenon by applying negative feedback. Sullivan has adopted a 'short to ground' approach through an NPN transistor, essentially a periodic reset of the input followed by a period of tolerable drift.

Plessey Semiconductors [32] have developed the Sullivan and Smith approaches and are in the process of launching the EPIC electrostatic-voltometer ASIC in the form of a non-contact ECG electrode. Plessey have also commercialised the EPIC technology as a wrist worn heart monitor [33] but have evidently run into problems of distal location and signal discrimination issues, as the product [34] requires the user to adopt the technique described in the Righter patent [26].

A further alternative to capacitive coupling to allow detection of the changes in the body's electric field, is a proximal impedance spectroscopy technique described in the industrial patent Lynn et al. US0178902A1 [35]. Although the spirit of the patent is biased toward the industrial monitoring of carbon fibre composites, the technique may lend itself to be effective for the detection of small changes in the body's electric field. Essentially, the system uses a plurality of transformer windings, displaced along a continuous ferrite core, to form a magnetic amplifier. The core is swept to determine its resonant frequency. The amplitude and frequency of the natural resonant frequency (F0) are indicative of the instantaneous shunt capacitance (Cp) and shunt resistance (Rp) of the proximal body. It is evident that this technique, although requiring substantial development, may also be capable of detecting an ECG without the requirement for a contact reference electrode.

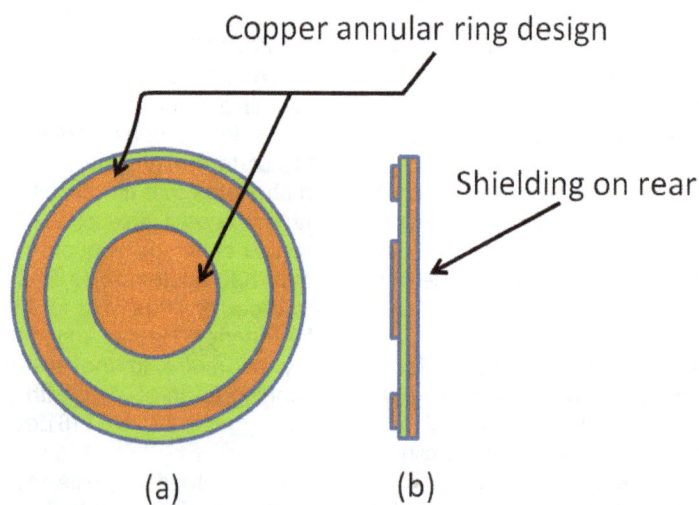

Fig. 5. Illustration showing annular ring electrode design cut from FR4 PCB material. (a) frontal elevation. (b) cross-section showing copper shielding layer

4. POWERING THE DEVICE

A body worn device is ultimately required to have a low mass, a problem for long term monitoring. Traditional battery capacity is proportional to mass, as can be seen in Fig. 6 [36]. The portable, body worn device must have a long term operation window in excess of 4 weeks, it must also record and process continuously. All of which requires a significant power delivery capacity. Existing extended period monitoring technologies have circumvented this challenge by either reducing the period where the device is in full operation, by increasing the size of the battery or making the battery replaceable/ rechargeable.

Periodic operation of the system is the usual industry technique for dealing with limited battery capacity. Devices such as implantable loop recorders and pacemakers run, the large majority of their life, in a semi-shutdown mode, only monitoring and processing the heart rhythm. The device is fully powered once an event is detected allowing the device to stay in use for 5 to 10 years [37]. The act of writing to flash memory, delivering a pacing pulse or communicating via a radio frequency link is particularly power hungry and unsustainable for long periods with today's battery technology.

Industry, in particular Supervisory Control and Data Acquisition (SCADA) systems [38], has lead the way on techniques for supporting the limited battery life available for sensing technology. The use of energy harvesting is widespread however, a direct transfer of technology to the biomedical industry is not straight forward. The energy quotients used in industry and those wasted and therefore available for harvesting, are many scales of magnitude greater than those available from the human body. Techniques in kinetic energy harvesting from the body have already been commercialised [39,40]; though able to produce considerable energy, are not sufficiently compact or ergonomic to suit long term wearing. Other possibilities are solar [40] and thermoelectric [41], both attractive due to their robustness and high reliability. However, availability of direct light in sufficient quantities for solar operation, traded off against the physical size of the solar panel, is a significant problem. Thermoelectric energy harvested from the human body was first commercialised in the form of the Seiko Thermic wrist watch in 1998 [42]. It is possible to recover approximately 1 mW of the 100W available from an adult at rest using today's technology. Generation is dependent on a thermal gradient between the skin contact and the outer surface of the thermoelectric generator, an issue if the device is worn under clothing.

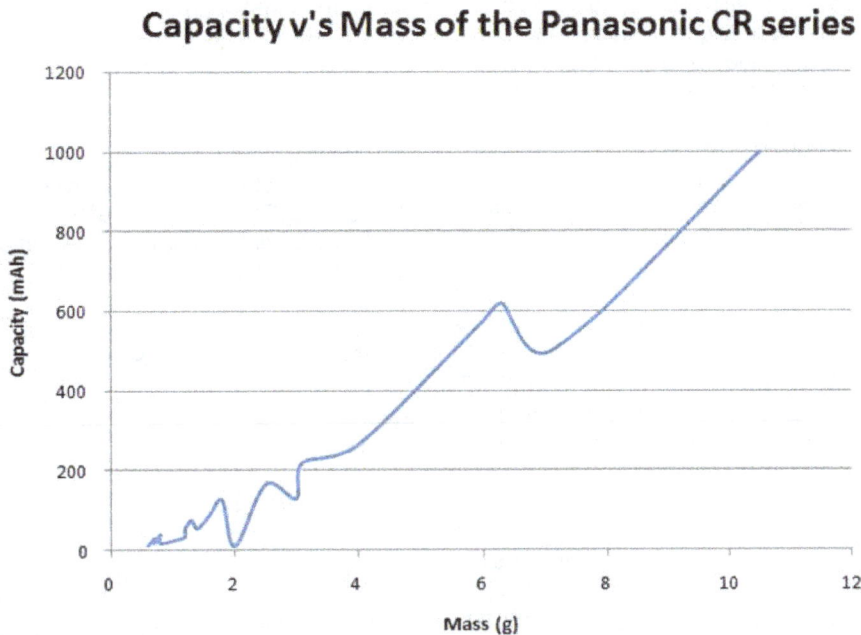

Capacity v's Mass of the Panasonic CR series

Fig. 6. Battery capacity plotted against mass for the panasonic CR lithium manganese dioxide cell range

5. SUMMARY

It is clear from the review that distal limb recovery of rhythm information is possible. Lynn [12] and Yang [13] have successfully recovered QRST ventricular electrical activity from the upper arm, showing that the signal is present, in some form, along the limb. Electrical noise is the confounding factor of recovery from the wrist, though it has been shown that the wrist may not be the most suitable place for a monitor of this type. A more stable platform may be the upper arm. That being the case, the techniques for successful recovery of rhythm information are in existence today.

The importance of high quality signal recording has been made clear. Low noise, high impedence differential amplifiers are becoming common place in the electronics world. Their reliability is increasing and size and cost are decreasing, all driven by demand from other sectors, mainly mobile electronics. A reduction in physical size and over all power consumption, allows the construction of an extremely efficient, low noise device, which is ideal for use in a body-worn monitor.

Low noise recovery techniques deal with environmental and general system noise. The recovered signal is still subject to additionally recovered biological signals such as EMG. These are also considered to be 'noise', as they are unwanted in this particular application. The removal of such is made complex by the fact that the frequency domains of the desired signal and that of the noise overlap, a factor which precludes bandwidth narrowing as a sole method of filtering and post processing. A review of non-syntactic algorithms showed that empirical mode decomposition and partial reconstruction can be used to improve the denoising of ECG signals recovered from the left arm. It is also worth noting that the syntactic approach, although successful has excessive latency and is therefore not suitable for dysrhythmia or complex morphology analysis in real time.

As with all mobile technology the limitations are mainly from battery power sources. The possible implementation of an energy harvesting technique could increase the operation time and reduce the amount of patient interaction with the device, providing a more stable recording platform.

6. CONCLUSION

Cardiac disease is a prevalent killer in the modern world. More worryingly, the root cause of sudden cardiac death in the young often goes undiagnosed due to the inconvenience of the currently available long term monitoring solutions. The propositions mentioned herein describe the possibility of producing a non-invasive long term monitor. The challenges presented are in the areas of positioning for comfort, electrode design, signal processing and power supply technology. All of which are discussed.

It is evident from the literature the current technological capacity is such that developing a long term, non invasive continuous monitoring device is possible.

CONSENT

All authors declare that 'written informed consent was obtained from the patient (or other approved parties) for publication of this case report and accompanying images.

ETHICAL APPROVAL

All authors hereby declare that all experiments have been examined and approved by the appropriate ethics committee and have therefore been performed in accordance with the ethical standards laid down in the 1964 Declaration of Helsinki."

The clinical study conducted by Lynn D. et al. (2013), had ethical approval from the Office of Research...(ORECNI), reference number 10/NIR02/6, date of favourable ethical opinion: 20/05/2010, sponsored by Southern Health and Social Care Trust.

COMPETING INTERESTS

Authors have declared that no competing interests exist.

REFERENCES

1.   Papadakis M, Sharma S, Cox S, Sheppard MN, Panoulas VF, Behr ER. "The magnitude of sudden cardiac death in the young: a death certificate-based review in England and Wales." Europace. 2009; 11(10):1353-1358.

2. Sami Viskin, MD et al. "The Response of the QT Interval to the Brief Tachycardia Provoked by Standing - A Bedside Test for Diagnosing Long QT Syndrome". American College of Cardiology. 2010;55(18):1955-61.

3. Lewis DC. "Predicting the future of health care," The Brown University Digest. of Addiction Theory & Application. 1999; 18(4):12-16.

4. Gemperle F, Kasabach C, Stivoric J, Bauer M, Martin R. Design for wearability. In The Second International Symposium on Wearable Computers, (ppll6- 122). Los Alamitos, CA: IEEE Computer Society; 1998.

5. MHRA. Drug Safety Update; 2012. Available:http://www.mhra.gov.uk/Safetyinf ormation/DrugSafetyUpdate/CON152725 Last accessed 31/07/14

6. NHS. Atrial Fibrillation; 2013. Available:http://www.nhs.uk/conditions/Atri al-fibrillation/Pages/Introduction.aspx Last accessed 30/07/14.

7. Omron. HCG-801 User Manual; 2011. Available:http://www.omron-healthcare.com/data/catalog/3/655/1/IM-HCG-801-E%2005-11-2011%20EN.pdf, Last accessed 31/7/14

8. Joshi AK, Kowey PR, Prystowsky EN, Benditt DG, Cannom DS, Pratt CM, McNamara A, Sangrigoli RM. First experience with a Mobile Cardiac Outpatient Telemetry (MCOT) system for the diagnosis and management of cardiac arrhythmia. Am J Cardiol. 2005;95:878–881.

9. Zimetbaum P, Goldman A. Ambulatory Arrhythmia Monitoring: Choosing the Right Device. Circulation. 2010;122(1):1629-1636.

10. Crouch MA et al. Clinical Relevance and Management of Drug-Related QT Interval Prolongation; 2003. Available:http://www.medscape.com/viewa rticle/458868_3 Last accessed 31/07/14

11. Shackel B, Chidsy KD, Shipley P. The assessment of chair comfort. Ergonomics. 1969;12(2):269-306.

12. Lynn WD, et al. "Arm and wrist surface potential mapping for wearable ECG rhythm recording devices: a pilot clinical study". Journal of Physics: Conference Series. 2013;450(1):1-8.

13. Yang H, et al. Study of Single-Arm Electrode for ECG Measurement Using Flexible Print Circuit; 2011.

Available:http://eshare.stust.edu.tw/Eshare File/2011_6/2011_6_7f351cdf.pdf, Last accessed 23/07/2014

14. Crone B. Common-Mode Rejection: How It relates to ECG subsystems and the techniques used to provide superior performance. Analogue Devices. MS-. 2011;2125 (1):1-4.

15. Horowitz P, Hill W. Precision circuits and low noise techniques. In: The Press Syndicate of the University of Cambridge The art of Electronics. 2nd ed. London: Cambridge University Press. 1989;286-315.

16. Escalona OJ. "Analog implementation of the single fiducial point alignment technique for real-time high resolution ECG analysis in the P-R interval." In Proceedings of Computers in Cardiology 1998, Cleveland, OH, USA. 1998;229–232.

17. William Craelius, et al. 'Criteria for optimal averaging of cardiac signals'. IEEE Transactions on Biomedical Engineering; 1986. BME No10.

18. Huang NE, et al. 'The empirical mode decomposition and Hilbert spectrum for non linear and non stationary time series analysis'. Proceeding of The Royal Society London. 1998;454.

19. Zhao Zhidong, et al. 'Adaptive noise removal of ECG signal based on ensemble empirical mode decomposition'. Hangzhou Dianzi University, China; 2011.

20. Lynn WD, et al. 'A Low Latency Electrocardiographic QRS Activity Recovery Technique for Use on the Upper Left Arm'. Electronics. 2014;3030409(3): 409-418.

21. Wu ZH, et al. 'Ensemble Empirical Mode Decomposition: A noise assisted data analysis method'. Advances in adaptive data analysis. 2009;1-40.

22. Mikhled Alfaouri, et al. 'ECG Signal denoising by wavelet transform thresholding'. Communication and electronics engineering Dept, Philadelphia University, Jordan. 2008;276-280.

23. Singh BN, et al. 'Optmal selection of wavelet basis functions applied to ECG signal denoising'. Digital Signal Processing. 2006;16:275-287.

24. Bahoura M, et al. 'DSP implementation of wavelet transform for realtime ECG waveforms detection and heart rate analysis', Computer Methods and Programs in Biomedicine. 1997;52:35-44.

25. Pan J, Tompkins WJ. 'A realtime QRS detection algorithm'. IEEE Transcript Biomedical Engineering. 1985;32:230-236.

26. Righter, William H, et al. US Patent 4938228, 'Wrist worn heart rate monitor'; 1990.

27. Escalona OJ, Mitchell RH. 'Frequency bandwidth limitations in the signal-averaged ECG by the maximum coherence matching technique'. Automedica. 1991;13:177-186.

28. Nagel, JH. 'The Biomedical Engineering Handbook: Second Edition', CRC Press LLC, C70.1 - 70.2; 2000.

29. Webster JG. 'Medical Instrumentation, Application and Design, second edition', Houghton Mifflin Co, Boston, MA; 1992.

30. Wayne J. Smith, et al. 'Non-contact Biopotential Measurement from the Human Body Using a Low-Impedance Charge Amplifier'. Dept of Electrical and Computer Engineering, Biomedical Laboratory, Durham, NH; 2004.

31. Thomas J. Sullivan, et al. 'A Low Noise, Non-Contact EEG/ECG Sensor'. Division of Biological Sciences, University of California, San Diego, CA; 2007.

32. Plessey Semiconductors, Application note PS25201B 'EPIC Ultra High Impedance Electrophysiological Sensor', Swindon, UK; 2012.
Available:www.plesseysemiconductors.com Accessed July 2014

33. Plessey Semiconductors, Press Release, 'Plessey uses its EPIC technology to create a heart monitor in a wrist watch', Swindon, UK; 2012.
Available:www.plesseysemiconductors.com, Accessed July 2014

34. Plessey Semiconductors, Application note 291465 'ECG using wrist mounted EPIC sensors', Swindon, UK; 2012.

Available:www.plesseysemiconductors.com, Accessed July 2014

35. Lynn WD, et al. US Patent 0178902A1 'Belt Monitoring Systems and Methods', Schrader Electronics Ltd., UK; 2009.

36. Micro Power Battery Company. Panasonic Lithium Coin Batteries Tech Specs; 2014. Available:http://www.microbattery.com/specs-panasonic-lithium-coin Last accessed 31/07/14

37. Mallela VS, et al. 'Trends in Cardiac Pacemaker Batteries'. Indian Pacing and Electrophysiology Journal - Technical Series. 2004;4(4):201-212.

38. Lynn WD. US Patent 0316525A1 'Power transmission monitoring and maintenance systems and methods', Schrader Electronics Ltd., UK; 2011.

39. Maxwell Donelan, J, Naing, V, Li, Q. Biomechanical Energy Harvesting, Proceedings of Power MEMS'08, Sendai, Japan. 2008;39–44.

40. Feenstraa J, Granstroma J, Sodano H. Energy harvesting through a backpack employing a mechanically amplified piezoelectric stack. Mechanical Systems and Signal Processing. 2008;22(3):721–734

41. Leonov V, Van Hoof C, Vullers RJM. Thermoelectric and hybrid generators in wearable devices and clothes. proceedings of body sensors networks. Berkeley, USA. 2009;195–200

42. Ozcanli OC. Turning body heat into electricity; 2010.

Available:http://www.forbes.com/2010/06/07/nanotech-body-heat-technology-breakthroughs-devices.html Last accessed 31/07/14

22

Antioxidant and Radical Scavenging Properties of β-Carotene on Cisplatin Induced Cardiotoxicity

B. Uday Kiran[1*], M. Sushma[1], K. V. S. R. G. Prasad[2], V. Uma Maheshwara Rao[1], D. Jhansi Laxmi Bai[1] and V. Nisheetha[3]

[1]Department of Pharmacology, CMR College of Pharmacy, Kandlakoya, Medchal, R R Dist, Hyderabad, 501 401, India.
[2]Department of Pharmacology, Institute of Pharmaceutical Technology, SPMVV, Tirupathi, Andhra Pradesh, India.
[3]Department of Pharmacology, Sri Sai Jyothi College of Pharmacy, Vattinagula pally, Gandipet, Ranga Reddy Dist, Hyderabad-500 075, India.

Authors' contributions

This work was carried out in collaboration between all authors. All authors read and approved the final manuscript.

<u>Editor(s):</u>
(1) Wilbert S. Aronow, University of California, College of Medicine, Irvine, USA.
<u>Reviewers:</u>
(1) Anonymous, Chiang Mai University, Thailand.
(2) Pratibha Ravindra Kamble, Division of Cardiac Surgery, Ohio State University Medical Centre, USA.

ABSTRACT

Objective: To investigate the protective role of β-Carotene against cisplatin induced cardiotoxicity in male albino rats.
Methods: Various biochemical parameters such as Creatine kInase-MB, Lactate dehydrogenase (LDH), Alkaline phosphatase (ALP), Aspartate aminotransferase (AST), Alanine aminotransferase (ALT), Triglycerides (TG) and Total cholesterol (TC) are being assessed. Also the levels of the *in vivo* antioxidants such as Reduced glutathione (GSH), Catalase (CAT), and Malondialdehyde (MDA) in the post mitochondrial supernatant of heart were measured. In addition, the histopathological studies were performed to study the protective activity of β-carotene.
Results: Cisplatin administration has shown the elevated levels of the cardiac markers and diminished the endogenous antioxidant levels when compared with the normal rats. β-carotene treatment showed the inhibitory effect on the free radicals showing decreased levels of the cardiac

Corresponding author: E-mail: udaykiran.bijja@gmail.com

markers like CK-MB, LDH, AST, ALT and ALP. The β-carotene treated rats showed significant (p<0.001) decrease in lipid peroxidation in both prophylactic and curative groups when compared to the cisplatin group. Also showed a significant (p<0.05, p<0.001) increase in the levels of GSH in prophylactic and curative group respectively when compared with the cisplatin group. Both prophylactic and curative groups have shown a significant (p<0.001) increase in the levels of CAT. Further, the histopathological studies confirm the protective effect of β-carotene.

Conclusion: These findings justify the biological and traditional uses of β-carotene as confirmed by its promising radical scavenging activity against cisplatin induced cardiotoxicity.

Keywords: β-Carotene; cardiotoxicity; lipid peroxidation; reduced glutathione; catalase; post mitochondrial supernatant.

1. INTRODUCTION

Cisplatin (CP) is widely used and highly effective antineoplastic agent. It remains as a standard component for the treatment of head and neck tumours. It is also used to treat many solid tumours, including those of the lung, testis, ovary and breast etc. The main dose limiting side effect is nephrotoxicity which was recognized since its introduction [1].

Besides, it also causes several dose dependent adverse effects, notably neurotoxicity, hepatotoxicity, and cardiotoxicity etc [2-3]. Administration of cisplatin with other antineoplastic drugs like methotrexate, 5-fluorouracil, bleomycin and doxorubicin are associated with lethal cardiomyopathy [4].

The emergence of the cardiotoxicity which includes the changes in the cardiac events such as arrhythmias, cardiomyopathy, electro-cardiographic changes and congestive heart failure is being reported in many case reports. Though intense efforts are made over decades to find the equally potent but less toxic drug, cisplatin is widely prescribed [5-6].

Carotenoids are a group of naturally occurring fat-soluble compounds. Over 700 naturally occurring carotenoids are identified so far. β-carotene (BC) is one of the most prominent natural antioxidants, orange-coloured carbon-hydrogen carotenoid and a precursor of vitamin A [7-8]. It is an organic hydrocarbon containing compound specifically referred as a terpenoid, reflecting its derivation from isoprene units. BC is a common substance abundant in yellow-orange fruits and vegetables (eg: carrots, pumpkins and sweet potatoes etc.) and in dark green leafy vegetables and also the most widely distributed carotenoid in foods that colours them orange [9]. It is known to induce hepatic enzymes that detoxify the carcinogens in a rat model [10], has strong inhibitory effect against DMH (1,2-dimethylhydraine) induced colon tumours [11]. Moreover, BC has an ability to function as a chain breaking antioxidant in the lipid environment at partial pressures of oxygen that are more likely considered in mammalian cells [12].

The BC molecule reacts with the free radical, resulting in the formation of a new much more stable radical possibly due to the presence of a conjugated double bond system which facilitates a resonance condition [13]. It is known that β-carotene can quench singlet oxygen with a multiple higher efficiency than α-tocopherol. The *in vitro* studies have shown the potent antioxidant activity of BC [7].

Nutrition has a prominent role in the prevention of many chronic disease such as cancers, degenerative brain diseases and cardiovascular diseases. The consumption of food based antioxidants including BC seems to be useful for the prevention of cataracts and macular degeneration. Several studies have revealed the protective effect of food based BC, along with diet rich in fruits and vegetables, on liver carcinogenesis as well the lung disease [7].

Earlier literature suggests the beneficial effects of use of antioxidants such as silymarin, acetyl-L-carnitine & DL-α-lipoic acid which are proven to be potential against the cardiotoxicity associated with cisplatin in experimental animals [4]. Most endogenous compounds exhibit antioxidant functions which often act synergistically with the antioxidants supplied through the dietary origin [14].

The role of BC in the prevention of cardiotoxicity, especially by CP has not been established yet; the focus on the most important non enzymatic antioxidant activity of BC in scavenging the oxygen free radicals released by the administration of cisplatin is being assessed. The protective effect of β-carotene on heart is studied by estimating various biochemical parameters, antioxidant parameters (on the post mitochondrial supernatant of the organ) and the histopathological findings. The rationale behind this is to study the cessation of adverse effects caused by ROS generated by the overdose of CP by using a natural antioxidant-carotenoid, β-carotene.

2. MATERIALS AND METHODS

2.1 Chemicals and Drugs

Cisplatin injection available as Cytoplatin 50 mg/50 ml manufactured by cipla is used. β-carotene was obtained from sigma aldich. The biochemical kits used are obtained from Coral, Excel and Span diagnostics. All the chemicals used were of analytical grade.

2.2 Animals and Experimental Design

Male albino Wistar rats were purchased from Teena labs, Hyderabad. The animals are subjected to acclimatization for one week provided with food and water *ad libitum*. The animals were maintained at a controlled temperature under 12hrs dark/light cycle in the animal house at CMR College of pharmacy, Hyderabad approved by CPCSEA (657/PO/a/12/CPCSEA -June, 2012).

The experimental animals weighing 200-250 g were used in the studies which were divided into five groups containing six in each. The treatment is followed according to the details mentioned in Table 1. Blood samples are collected after 2 hrs of the treatment on the last day. The blood was withdrawn by retro-orbital puncture and the animals were sacrificed by spinal dislocation [15]. The changes in body weights are noted. Olive oil is used as vehicle for administration of BC.

2.3 Biochemical Estimations

The blood samples obtained are centrifuged at 3000 g for 10 mins at 4℃ and the serum obtained from the blood was used for the evaluation of biochemical parameters such as CK-MB, LDH, AST, ALT, ALP, TG and TC.

Hearts were rapidly excised, trimmed of connective tissue and weighted, subjected to washing with ice-cold normal saline to make free from blood and were used for the preparation of post mitochondrial supernatant for *in vivo* antioxidant studies and histopathological studies. The hearts of the animals were dissected out soaked in 10% formalin solution, stained with eosin and haematoxylin. 5 μm thick sections were observed under light microscope with magnification 100x.

2.3.1 *In vivo* antioxidant studies

The tissue homogenates (10% w/v) were prepared with a Teflon homogenizer using ice-cold 1.15% KCl [16]. The homogenates were centrifuged at 800 g for 5 min at 4℃ (REMI C-24) to separate the molecular debris. The Post mitochondrial supernatant is collected after centrifuging at 10000 g for 20 mins which was used for *in vivo* antioxidant parameters like lipid peroxidation (LPO), Catalase (CAT) and reduced glutathione (GSH).

2.3.2 Estimation of lipid perioxidation (LPO)

The procedure was followed according to the modified method of [17]. The PMS of volume 0.5 ml was allowed to react with 0.5ml tris HCl buffer (pH 7.4) and incubated at 37℃ for 2 hrs followed by addition of 1ml of 10% ice cold trichloroacetic acid and centrifuged at 1000rpm for 10 mins and 1 ml supernatant was added to 1ml of 0.67% w/v thiobarbituric acid and boiled for 10 mins. After cooling 1 ml distilled water is added and the absorbance was measured at 532 nm against the blank without tissue homogenate.

Table 1. Treatment schedule

Group	Drug Treatment	Dose	Duration in days	Day of withdrawal of blood/ sacrifice	Purpose
I	Vehicle	1 ml/kg	1-7	7th	Normal control
II	Cisplatin	7 mg/kg	1st	5th	Disease control
III	β-carotene	10 mg/kg	1-7	7th	BC control
IV	β-carotene	10 mg/kg	1-7	7th	Prophylactic
	Cisplatin	7 mg/kg	3rd		
V	Cisplatin	7 mg/kg	1st	11th	Curative
	β-carotene	10mg/kg	5-11		

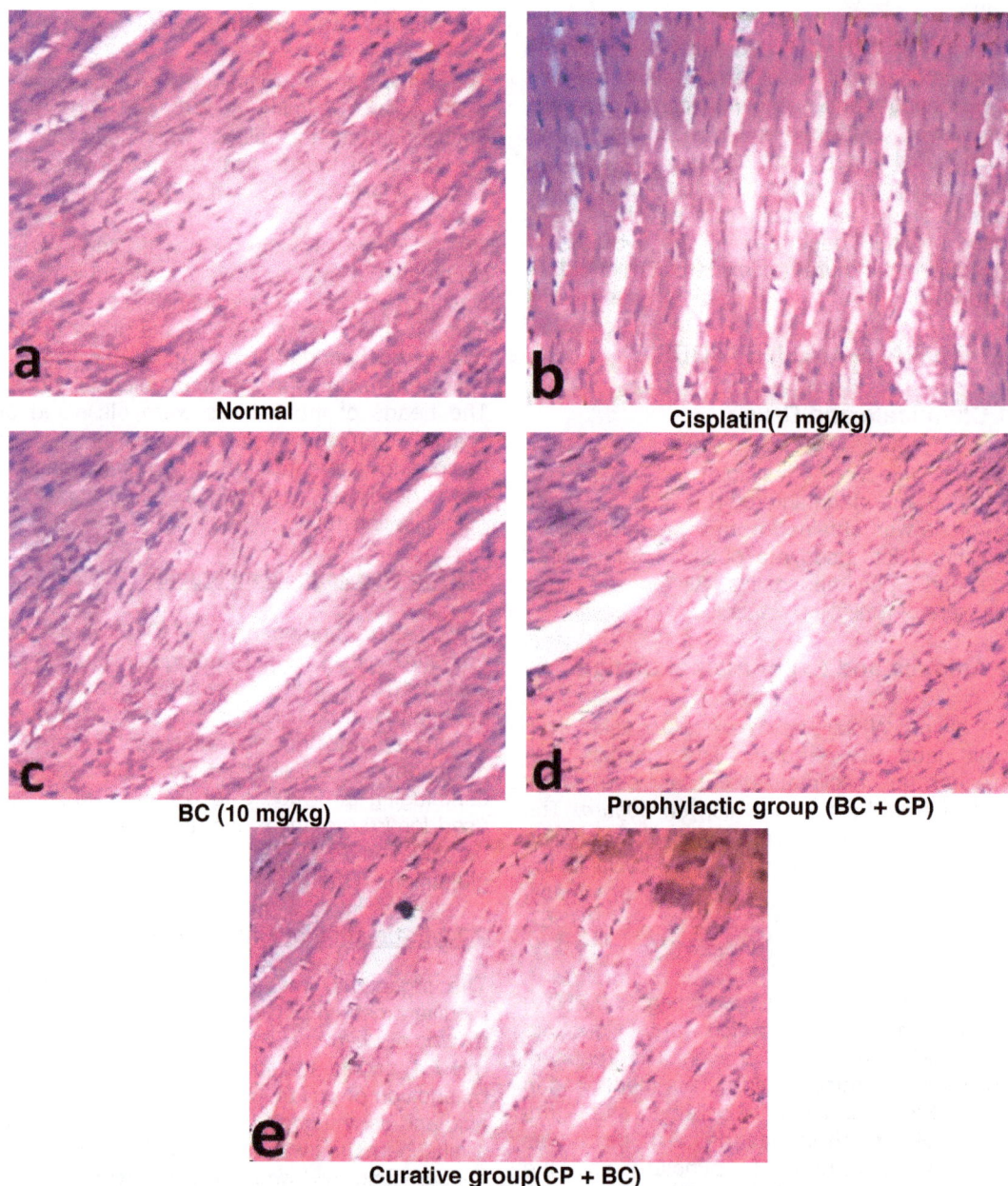

Fig. 1. Photomicrographs of histological changes of cardiac tissue under light microscopy with magnification 100X

The Cardiac damage produced by cisplatin showing the degenerative changes and necrosis of cardiac muscle fibre cells. Prophylactic (d) and curative (e) groups showing decreased myocardial necrosis.

The malondialdehyde (MDA) content, a measure of lipid peroxidation was assayed in the form of TBARS.

2.3.3 Estimation of reduced glutathione (GSH)

Modified method of [18], the PMS of volume 0.75 ml is mixed with equal volume of 4% sulfosalicylic acid and centrifuged at 1200 g for 5

mins at 4°C. 0.5 ml of supernatant was added with 4.5 ml of 0.01 M DTNB and the absorbance was measured at 412 nm against the blank without tissue homogenate.

2.3.4 Estimation of catalase (CAT)

According to the modified method of [19], the tissue homogenate in volume 0.05 ml was diluted with 1.95 ml of 0.05 M phosphate buffer (pH 7.0) and for 2 ml of the diluted homogenate 1 ml of 0.019 M hydrogen peroxide (prepared using 0.05 M phosphate buffer) was added and immediately the absorbance was measured at 240 nm against the blank without tissue homogenate for 2 minutes with 60 seconds intervals and the average is considered.

2.3.5 Statistical analysis

The statistical analysis was carried out using one way ANOVA followed by tukey's multiple comparison test and the values were expressed as mean ± SEM. Values at P<0.05 are considered statistically significant.

3. RESULTS

Protective effects of BC against CP induced cardiotoxicity was established by observing the parameters such body weight, heart weight, cardiac biomarkers such as CK MB and endogenous antioxidants.

3.1 Body Weight and Heart Weight

The animals treated with CP significantly (p<0.001) decreased the body weight when compared to the normal rats. Also, significant (p<0.001) decrease in the weight of the heart when compared with the normal rats as mentioned in the Table 2.

3.2 Biochemical Estimation

The animals treated with CP have shown the elevated levels of the enzymatic markers such as CK MB, LDH, AST, ALT and ALP when compared to normal rats. It also has shown the elevated levels of Triglycerides (TG) and Total cholesterol (TC). The treatment groups both prophylactic and curative has shown significant reduction of the markers in serum as represented in the Tables no. 2 and 3.

3.3 Antioxidant Biomarkers

The elevated levels of MDA clearly indicate the myocardial damage with a significant reduction in the non-enzymatic antioxidants such as GSH and CAT. Upon treatment, both groups (prophylactic and curative) showed a significant decrease in lipid peroxidation levels and would have successfully defended in the depletion of GSH and CAT as the details mentioned in Table 4.

3.4 Histopathological Observations

The histopathological studies according to [6] [20], have shown the cardiac damage including, degenerative changes and necrosis of cardiac muscle fibre cells with fibrous tissue reaction in cisplatin group (Fig. 1). The hearts of the Prophylactic and curative groups showed decreased myocardial necrosis.

4. DISCUSSION

Chemotherapy, especially using CP declines the normal homeostasis of the body [21]. Cisplatin is still a frequently used chemotherapeutic agent due to its potential activity on carcinoma cells, despite of its frequent adverse effects. There are various outcomes to attenuate its toxicity which includes dose optimization, excess hydration therapy, use of osmotic diuretics etc though of limited usefulness [22].

During the physiological process the electrons continuously escape from respiratory chain partially reduces the molecular oxygen generating the superoxide anions, precursors of ROS which are continuously produced in mitochondria. The efficient mitochondrial antioxidant defense system maintains the balance between the generation of ROS and detoxification.

Table 2. Effect of BC on CP induced changes in body weights, heart weights and various biochemical markers

Group	Treatment	Changes in body weight (gms)	Heart Weight (mg)	Body weight/Heart weight ratio	CK MB (U/L)	LDH (U/L)
I	Normal	12.3 ±1.59	739.2±17.19	1/0.0035	667.4±29.03	408.9±17.47
II	CP	-23.67±2.51^x	559.3±19.23^x	1/0.0032	2560.0±110.00^x	1760.0±57.19^x
III	BC	19.33±2.06^a	774.3±10.82^a	1/0.0035	635.4±53.26^a	368.7±12.66^a
IV	BC + CP	-2.00±2.78^a	658.2±9.20^a	1/0.0033	705.9±59.18^a	586.7±36.16^a
V	CP + BC	-13.8±1.22^c	604.3±19.00^a	1/0.0033	1147.0±71.07^a	724±44.64^a

Values are expressed as (Mean ± SEM). ^{x} p<0.001, ^{y} p<0.01 when compared to normal group ^{a} p<0.001, ^{b} p<0.01, ^{c} p<0.05 when compared to cisplatin control group

Table 3. Effect of BC on CP induced changes in various biochemical markers

Group	Treatment	TG (mg/dl)	TC (mg/dl)	ALP (U/L)	AST (U/L)	ALT (U/L)
I	Normal	48.7±3.75	49.6±3.45	308.2±8.45	151.4±12.67	26.7±1.17
II	CP	68.7±3.05^y	71.1±3.26^x	650.4±12.72^x	271.9±15.98^x	78.5±5.01^x
III	BC	46.3±3.00^a	42.3±3.54^a	292.5±15.90^a	149.1±7.70^a	24.4±1.90^a
IV	BC + CP	54.6±3.53^c	51.3±1.63^a	329.0±17.89^a	163.8±4.14^a	29.3±2.28^a
V	CP + BC	56.5±2.36^{ns}	58.6±3.14^c	441.0±14.07^a	199.6±5.04^a	33.1±1.10^a

Values are expressed as (Mean ± SEM). $^x p<0.001$, $^y p<0.05$ compared to normal group.
$^a p<0.001$, $^b p<0.01$, $^c p<0.05$ when compared to cisplatin control group

Table 4. Effect of BC on CP induced changes in various antioxidant biomarkers

Group	Treatment	MDA (nmol/g)	GSH (nmol/g)	CAT (nmol/g)
I	Normal	1.1±0.05	4.2±036	16.7±0.64
II	CP	9.7±0.41^x	1.6 ±0.20^x	3.4±0.23^x
III	BC	1.4±0.36^a	4.3 ±0.36^a	17.3±1.52^a
IV	BC + CP	2.2±0.58^a	3.9±0.45^a	16.0±1.40^a
V	CP + BC	3.5±0.49^a	3.7±0.23^b	18.0±1.97^a

Values are expressed as (Mean ± SEM). $^x p<0.001$ compared to normal group $^a p<0.001$, $^b p<0.01$,
$^c p<0.05$ when compared to cisplatin control group

GSH is low molecular weight endogenous radical scavenger in the cytoplasm and is one of the important inhibitors of free radical generation mediated by lipid peroxidation [20]. The reduction in the GSH and other related endogenous antioxidants by cisplatin, shifts the cellular redox status leading to the accumulation of endogenous ROS within the cells enhancing the lipid peroxidation which is another pathway for the cardiac cells damage [23,24]. The oxidative stress reflects a shift towards the imbalance of the antioxidant defense system leading to the damage of the cellular components, notably proteins, membrane lipids and nucleic acids, leading to the leakage of cardiac markers which indicate the cardiac injury [25,26].

The loss of weight is might be due to the gastrointestinal toxicity and by reduced ingestion of food [27]. The body weight/heart weight ratio is decreased in Cisplatin treated group which has increased in the BC treatment groups when compared with the toxic group which might be due to the prevention of oxidative stress induced cell death.

In the present study the administration of single intraperitoneal dose of CP (7 mg/kg) [28] imbalanced the ratio of ROS and detoxifiction by enhancing the ROS generation and depletion of the endogenous enzymatic antioxidants such as GSH, and CAT [29]. The ROS generated by cisplatin during this process triggers the mitochondrial permeability transition pore opening which permits the release of cytochrome c from mitochondria to cytosol activating the mitochondrial pathway leading to apoptosis. Also, cisplatin is converted to highly reactive form, which reacts with thiol containing compounds such as glutathione and causes its depletion [4]. In the present has shown the significant elevation of the serum cardiac markers such as CK MB, LDH, AST, ALT and ALP when compared to the normal rats [20]. CK-MB is the main marker indicating cardiac damage, the other enzymes also represent the extent of damage. Although, the endogenous enzymes are also present in various other tissues, the elevated levels of *in vivo* antioxidants such as MDA and the decline of GSH and CAT clearly indicate the cardiac damage. The ROS generated due to the administration of CP (7 mg/kg) might have caused the membrane injury indicated by the lipid peroxidation causing the loss of function and integrity of myocardial membrane leading to the leakage of the cardiac markers into the circulation. The administration of BC protected the myocytes against CP by decreasing their susceptibility to the free radicals.

BC is one the most prominent natural compound with lipophilic nature which contains an extended system of conjugated double bonds which are responsible for their antioxidant activity. The mechanisms by which BC protect biological systems, against cisplatin induced damage is associated with lowered DNA damage, decreased lipid peroxidation against oxidative damage tends to depend largely on the polyene chain in the center of the molecule which is responsible for physical quenching [30,31]. BC undergoes oxidation by the ROS, which involves the interruption of conjugated double bond system either by cleavage or by addition to one of the double bonds of BC molecule. The possible mechanisms by which BC scavenge free radicals include either radical addition, electron transfer to the radical or the allylic hydrogen abstraction leads to the formation of stable metabolites [32].

Singlet oxygen, though it is short lived, can be intercepted by reactions occurring near diffusion control, the process of physical quenching which is the main domain for carotenoids [14]. The phenolic antioxidants like Flavanoids, phenolic acids (cinnamic acid and hydroxylated benzoic acid), tocopherols and ascorbic acid exerts their radical scavenging activity by their hydroxyl groups (combined with a conjugated double bond system) at the outer part of the molecule reacting with the radicals to form a resonance-stabilized radical [31-34].

The biological defense developed can be classified as prevention, interception and repair. The defense against the highly reactive hydroxyl radical can only be by prevention or repair because any agent capable of interception would have to be present at very high concentrations, which would be biologically intolerable simply for osmotic reasons [14]. Generally, the repair occurs via enzymatic mechanisms, which are important for the repair of DNA damage before it is fixed as mutation. Also, the reacylation is the main pathway by which the repair of phospholipids and repair or synthesis of proteins occur [14].

The increase in the levels of LPO and the decrease in the levels of GSH and CAT in the present study clearly indicate the oxidative stress induced by CP. The increased lipid peroxidation leads to the increased utilisation of GSH in the heart, as observed in our study. The prophylactic and curative groups have shown the significant reduction in lipid peroxidation levels which is indicated by the recovered levels of GSH and CAT. The leakage of the markers such as CK MB, LDH, AST, ALT and ALP from the cardiac myocytes significantly reduced possibly due to the protective effect of BC against free radicals when compared to CP group.

5. CONCLUSION

In conclusion, the results of the study suggest that the suppression of the oxidative stress by

BC could be an effective strategy for the treatment of CP induced cardiomyopathy. However, further studies have to be performed to confirm the therapeutic activity of BC in the patients receiving CP chemotherapy.

CONSENT

It is not applicable.

ETHICAL APPROVAL

All authors hereby declare that "Principles of laboratory animal care" (NIH publication No. 85-23, revised 1985) were followed, as well as specific national laws where applicable. All experiments have been examined and approved by the appropriate ethics committee.

All authors hereby declare that all experiments have been examined and approved by the appropriate ethics committee and have therefore been performed in accordance with the ethical standards laid down in the 1964 Declaration of Helsinki.

COMPETING INTERESTS

Authors have declared that no competing interests exist.

REFERENCES

1. Miller RP, Tadagavadi RK, Ramesh G, Reeves WB. Mechanisms of cisplatin nephrotoxicity. Toxins. 2010;2(11):2490-518.

2. Al-Majed AA. Carnitine deficiency provokes cisplatin-induced hepatotoxicity in rats. Basic & Clinical Pharmacology & Toxicology. 2006;100:145-150.

3. Hussein A, Ahmed AA, Shouman SA, Sharawy S. Ameliorating effect of DL-α-lipoic acid against cisplatin-induced nephrotoxicity and cardiotoxicity in experimental animals. Drug Discov Ther. 2012;6(3):147-56.

4. El-Awady el-SE, Moustafa YM, Abo-Elmatty DM, Radwan A. Cisplatin-induced cardiotoxicity: Mechanisms and cardio-protective strategies. Eur J Pharmacol. 2011;650(1):335-41.

5. El-sayed EM, EL-azeem ASA, Afify AA, Shabana MH, Ahmed HH. Cardioprotective effects Curcuma longa L.

extracts against doxorubicin-induced cardiotoxicity in rats. J Med Plants Res. 2011;5(17):4049-58.

6. Attyah AM, Ismail SH. Protective effect of ginger extract against cisplatin-induced hepatotoxicity and cardiotoxicity in rats. Iraqi J Pharm Sci. 2012;21(1):27-33.

7. Mueller L, Boehm V. Antioxidant activity of β-carotene compounds in different in vitro assays. Molecules. 2011;16:1055-69.

8. Morakinyo AO, Iranloye BO, Oyelowo OT, Nnaji J. Anti-oxidative and hepato-protective effect of beta-carotene on acetaminophen-induced liver damage in rats. Biol & Med. 2012;4(3):134-40.

9. Van Arnum SD. Vitamin A. Kirk-Othmer Encyc Chem Tech. 2000;45:99-107.

10. Patrick L. Beta-carotene: The controversy continues. Alt med Rev. 2000;5(6):530-45.

11. Temple NJ, Basu TK. Protective effect of β-carotene against colon tumors in mice. JNCI. 1987;78(6):1211-4.

12. Azeim BHA, Abd-Ellah HF, Mohamed NE. Prophylactic role of β-carotene against acrylonitrile-induced esticular toxicity in rats: Physiological and microscoical studies. J Bas & App Zoolo. 2012;65:257-66.

13. Bendich A. From 1989 to 2001: What have we learned about the biological actions of beta-carotene? J Nutr. 2004;134(1):225S-30S.

14. Sies H, Stahl W. Vitamins E and C, β-carotene, and other carotenoids as antioxidants. Am J Clin Nutr. 1995;62:1315S-21S.

15. Khanam S, Mohan NP, Devi K, Sultana R. Protectiv role of Tinospora cordifolia against cisplatin induced nephrotoxicity. Int J Pharm & Pharm Sci. 2011;3(4):268-70.

16. Katalinic V, Modun D, Music I, Boban M. Gender differences in antioxidant capacity of rat tissues determined by 2,2V-azinobis (3-ethylbenzothiazoline 6-sulfonate; ABTS) and ferric reducing antioxidant power (FRAP) assays. Comp Biochem & Physiol. 2005;140:47-52.

17. Niehaus WG, Samuelsson B. Formation of malondialdehyde from phospholipids arachidonate during microsomal lipid peroxidation. Eur J Biochem. 1968;6:126-30.

18. Jollow D, Mitchell L, Zampaglione N, Gillete J. Bromobenzene induced liver necrosis: Protective role of glutathione and evidence for 3, 4-bromobenzenoxide as the hepatotoxic intermediate. Pharmacol. 1974;11:151-169.

19. Hugo EB. Oxidoreductases acting on groups other than CHOH: Catalase. In: Colowick SP, Kalpan NO, Packer, L. (editors). Methods in enzymology. London: Academic Press. 1984;121-25.

20. Viswanatha Swamy AH, Patel UM, Koti BC, Gadad PC, Patel NL, Thippeswamy AH. Cardioprotective effect of Saraca indica ag ainst cyclophosphamide induced cardiotoxicity in rats: A biochemical, electrocardiographic and histopathological study. Ind J Pharmacol. 2013;45(1):44-8.

21. Yousef MI, Saad AA, El-Shennawy LK. (2009). Protective effect of grape seed proanthocyanidin extract against oxidative stress induced by cisplatin in rats. Food Chem. Toxicol. 2009;47:1176–83.

22. Domitrović R, Potočnjak I, Crnčević-Orlić Z, Škoda M. Nephroprotective activities of rosmarinic acid against cisplatin-induced kidney injury in mice. Food Chem Toxicol. 2014;66:321-8.

23. Arany I, Safirstein RL. Cisplatin nephrotoxicity. Semin. Nephrol. 2003;23:460–64.

24. Karthikeyan K, Bai BR, Devaraj SN. Cardioprotective effect of grape seed proanthocyanidins on isoproterenol-induced myocardial injury in rats. Int. J. Cardiol. 2007;115:326–33.

25. Conklin KA, Nicolson GL. Molecular replacement in cancer therapy: reversing cancer metabolic and mitochondrial dysfunction, fatigue and the adverse effects of cancer therapy. Curr Cancer Ther Rev. 2008;4:66-76.

26. Satoh M, Kashihara N, Fujimoto S, Horike H, Tokura T, Namikoshi T, et al. A novel free radical scavenger, edarabone, protects against cisplatin-induced acute renal damage in vitro and in vivo. J Pharmacol Exp Ther. 2003;305:1183–90.

27. Mora Lde O, Antunes LM, Francescato HD, Bianchi Mde L. The effects of oral glutamine on cisplatin-induced nephrotoxicity in rats. Pharmacol Res. 2003;47:517-22.

28. El-Sawalhi MM, Ahmed LA. Exploring the protective role of apocynin, a specific NADPH oxidase inhibitor, in cisplatin-induced cardiotoxicityin rats. Chem Biol Interact. 2014;207:58-66.

29. Hadi AA, Thamir SNA. Evaluation of the protective properties of amlodipine, on cisplatin induced cardiotoxicity in male rats. Glo J Med Res Interd. 2013;13(2):23-8.

30. Mayne ST. Beta-carotene, carotenoids, and disease prevention in humans. The FASEB Journal. 1996;10:690-701.

31. Müller L, Fröhlich K, Böhm V. Comparative antioxidant activities of carotenoids measured by ferric reducing antioxidant power (FRAP), ABTS bleaching assay (αTEAC), DPPH assay and peroxyl radical scavenging assay. Food Chemistry. 2011;129:139-48.

32. Miller NJ, Sampson J, Candeias LP, Bramley PM, Rice-Evans CA. Antioxidant activities of carotenoids and xanthophylls. FEBS Letters. 1996;384:240-42.

33. Kamal-Eldin A, Appelqvist LA. The chemistry and antioxidant properties of tocopherols and tocotrienols. Lipids. 1996;31:671-701.

34. El-Agamey A, Lowe GM, McGarvey DJ. Mortensen A, Phillip DM, Truscott TG, et al. Carotenoid radical chemistry and antioxidant/pro-oxidant properties. Arch. Biochem Biophys. 2004;430:37-48.

23

Factors Influencing the Risk of Death among Patients with Heart Failure

Muzeyin Ahmed Berarti[1] and Ayele Taye Goshu[2*]

[1]*Department of Statistics, Wolaita Sodo University, Ethiopia.*
[2]*Department of Statistics, School of Mathematical and Statistical Sciences, Hawassa University, Ethiopia.*

Authors' contributions

This work was carried out in collaboration between both authors. Author MAB conceptualized, proposed and designed the research, design R-code and existing library routines and software packages in combination, analyzed the data and wrote the draft manuscript. Author ATG commented with dedication on the draft, participated in editing design of the study, performed the statistical analysis and approved the final manuscript. Both authors conventionally read and approved the final manuscript.

Editor(s):
(1) Francesco Pelliccia, Department of Heart and Great Vessels University La Sapienza, Rome, Italy.
Reviewers:
(1) Kuipo Yan, Department of Cardiology, Hospital of Henan College of TCM, China.
(2) Alexander Berezin, Internal medicine Department, Zaporozhye Medical University, Ukraine.

ABSTRACT

The purpose of this study was to investigate the impact of risk factors on the death of patients with heart failure in a cohort of patients hospitalized with heart failure disease. In this paper we used chi-square tests with the aim of studying the relationship of each factor with survival. Generalized Additive Models (GAM), particularly Generalized Additive Logistic Regression Model, was used to examine the impact of risk factors on the death of patients with heart failure out of 263 patients considered in the analysis, 18.6% patients died of heart failure. A death proportion for female was 19.6% and that of male patients was 17.5%. From the GAM analysis the predictors: age, anemia, Tuberculosis, HIV status, renal inefficiency, diabetes, hypertension and sinus were found to significantly affect the death status of a patient. Being older age, anemic, renal inefficient, TB positive, HIV positive, diabetic, hypertensive and sinus positive increase the risk of death of a heart failure patient.

Keywords: Heart failure; generalized additive model; smoothing method; splines.

*Corresponding author: E-mail: ayele_taye@yahoo.com

1. INTRODUCTION

Cardiovascular diseases are among the most frequent causes of death worldwide. Heart failure is an enormous medical and societal burden and a leading cause of hospitalization among cardiovascular diseases. It is a very common disease, with severe morbidity and mortality, and a frequent reason of hospitalization. Heart failure is the end stage of many cardiac and non cardiac pathological processes, from ischemic heart disease and the range of cardiomyopathies to respiratory disease and severe anemia (Ahern et al. [1]). As such, heart failure is not an underlying cause of death according to the WHO (World Health Organization) definition, but rather an intermediate cause of death with a diverse range of possible underlying causes of death. Anemia in heart failure is complex and multi factorial. Anemia resulting from a lack of sufficient Iron for synthesis of hemoglobin is by far the most frequent hematological disease of infancy and childhood (Lulu et al. [2]).

Using the historical definition by the World Health Organization, anemia is defined when Hemoglobin concentration is less than 13 g/dl for men or less than 12 g/dl for women (Oliva et al. [3]). Anemia is not a specific entity but an indication of an underlying pathologic process or disease (Lulu et al. [2]).

2. METHODS

2.1 Design of the Study

The study was a retrospective cohort study, which reviews the patient's card and information sheet. In this study secondary data was incorporated. The hospital's registry was used to retrieve data on Heart failure.

2.2 Variables in the Study

Outcome Variables: The response or outcome variable in this study is the binary response variable: Death status of patients during Hospital stay due to heart failure. This status of patient is coded as 1 if the patient died in hospital and 0 if the patient alive.

Independent Variables: The prognostic variables which were expected to be the risk factors of heart failure are categorical and continuous (see Table 1).

2.3 Statistical Methods

In this study, Chi-square analysis w as used to find out whether there is an association between each predictor variables and death status and the Generalized Additive Logistic Regression Model was used to assess the impact of various risk factors on the death in patients with heart failure[1].

In this section the flexible statistical methods (which are the extension of the traditional linear models) have been described which may be used to identify and characterize the effect of potential prognostic factors on an outcome variables. These methods are called Generalized Additive Models.

Here the logistic regression model which is among the most commonly used statistical methods in medical researches was used as specific illustration of Generalized Additive Model.

2.3.1 Generalized additive models (GAMs)

A generalized additive model is a generalized linear model with a linear predictor involving a sum of smooth functions of covariates (Hastie and Tibshirani, [4] and [5]). Generalized additive models (GAMs) follow from additive models, as generalized linear models (GLM) follow from linear models. The response may follow any exponential family distribution, or simply have a known mean variance relationship, permitting the use of a quasi-likelihood approach as described (Wood [6]). The model allow s for rather flexible specification of the dependence of the response on the covariates, but by specifying the model only in terms of smooth functions, rather than detailed parametric relationships.

To use GAMs in practice require s some extensions to GLM methods:

1. The smooth functions must be represented somehow.
2. The degree of smoothness of the functions must be made controllable, so that models with varying degrees of smoothness can be explored.
3. Some means for estimating the most appropriate degree of smoothness from data is required, if the models are to be useful for more than purely exploratory work.

---

[1]R version 3.0.3 (2014-03-06) Statistical software have been used to analyze the data throughout the paper

In general the model has the following structure

$$g(\mu_i) = X_i^* \theta + f_1(x_{1i}) + f_2(x_{2i}) + f_3(x_{3i}, x_{4i}) + \ldots\ldots \text{ (1)}$$

Where, $\mu_i \equiv E(Y_i)$ and $Y_i \sim$ some exponential family distribution. Y_i is a response variable, $\mathbf{X}^*_i$ is a row of the model matrix for any strictly parametric model components, $\boldsymbol{\theta}$ is the corresponding parameter vector, and the f_j are smooth functions of the covariates, x_k.

Logistic model for binary data is one of the most widely used models in medical research. Here the dependent (outcome) variable Y_i is 0 or 1, with 1 indicating an event (like death or relapse of a disease) and 0 indicating no event. Our goal is modeling $p(y_i \mid x_{i1}, x_{i2}, \ldots\ldots x_{ip})$ the probability of an event given prognostic factors $x_{i1}, x_{i2}, \ldots\ldots x_{ip}$. The linear logistic model assumes that the log-odds are linear:

$$\log\left(\frac{p(y_i \mid x_{i1}, x_{i2}, \ldots\ldots x_{ip})}{1 - p(y_i \mid x_{i1}, x_{i2}, \ldots\ldots x_{ip})} \right) = \beta_0 + \quad (2)$$
$$\beta_1 x_{1i} + \beta_2 x_{2i} + \ldots\ldots + \beta_p x_{pi}$$

whereas the generalized additive logistic model (Hastie and Tibshirani, [7]) is:

$$\log\left(\frac{p(y_i \mid x_{i1}, x_{i2}, \ldots\ldots x_{ip})}{1 - p(y_i \mid x_{i1}, x_{i2}, \ldots\ldots x_{ip})} \right) = \beta_0 + \quad (3)$$
$$f_1(x_{1i}) + f_2(x_{2i}) + \ldots\ldots + f_p(x_{pi})$$

The functions $f_1, f_2, \ldots\ldots, f_p$ are unspecified (non-parametric) smoothing functions. The generalized additive model replaces $\sum \beta_j x_j$ with $\sum f_j(x_j)$ where f_j is an unspecified ('nonparametric') function. This function is estimated in a flexible manner using a scatter plot smoother. The estimated function $f(x_j)$ can reveal possible nonlinearities in the effect of the x_j.

2.3.2 Smoothing Methods

A spline curve is a piecewise polynomial curve, i.e., it joins two or more polynomial curves. The locations of the joins are known as "knots". In addition, there are boundary knots which could be located at or beyond the limits of the data. Smoothing splines arise as the solution to the following simple-regression problem: Find the function $\hat{f}(x)$ with two continuous derivatives that minimizes the penalized sum of squares (Wood, [8] and [6] , Fox & Weisberg, [9] and Hastie & Tibshirani, [7], Maindonald, [10]),

$$SS^*(h) = \sum_{i=1}^{n} [y_i - f(x_i)]^2 + \lambda \int_{x_{\min}}^{x_{\max}} [f''(x)]^2 dx \quad (4)$$

Table 1. Explanatory variables and their coding

Variables	Category and coding
Sex	Male= 1, Female= 0
Age at the start of treatment	Continues
Renal inefficiency	Yes= 1, No= 0
Place of residence	Rural= 0, Urban = 1
Pneumonia	Positive= 1, Negative= 0
Tuberculosis (TB)	Positive= 1, Negative= 0
Pulse rate at the start of treatment	Regular (60 − 80 bpm)=1, Irregular (≥ 80 bpm)=2
Diabetes mellitus	Positive= 1, Negative= 0
Human Immune Deficiency Virus (HIV)	Reactive= 1, Nonreactive= 0
Anemia	Anemic= 1, Non- anemic= 0
Hyper tension	Positive= 1, Negative= 0
Blood pressure at the star t of treatment	Nor mal (below1 20 /80 mm Hg)=1
	High(between12 0/80 -1 79 /1 09 mm Hg)=2
	Uncontrollable(above 1 80/1 10 mm Hg)=3
Sinus	Positive= 1, Negative= 0

Where, λ is a smoothing parameter, analogous to the neighborhood-width of the local polynomial estimator. Here y is a response or outcome variable, and x is a prognostic factor. The interest is to fit a smooth curve $f(x)$ that summarizes the dependence of y on x. If we were to find the curve that simply minimizes $\sum_{i=1}^{n}[y_i - f(x_i)]^2$, the result would be an interpolating curve that would not be smooth at all. In statistical work, y_i is usually measured with noise, and it is generally, more useful to smooth (x_i , y_i) data, rather than interpolating them. Notice that $\int_{x_{\min}}^{x_{\max}}[f''(x)]^2$ measures the "wiggliness" of the function f. linear f s have $\int_{x_{\min}}^{x_{\max}}[f''(x)]^2 = 0$, while non-linear f s produce values bigger than zero.

- The first term in Equation (4) is the residual sum of squares. The second term is a roughness penalty, which is large when the integrated second derivative of the regression function $f''(x)$ is large that is, when $f(x)$ is 'rough' (with rapidly changing slope). The endpoints of the integral enclose the data.
- At one extreme, when the smoothing constant is set to $\lambda = 0$ (and if all the x-values are distinct), $f'(x)$ simply interpolates the data; this is similar to a local-regression estimate with $span = 1/n$. At the other extreme, if λ is very large, then $\hat{f}$ will be selected so that $\hat{f}''(x)$ is everywhere 0, which implies globally linear least-squares fit to the data (equivalent to local regression with infinite neighborhoods).

2.4 Model Selection

Choosing an appropriate model is the major issue in statistical investigations. Omitting relevant variables that are correlated with regressors causes least square s to be biased and inconsistent. Including irrelevant variables reduces the precision of least squares. So, from a purely technical point, it is important to estimate a mo de l that has all of the necessary relevant variables and no ne that are irrelevant. It is also important to u se a suitable functional form.

The mgcv-package of R Statistical software selects the degrees of freedom for each term automatically. However, it cannot automatically decide whether to drop a term all together or not. Hence the term must be removed by the investigator. The criteria for removal of a term are the following based on Wood [11]:

- If the effective degrees of freedom (edf) for the smooth term close to 1 and large p.value for parametric term.
- If the plotted confidence limit includes zero everywhere.
- If the Generalized Cross Validation (GCV) / Un-Biased Risk Estimator (UBRE) dropped when the term is dropped.

2.5 Goodness of Fit of the Model

The goodness of fit or calibration of a model mea sures how well the model describes the response variable.Assessing goodness of fit involves inves tigating how close values predicted by the model with that of observed values (Bewick and Jonathan, [12]).

After fitting the logistic regression model or once a model has been developed through the various steps in estimating the coefficients, there are several techniques involved in assessing the appropriateness, adequacy and usefulness of the model. The Pearson's Chi-square, the likelihood ratio tests (LRT), Hosmer and Lemeshow Test and the Wald tests are the most commonly used measures of goodness of fit for categorical data (Hosmer and Lemeshow, [13]). Besides these, different diagnostic plots can be used based on the model class.

The *gam.check* function of mgcv-package of R Statistical software returns four diagnostic plots for Generalized Additive Models:

1. A quintile-comparison plot of the residuals allows us to look for outliers and heavy tails.
2. Residuals versus linear predictors (simply observed y for continuous variables) helps detect non constant error variance.
3. Histogram of the residuals are good for detecting non normality
4. Response versus fitted value.

2.6 Ethical Considerations

Ethical clearance was obtained from the Hospital.

3. RESULTS AND DISCUSSION

The main objective of this study has been to assess the impact of risk factors in the death of patients with heart failure. The data of size 263 were obtained from record reviews of all inpatient heart failure patients admitted to Asella Referral Hospital from February, 2009 to March, 2012. The mean age of patients is 41.51 with standard deviation 19.784 ranging from 15 to 91.25% of patients were less than 24 years old the median age is 40 and 75% of the patients were aged below 58 years.

The output on Table 2 shows the proportions of death among patient of heart failure, frequency distribution, Chi-square, p-value and degrees of freedom with respect to each category of the categorical explanatory variables.

The results reveal that out of 263 patients considered in the analysis, 18.6% patients have died of heart failure while 81.4% were alive. A death proportion for female was 19.6% and that of male patients was 17.5%.

Hypertensive patients have higher Risk of death than any other groups. Anemia status was found significantly associated with death status of patients.

Moreover, the Table 2 shows that anemia, diabetes mellitus, HIV, hypertension, pneumonia, blood pressure, renal inefficiency, sinus and tuberculosis were found to have significant association with death status of heart failure patients. In contrast, no association was found between death status and the independent variables: sex, pulse rate and residence of patients.

Table 2. Test of association between death status and explanatory variables
(Asella Referral Hospital, April 2012)

Variable	Category	Patient (N=49)				
		Alive N(%)	Dead N(%)	Total N(%)	Chi-square value (p-value)	Df
Sex	Male	99(82.5)	21 (17.5)	120 (45 .6)	0.1863(0.666)	1
	Female	115(80.4)	28 (19.6)	143 (54 .4)		
Residence	Urban	95(81.2)	22(18.8)	117(44.5)	0.0041(0.9488)	1
	Rural	119(81.5)	27(18.5)	146(55.5)		
Anemia	Anemic	45(65.2)	24(34.8)	69(26.2)	16.09(0.0000)	1
	Non-anemic	169(87.1)	25(12.9)	194(73.8)		
Diabetes	Positive	30(53.6)	26(46.4)	56(21.3)	36.27(0.000)	1
	Negative	184(88.9)	23(11.1)	207(78.7)		
HIV	Reactive	27(61.4)	17(38.6)	44(16.7)	13.9499(0.0001)	1
	Nonreactive	187(85.4)	32(14.6)	119(83.3)		
Hypertn.	Positive	41(51.9)	38(48.1)	79(30)	64.69(0.000)	1
	Negative	173(94.0)	11(6.0)	184(70)		
Pneumonia	Positive	83(73.5)	30(26.5)	113(43)	8.19(0.004)	1
	Negative	131(87.3)	19(12.7)	150(57)		
Pressure	Normal	117(90.0)	13(10.0)	130(49.4)	39.31(0.000)	1
	High	59(96.4)	6(3.6)	65(24.7)		
	Uncontrol	38(55.9)	30(44.1)	68(25.9)		
Pulse rate	Regular	111(83.5)	22(16.5)	133(50.6)	0.7751(0.3786)	1
	Irregular	103(79.2)	27(20.8)	130(49.4)		
Renal ineffi.	Yes	31(53.4)	27(46.6)	58(22.1)	38.263(0.000)	1
	No	183(89.3)	22(10.7)	205(77.9)		
TB	Positive	54(65.1)	29(34.9)	83(31.6)	21.28(0.000)	1
	Negative	160(88.9)	20(11.1)	180(68.4)		
Sinus	Positive	28(56.0)	22(44.0)	50(19)	26.21(0.000)	1
	Negative	186(87.3)	27(12.7)	213(81)		

3.1 Analysis of Generalized Additive Logistic Regression

Here Generalized Additive Logistic regression is illustrated. For each of the predictors, a smoother was fit by the *f* functions. The default spline used in the function *f* that does the smoothing is thin plate regression splines, which are slightly different from the B-splines, but are apparently preferred because they don't depend on the number of knots selected and also they generalize to smooth's of more than one variable at a time.

3.1.1 Full model

```
Data <- read.table("mom.dat", header =T)
library(mgcv)
model <-
 gam(death ~ s(age) + as.factor(pulserate)
+ as.factor(sex) + as.factor(anemia) +
as.factor(pneumonia) + as.factor(HIV) + as.
factor(TB) + as.factor(pressure) +
as.factor(renalineffeciency) + as.factor(diab
etes) + as.factor(residence) + as.factor(hyp
ertension) + as.factor(sinus), family = bino
mial(link = logit), data =Data)
summary(model)
```

Approximate significance of smooth terms:

```
edf   Ref. df  Chi.sq  p-value
s(age)  2.27  2.84  13.5  0.0033 **
Signif. codes: 0 '***' 0.001 '**' 0.01 '*'
0.05 '.' 0.1 '' 1
R-sq. (adj) = 0.705 Deviance explained =
```

69.7%
UBRE = -0.585 Scale est. = 1 n = 263

Graphical presentation of the data is carried out through R-code below.

```
>   library(lattice )
>   par(mfrow=c(4,4))
>   plot(model,all.terms=T,residual=T)
```

The model consists of smooth and parametric linear terms. As it can be seen from the output of the parametric model, in Table 3, anemia, Human Immune deficiency Virus (HIV), Tuberculosis (TB), renal inefficiency, Diabetes mellitus hypertension and sinus were significantly related to death of a patient. The smooth term age was significant as effective degrees o f freedom is much greater than 1 and p- value is very small.

The plot (Fig. 1) of the model shows, a semi-parametric model of death status o f Heart failure patients at follow- up Clinic of Asella Hospital, with factor for discrete variables and a smooth term for the dependence o n age. The first plot shows the smooth of age, with 95% confidence interval, while the other plots show the estimated effect, for e ach level of discrete variables.

The rug plots, along the bottom of the first plot, show the observed values of the covariate age, while the other plots show the levels (factor) of each explanatory variable. Number in y-axis caption is the effective degrees of freedom of the term being plotted for the continuous variables (age in the case of this research paper) and partial for discrete variables.

Table 3. The output of GAM when all variables are considered

	Estimate	Std. error	z value	Pr(>|z |)
(Intercept)	-8.2983	1.4530	-5.71	1.1e-08
as.factor(pulserate)2	0.0348	0.6701	0.05	0.95855
as.factor(sex)1	-0.5132	0.6796	-0.76	0.45017
as.factor(anemia)1	1.9846	0.7573	2.62	0.00878
as.factor(pneumonia)1	1.0641	0.6518	1.63	0.10255
as.factor(HIV)1	3.2934	0.9146	3.60	0.00032
as.factor(TB)1	1.7795	0.6695	2.66	0.00786
as.factor(pressure)2	-0.1340	0.8837	-0.15	0.87942
as.factor(pressure)3	-1.0965	1.1173	-0.98	0.32641
as.factor(renalineffeciency)1	2.4045	0.7279	3.30	0.00095
as.factor(diabetes)1	2.4856	0.7610	3.27	0.00109
as.factor(residence)1	0.6671	0.7177	0.93	0.35268
as.factor(hypertension)1	3.4242	1.0830	3.16	0.00157
as.factor(sinus)1	1.9232	0.7700	2.50	0.01250

The solid lines/curves represent the estimated effects, with 95% Bayesian confidence limits shown as dashed lines. If the confidence limits includes zero everywhere and the estimated straight line comfortably and fully laid confidence limit, at the point where the line passes through zero on the vertical axis, then the explanatory variable under consideration is unrelated with the response variable. The points shown on the first plot are Pearson partial residuals. For a well fitting model the partial residuals should be evenly scattered around the curve to which they relate. The plot shows anemia, Human Immune deficiency Virus (HIV), Tuberculosis (TB), renal inefficiency, diabetes mellitus, hypertension and sinus are relate d with death of patients with

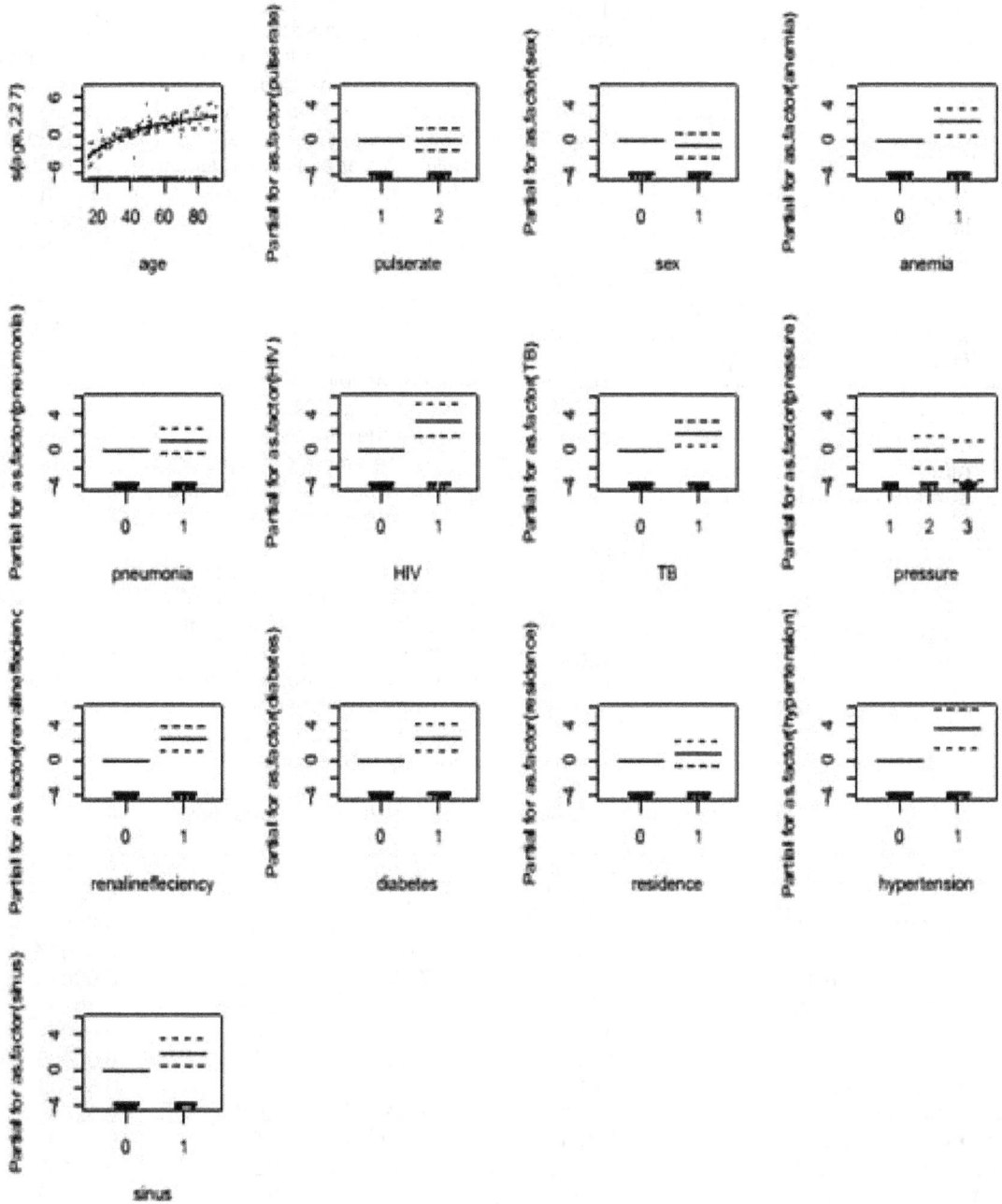

Fig. 1. Components of GAM model including all variables

Heart failure. That is, a patient with positive status of anemia, Human Immune deficiency Virus (HIV), Tuberculosis (TB), renal inefficiency, diabetes mellitus, hypertension and/or sinus was more likely had risk of death than that with respective opposite tests.

3.1.2 Variable selection

In statistical modelling, the choice of an optimal predictive model from a set of competing models is of extreme importance problem. There are a great deal of algorithms and procedures for searching the model space and selection criteria for choosing between competing models.

If all the three criteria stated under section 2.4 are satisfied, the term should be dropped (re moved). Hence, from Fig. 1, pulse rate, pressure,

sex, residence and pneumonia are candidates to be dropped. Let us examine each of them dropping a term per step. It makes sense to start with the term for which the zero line is most comfortably lie within confidence band. Alternatively we can start dropping the term having largest p-value first. Accordingly pulse rate looks like the first candidate for removal.

Model <**gam**(death ~ **s**(age) + **as.factor**(sex) + **as.factor**(anemia) + **as.factor**(pneumonia) +**as.factor**(HIV) + **as.factor**(TB) + **as.factor**(pressure) + **as.factor**(renalineffeciency) +**as.factor**(diabetes) + **as.factor**(residence) + **as.factor**(hypertension) + **as.factor**(sinus), family = **binomial**(link =logit),data =Data)
model

Estimated degrees of freedom:
2.2744   total = 15.27437
UBRE score: -0.5924804
> **pdf**(file="gamplot07.pdf")
> **par**(mfrow=**c**(4,3))
>
plot(model,all.terms=T,residual=T)
> **dev.off**()
pdf

2
Un-Biased Risk Estimator (UBRE) score has decreased from -0.585 to -0.5925 supporting the decision to remove the pulse rate term. Still from Fig.2 pressure, sex, residence and pneumonia are candidates to be dropped and pressure seem the second variable to remove.

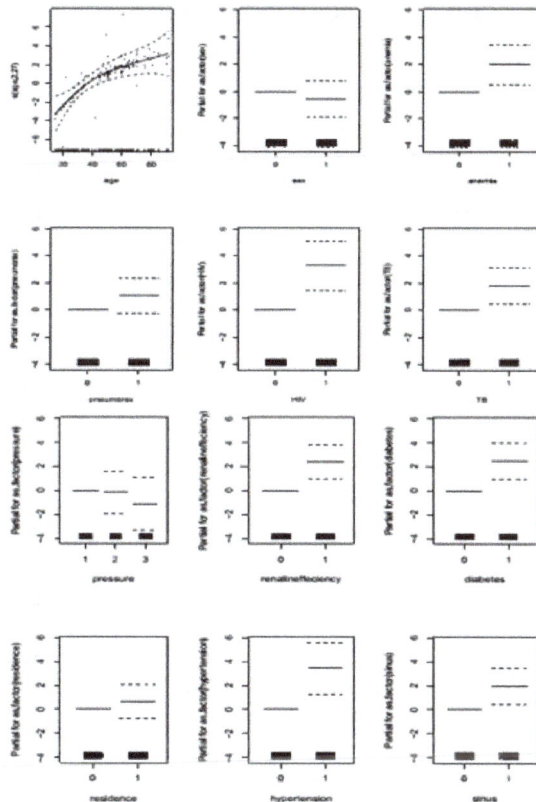

Fig. 2. Components of GAM model excluding pulse rate

model <- **gam**(death ~ **s**(age) + **as.factor**(sex) + **as.factor**(anemia) + **as.factor**(pneumonia) + **as.factor**(HIV) + **as.factor**(TB) + **as.factor**(renalineffeciency) + **as.factor**(diabetes) + **as.factor**(residence) + **as.factor**(hypertension) + **as.factor**(sinus), family = **binomial**(link = logit), data = Data)
model

Estimated degrees of freedom:
2.1303 total = 13.13026
UBRE score: -0.6034817
> **pdf**(file="gamploto3.pdf")
> **par**(mfrow=**c**(4,4))
> **plot**(model,all.terms=T,residual=T)
> **dev.off**()
pdf
2

- Fig. 3 (plot for Components of GAM Model excluding pulse rate & pressure) shows sex, residence and pneumonia are candidates to be dropped and sex is the third covariate to be dropped and we were right in dropping pressure since UBRE has dropped.

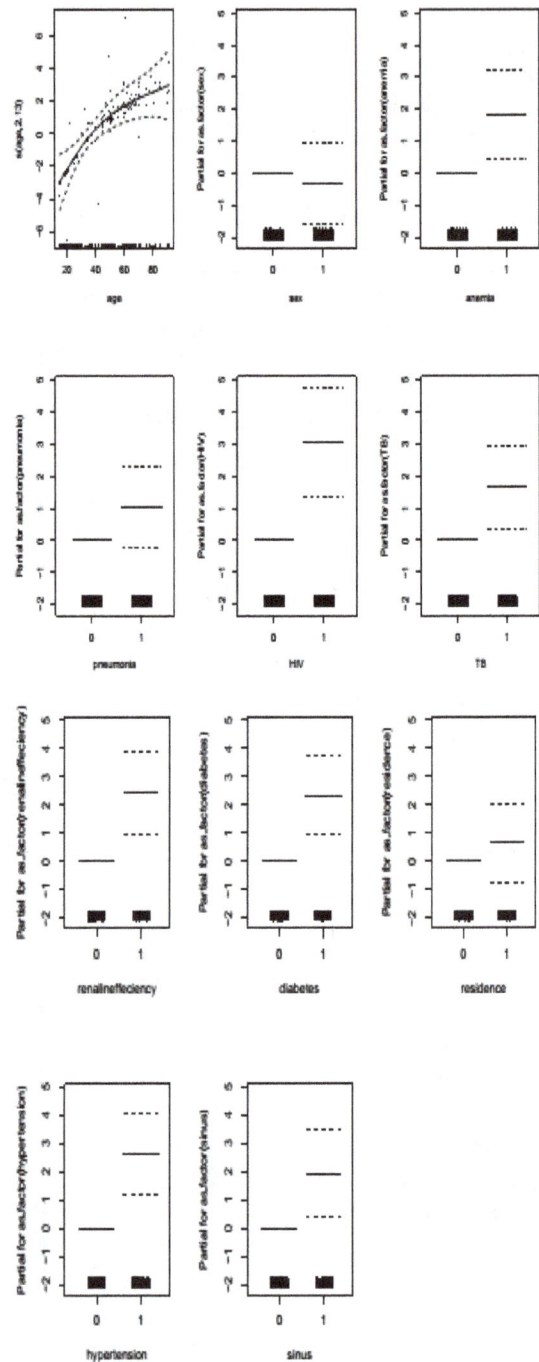

Fig. 3. Components of AM model excluding pulse rate & pressure.

```
model <- gam(death ~ s(age) + as.factor(anemia) + as.factor(pneumonia) + as.factor(HIV) +
        as.factor(TB) + as.factor(renalineffeciency) + as.factor(diabetes) + as.factor(residence) +
        as.factor(hypertension) + as.factor(sinus), family = binomial(link = logit), data = Data)
model
```

Estimated degrees of freedom:
2.0734   total = 12.0734
UBRE score: -0.6099116
> **pdf**(file="gamplot04.pdf")
> **par**(mfrow=**c**(4,3))
> **plot**(model,all.terms=T,residual=T)
> **dev.off**()
pdf
2

Here also UBRE is dropped and from Fig. 4 all the three conditions are satisfied for the removal of the variable sex from the model.

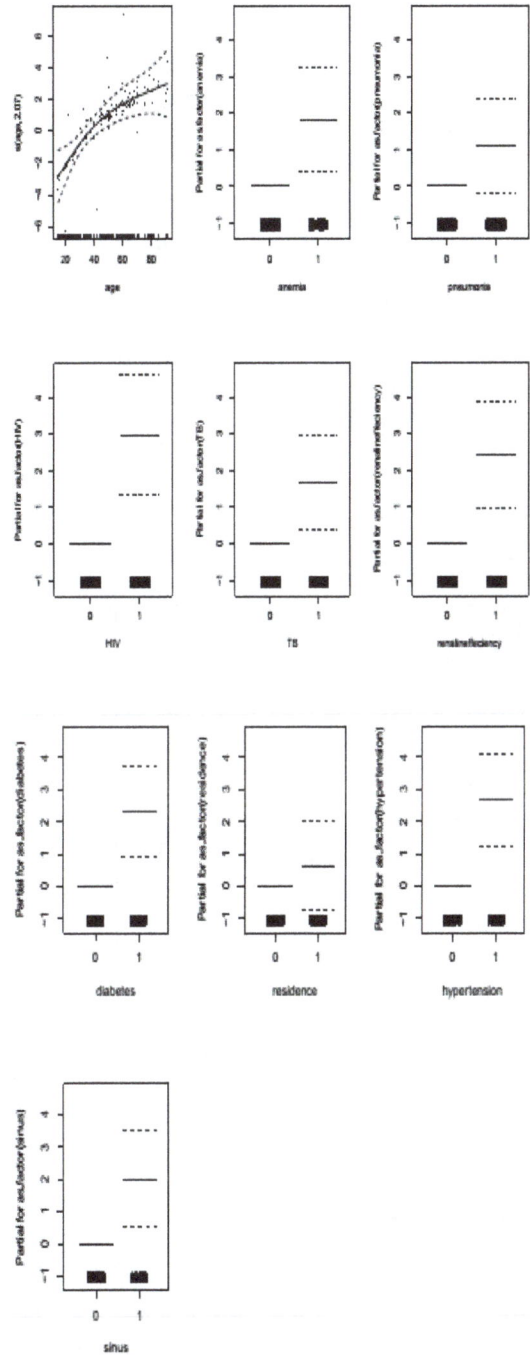

Fig. 4. Components of GAM model excluding pulse rate, pressure & sex

model <- **gam**(death ~ **s**(age) +
    as.factor(anemia) +
    as.factor(pneumonia) + **as.factor**(HIV)
    + **as.factor**(TB) +
    as.factor(renalineffeciency) +
    as.factor(diabetes) +
    as.factor(hypertension) +

as.factor(sinus), family = **binomial**(link
= logit), data = Data)
model

UBRE is dropped and looking at Fig. 5 , all the three criteria are satisfied for removal of Residence.

```
library(mgcv)
        model1  <-  gam(death  ~  s(age)  +
        as.factor(anemia) + as.factor(HIV) +
        as.factor(TB)                      +
        as.factor(renalineffeciency)       +
        as.factor(diabetes)                +
        as.factor(hypertension)            +
        as.factor(sinus), family = binomial(link
        = logit), data = Data)
model1
```

Considering Fig. 6, the first two criteria are satisfied for removal of pneumonia, but the third is not since UBRE increased. However, very small increases in UBRE should not prevent a term from being dropped. Thus pneumonia should be dropped. We can test the statistical significance of a term in the model by dropping it and noting the change in the deviance (Fox &

Weisberg, [4]). To confirm the removal of pneumonia lets test it using analysis of deviance:

```
library(mgcv)
        model< gam(death ~ s(age) + as.factor
        (anemia) + as.factor(pneumonia) + as.facto
        r(HIV) +
        as.factor(TB) + as.factor(renalineffeciency)
        + as.factor(diabetes) + as.factor(hyperte
        nsion) +
        as.factor(sinus), family =binomial(link = logi
        t), data = Data)
        model2 <gam(death ~ s(age) + as.factor(an
        emia) + as.factor(HIV) + as.factor(TB) + as.
        factor (renalineffeciency) + as.factor(diabet
        es) + as.factor(hypertension) + as.factor(sin
        us),

        family = binomial(link = logit), data = Data)
        anova(model2, model, test = "Chisq")
```

```
Estimated degrees of freedom:
1.9467  total  = 10.94673
UBRE score: -0.61396
> pdf(file="gamplot05.pdf")
> par(mfrow=c(3,3))
>
plot(model,all.terms=T,residual=T)
> dev.off()
 pdf
 2
```

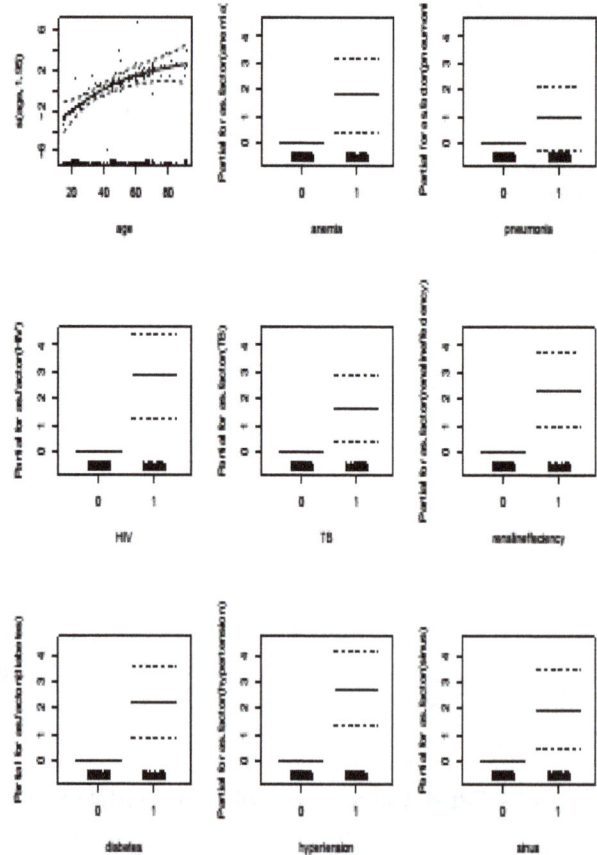

Fig. 5. Components of GAM model when pulse rate, pressure, sex & residence are excluded

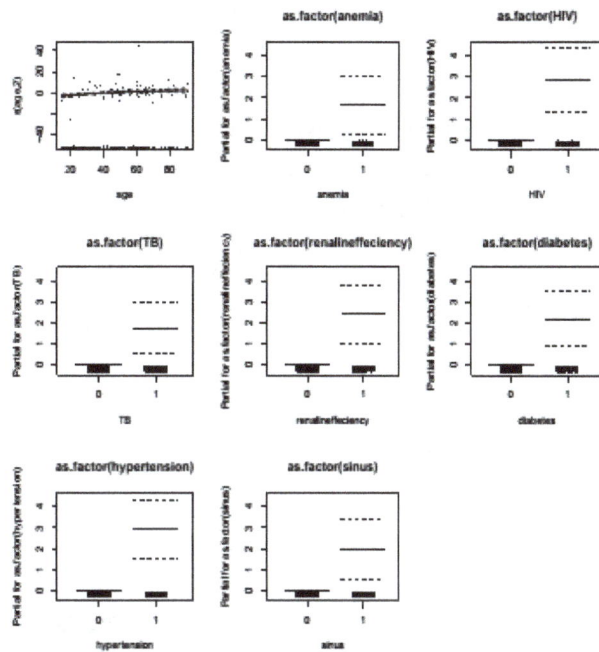

Fig. 6. Components of GAM model when pulse rate, pressure, sex, Residence & pneumonia are excluded

Analysis of Deviance Table

Resid. Df Resid. Dev Df Deviance Pr(>Chi)

1	253	81.9			
2	252	79.6	0.944	2.25	0.12

Signif. codes: 0 '***' 0.001 '**' 0.01 '*' 0.05 '.' 0.1 '' 1

Thus, the term pneumonia is statistically insignificant at 5% level of significance and should be dropped.

```
library(mgcv)
model <gam(death ~ s(age) + as.factor(anemia) + as.factor(HIV) + as.factor(TB) +
    as.factor(renalineffeciency) + as.factor(diabetes) + as.factor(hypertension) + as.factor(sinus),
    family = binomial(link = logit), data = Data)
summary(model)
```

	Estimate	Std. error	z value	Pr(>|z |)	
(Intercept)	-7.421	1.104	-6.72	1.8e-11	***
as.factor(anemia)1	1.664	0.691	2.41	0.01606	*
as.factor(HIV)1	2.837	0.779	3.64	0.00027	***
as.factor(TB)1	1.759	0.616	2.85	0.00431	**
as.factor(renalineffeciency)1	2.412	0.694	3.47	0.00051	***
as.factor(diabetes)1	2.201	0.664	3.32	0.00091	***
as.factor(hypertension)1	2.905	0.702	4.14	3.5e-05	***
as.factor(sinus)1	1.956	0.728	2.69	0.00723	**

Approximate significance of smooth terms:

edf   Ref.df   Chi.sq   p-value
s(age) 2   2.51   16.5   0.00062 ***

Signif. codes: 0 ' *** ' 0.001 ' ** ' 0.01 ' * ' 0.05 '.' 0.1 ' ' 1
R- **sq.** (adj) = 0.694   Deviance explained = 67.6%
UBRE = -0.61257 Scale est. = 1   n = 263

The graph is produced as stated below.

```
> pdf(file="gamplot06.pdf")
> par(mfrow=c(3,3))
> plot(model,all.terms=T,residual=T)
> dev.off()
```

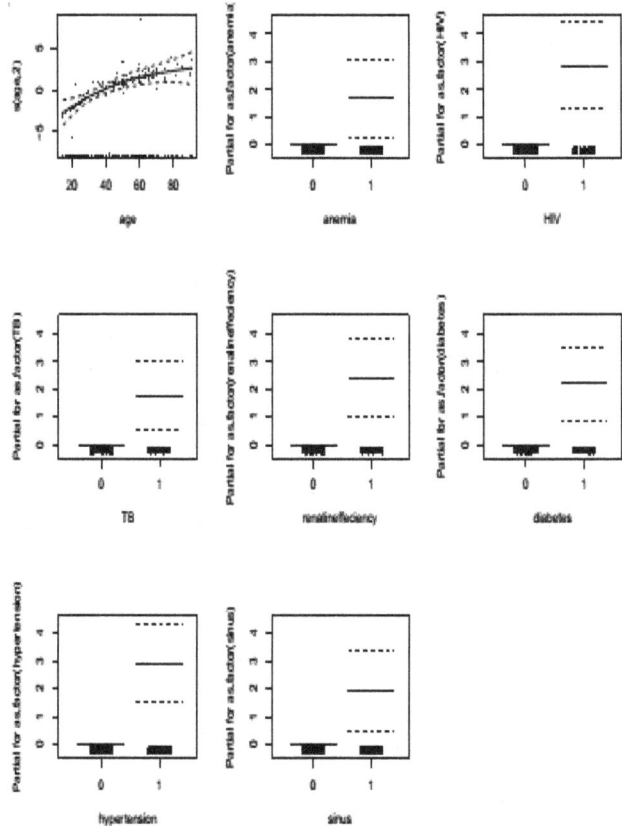

Fig. 7. Components of GAM Plot for the best fitted model: Partial-regression functions for the additive regression of overall significant variables

Both the last output and the plot (above Fig. 7) imply no further terms to delete; the model can be used for prediction. Hence, this is the best model. Therefore, the effects of the predictors age, anemia, Human Immune deficiency Virus (HIV), TB, renal inefficiency, diabetes, hypertension and sinus on the death status of the patients are found to be significant. A patient with positive status in anemia, Human Immune deficiency Virus (HIV), TB, renal inefficiency, diabetes, hypertension and/or sinus was more likely had risk of death than that with respective negative tests.

For continuous variable (age) case: The risk of death of a patient increases with increasing his/her age, after controlling all other covariates.

3.2 Goodness of Fit of the Model

After finding results, the overall adequacy of the model should be checked. There are several alternative methods to check the adequacy of the fitted model. Among many alternative methods, we used the following Diagnostic Plots to assess the model.

The normal Q-Q plot on the figure below resembles a (nearly) straight line and shows that there is no powerful outlier and influential value in the data respectively.

Residual s versus linear predictors above indicate, the standardized residuals are uncorrelated With the linear predictors; as this plot is a random scatter of points.

```
pdf(file = "modelcheck.pdf")
par(mfrow = c(2, 2))
gam.check(model)
dev.off()
```

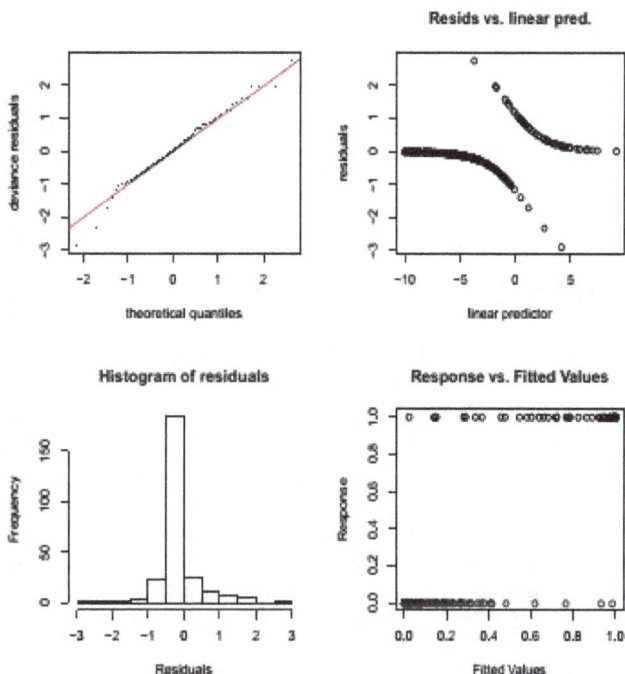

Fig. 8. Goodness of GAM Model

Histogram of the residuals approximately resemble s standard normal curve implying normality assumption is satisfied. Therefore, from the plot above, we can generalize that the model fits the data well.

3.3 Discussion

This study investigated the effect of predictor of mortality in group of hospitalized patients with heart failure. From the results, it was found that the survival of a patient is significantly related with age, anemia, TB, HIV status, hypertension, positive history of diabetics, renal inefficiency and sinus.

The findings obtained from this study were found to be comparable with similar studies in different countries. In this study renal inefficiency was related to both prevalence of anemia and death of heart failure patients. This result is highly comparable with the result obtained (Villacorta et al. [14] which found that renal dysfunction was associated with prevalence of anemia and risk of death of patients from Heart failure. According to the result of this study, hypertensive patients had higher Risk of death (48.1%) than any other groups followed by renal inefficiency (46.6%) and diabetes mellitus (46.4%), respectively. This result can best compared with the result obtained (Kosiborod et al. [15]) which found that the majority of patients had a history of hypertension (60%) and a substantial minority had diabetes (37%), and a history of renal insufficiency (20%).

Several previous studies have identified other adverse prognostic factors among patients with heart failure, including age, anemia, hypertension, positive history of diabetics, renal dysfunction and sinus. Our study suggests that Tuberculosis (TB), Human Immune deficiency Virus (HIV) status, should be added to this group of clinical variables.

4. CONCLUSIONS

The main objective of this study was to investigate effect of risk factors of death in patients with Heart failure at Asella Referral Teaching Hospital. The results revealed that out of 263 patients considered in the analysis, 18.6% patients had died of heart failure while 81.4% were alive. Hypertensive patients had higher risk of death than any other groups followed by renal inefficiency and diabetes respectively. The GAM analysis showed that the predictors: age, anemia, HIV status, renal inefficiency, diabetes, hypertension and sinus significantly affect the death status of a patient.

CONSENT

It is not applicable.

COMPETING INTERESTS

Authors have declared that no competing interests exist.

REFERENCES

1. Ahern R, Lozano R, Naghavi M, Foreman K, Gakidou E, Murray C. Improving the public health utility of global cardiovascular mortality data: The rise of ischemic heart disease. Population Health Metrics. 2011;9:8.

2. Lulu M, Birhane O, Hirut D, Shabbar J, Weber MW. Evaluation of clinical pallor in the identification and treatment of children with moderate and severe anaemia. Tropical Medicine and International Health. Addis Ababa University. 2000;11(5):805-810.

3. Oliva EN, Schey C, Hutchings AS. A review of anemia as a cardiovascular risk factor in patients with myelodysplastic syndromes. 2011;1/2:160-166.

4. Hastie T, Tibshirani R. Generalized additive models. Statistical Science. 1986;1(3):187-196.

5. Hastie T, Tibshirani R. Generalized additive models. London: Chapman and Hall; 1990.

6. Wood SN. Generalized additive models, An introduction with R. London: Chapman & Hall; 2006.

7. Hastie T, Tibshirani R. Generalized additive models for medical research. Statistical Methods in Medical Research. 1995;4:187-196.

8. Wood SN. Thin plate regression splines. Journal of Royal Statistical Society, Ser. B. 2003;65:95-114.

9. Fox J, Weisberg S. Nonparametric regression in R: An appendix to an R companion to applied regression, 2nd ed.; 2010.

10. Maindonald J. Smoothing terms in GAM models, centre for mathematics and its applications. Australian National University; 2010.

11. Wood SN. GAMs and generalized ridge regression for R. Martin Schlather University of Bayreuth, Germany. 2001;1/2.

12. Bewick L, Jonathan B. Statistics review 14: Logistic Regression; 2005.

13. Hosmer D, S. Lemeshow. Applied logistic regression. John Wiley and Sons, Inc., Newyork; 1989.

14. Villacorta H, Tello SB, Barcellos Dos Santos E, Steffen R, Wiefels C, Sales LA, Soares P, Mesquita TE. Renal dysfunction and anemia in heart failure. Arq Brascardiol. 2010;94(3):357-363.

15. Kosiborod M, Smith GL, Radford MJ, Foody JM, Krumholz HM. The prognostic importance of anemia in patients with heart failure. The American Journal of Medicine. 2003;114.

24

Learning Bayesian Networks Using Heart Failure Data

Muzeyin Ahmed Berarti[1] and Ayele Taye Goshu[2*]

[1]*Department of Statistics, Wolaita Sodo University, P.O.Box 138, Ethiopia.*
[2]*Department of Statistics, School of Mathematical and Statistical Sciences, Hawassa University, P.O.Box 05, Ethiopia.*

Authors' contributions

This work was carried out in collaboration between both authors. Author MAB conceptualized, proposed and designed the research, design R-code and existing library routines and software packages in combination, analyzed the data and wrote all drafts of the manuscript. Author ATG commented with dedication on the drafts, participated in editing design of the study, performed the statistical analysis, managed the literature searches and approved the final manuscript. Both authors conventionally read and approved the final manuscript.

Editor(s):
(1) Francesco Pelliccia, Department of Heart, Great Vessels University La Sapienza, Rome, Italy.
Reviewers:
(1) Loc Nguyen, University of Science, Ho Chi Minh, Vietnam.
(2) Cliff Richard Kikawa, Mathematics and Statistics, Tshwane University of Technology, Republic of South Africa.

ABSTRACT

Background: Several factors may affect heart failure status of patients. It is important to investigate whether or not the effects are direct. The purpose of this study was learning Bayesian networks that encode the joint probability distribution for a set of random variables.

Methods: The design was a retrospective cohort study. The target population for this study was heart failure patients who were under follow- up at Asella referral teaching Hospital from February, 2009 to March, 2012. Bayesian Network is used in this paper to examine causal relationships between variables via Directed Acyclic Graph (DAG).

Results: Death of patients can be determined using HIV, hypertension, diabetes, anemia, renal inefficiency and sinus. Hypertension and sinus were found to have direct effects while TB had only indirect effect. Age did not have an effect.

Conclusion: Anemia, HIV, diabetes mellitus renal inefficiency and sinus directly affect the death of heart failure patient. Death is conditionally independent on TB and age, given all other variables.

Keywords: Bayesian network; parameter learning; structure learning; causal relationships.

*Corresponding author: E-mail: ayele_taye@yahoo.com

1. INTRODUCTION

Graphs, as stated in [1], provide a comprehensive picture of a problem that makes for a more complete and better balanced understanding than could be derived from tabular or textual forms of presentation. Moreover, graphs can bring out hidden facts and relationships and can stimulate, as well as aid, analytical thinking and investigation.

The main focus of this paper is to describe and drive conditional independence relations existing among random variables through Directed Graphical model called Bayesian networks. Bayesian networks are among the leading techno logies to investigate such relations.

A Bayesian network [2] is a graphical model that encodes the joint probability distribution for a set of random variables and a way of finding important relationships between variables. Bayesian Networks provide a power full technique to understand causal relationships between variables via Directed Acyclic Graph (DAG). Directed graphical models represent probability distributions that can be factored into products of conditional distributions, and have the potential for causal interpretations. The nodes in the graph represent the random variables and missing arrows between the nodes, specify properties of conditional independence between the variables. We refer the reader [3] for detailed understanding of Undirected Graphical Models counterpart and comprehensive comparison with Directed Graphical Models.

A method for learning the parameters and structure of such Bayesian networks has recently been described by in [4]. [5] described a modern method for learning the parameters and structures of Bayesian networks in deal package of R statistical Software.

Bayesian networks are designed for making decisions in systems with uncertainties [6].

Bayesian networks are therefore suitable for problems where the variables exhibit a complicated dependency structure.

2. METHODS

2.1 Data Description

The design was a retrospective cohort study, which reviews the patient's card and information sheet. The data of size 263 were obtained from record reviews of all inpatient heart failure patients admitted to Asella Referral Hospital from February, 2009 to March, 2012.

2.2 Response Variables

Death status of patients during hospital stays due to heart failure. This status of patient is coded as 1 if the patient died in hospital and 0 if the patient alive.

2.3 Independent Variables

The prognostic variables which are expected to be the risk factors of heart failure are categorical and continuous (see Table 1).

Table 1. Independent variables and their coding

Variables	Category and coding
Age at the start of treatment	Continues
Renal inefficiency	Yes= 1, No= 0
TB	Positive= 1, Negative= 0
Diabetes mellitus	Positive= 1, Negative= 0
HIV	Reactive= 1, Nonreactive= 0
Anemia	Anemic = 1, Non-anemic = 0
Hypertension	Positive= 1, Negative= 0
Sinus	Positive= 1, Negative= 0

2.4 Bayesian Networks

A Bayesian network is a graphical model that encodes the joint probability distribution for a set of random variables. Bayesian network, [7], is a specific type of graphical model which is a directed acyclic graph (DAG). [8] described A Bayesian network as a compact, graphical model of a probability distribution. It consists of two parts: a directed acyclic graph which represents direct influences among variables, and a set of conditional probability tables that quantify the strengths of these influences. A graph consists of a set of vertices (nodes), along with a set of edges joining some pairs of the vertices. However, the edges have directional arrows (but no directed cycles) [3]. The nodes in the graph represent the random variables and missing arrows between the nodes, specify properties of conditional independence between the variables. Bayesian networks are designed for making decisions in systems with uncertainties. Here we perform the analysis using Bayesian networks for discrete and continuous variables in which the joint distribution of all the variables are Conditional Gaussian (CG).

Let D = (V, E) be a Directed Acyclic Graph (DAG), where V is a finite nonempty set of nodes and E is a finite set of directed edges (arrows) between the nodes. The DAG defines the structure of the Bayesian network. To each node $v \in V$ in the graph corresponds to a random variable X_v. The set of variables associated with the graph D is then $X = (X_v)$, $v \in V$. Often, we do not distinguish between a variable X_v and the corresponding node v. To each node v with parents pa(v), a local probability distribution, $p(x_v \mid x_{pa(v)})$ is attached. The set of local probability distributions for all variables in the network is P. A Bayesian network for a set of random variables X is then the pair (D, P). The possible lack of directed edges in D encodes conditional independences between the random variables X through the factorization of the joint probability distribution,

$$p(X) = \prod_{v \in V} p(x_v \mid x_{pa(v)}) \qquad (1)$$

Here, Bayesian networks with both discrete and continuous variables are allowed as treated in [4] So the set of nodes V is given by $V = \Delta \cup \Gamma$, where Δ and Γ are the sets of discrete and continuous nodes, respectively. The corresponding random variables X can then be denoted by

$$X = X_{(v)}, v \in V = (I, Y) = ((I_\delta), \delta \in \Delta, (Y_\gamma), \gamma \in \Gamma$$

,i.e. I and Y used for the sets of discrete and continuous variables, respectively. The set of levels for each discrete variable $\delta \in \Delta$ is denoted as I_δ. To ensure availability of exact local computation methods, we do not allow discrete variables to have continuous parents. The joint probability distribution then factorizes into a discrete part and a mixed part, so

$$p(x) = p(i, y) = \prod_{\delta \in \Delta} p(i_\delta \mid i_{pa(\delta)}) \prod_{\gamma \in \Gamma} p(y_\gamma \mid y_{pa(\gamma)}, i_{pa(\gamma)})$$

Where $i_{pa(\gamma)}$ and $y_{pa(\gamma)}$ denote observations of the discrete and continuous parents respectively. A method for estimating the parameters and

learning the dependency structure of a conditional Gaussian networks with mixed variables is presented in [4] and implemented in the software package deal in [5] and [9].

2.4.1 Inference

A substantial feature of Bayesian networks is that it enables us to infer conditional dependencies between variables by visually inspecting the network's graph. Therefore we can divide the set of Bayesian network nodes into nonoverlapping subsets of conditional independent nodes. Decomposition is very important when doing inference. Inference is the task of computing the probability of each state of a node in a Bayesian network when other variables are known. To perform inference we first need to be familiar with the belief propagation. Belief propagation is the action of updating the beliefs in each variable when observations are given to some of the variables. Inference in Bayesian networks is performed using Bayes' theorem. Variables in BNs can be divided into groups depending on their position in BNs and taking into account the meaning of real world state that they represent including their observability. Consider a network for a set of random variables X and assume that some of the variables, B, are observed (visible variable) and the rest, A, are not (hidden variable). Let Uk be any arbitrary subset of X. The goal of inference is to find the conditional probability density functions (pdfs) over U given the observed variable B Which can be written using Bayes' theorem as

$$p(U_k \mid B) = \frac{p(U_k, B)}{p(B)} = \frac{p(U_k) p(B \mid U_k)}{p(B)}$$

Thus $p(U_k)$ is the prior distribution of U_k, i.e. the distribution of U_k before we observe B, $p(B \mid U_k)$ is the likelihood of U_k and $p(B \mid U_k)$ is the posterior distribution of U_k, i.e. the distribution of U_k, when we have observed B.

Generally, finding these distributions are computationally demanding as it involves calculating huge joint distributions, especially if there are many variables in the network. The marginal or conditional distributions of interest can then be found by a series of local computations, involving only some of the variables at a time. For a thorough treatment of these methods see [2].

2.4.2 Parameter and structure learning

To estimate the parameters in the network and to find the structure of the network, a Bayesian approach has been used. So, regarding the parameters, uncertainty about µ is encoded in a prior distribution $p(\theta)$, using data d to update this distribution (see equation 2), i.e. learn the parameters, and here by obtain the posterior distribution $p(\theta \mid data)$. The section is based on [4] and [10]. Consider a situation with one random variable X. Let θ be the parameter to be assessed and Θ be the parameter space and d a random sample of size n from the probability distribution $p(x \mid \theta)$. We call d our database and $x^c \in d$ a case. Then, according to Bayes' theorem,

$$p(\theta \mid d) = \frac{p(d \mid \theta)p(\theta)}{p(d)}, \theta \in \Theta \qquad (2)$$

where $p(d \mid \theta) = \prod_{x^c \in d} p(x^c \mid \theta)$ is the joint probability distribution of d, also called the likelihood of θ. As prior parameter distributions, the Dirichlet distribution and the Gaussian inverse Gamma distribution have beenused for the discrete variables and for the continuous variables respectively. These distributions are conjugate to observations from the respective distributions and this ensures simple calculations of the posterior distributions. Now, to learn the structure of the network, we calculate the posterior probability o f the D AG, $p(D \mid d)$, which from Bayes' theorem is given by

$$p(D \mid d) = \frac{p(d \mid D)p(D)}{p(d)}$$

Where $p(d \mid D)$ is the likelihood of D and $p(D)$ is the prior probability of D. As the normalizing constant $p(d)$ does not depend upon structure, another measure, which gives the relative probability, is

$$p(D,d) = p(d \mid D)p(D)$$

We use the above measure and refer to it as the network score. For simplicity, we choose to let $p(D)$ be the same for all DAGs, so we are only interested in calculating the likelihood $p(d \mid D)$. So learning the DAG from data, we can in principle first calculate the network scores for all possible DAGs and then select the DAG with the highest network score. If many DAGs are possible, it is computationally infeasible to calculate the network score for all these DAGs. In this situation it is necessary to use some kind of search strategy to find the DAG with the highest score. In some cases it can be more accurate to average over the possible DAGs for prediction, instead of just selecting a single DAG. So if x is the quantity we are interested in, we can use the weighted average,

$$p(x \mid d) = \sum_{D \in DAG} p(x \mid d, D)p(D \mid d),$$

Where $D\,AG$ is the set of all DAGs and $p(D \mid d)$ is the weight. Again, if many DAGs are possible, this sum is too hard to compute, so instead, by using a search strategy, we can find a few DAGs with high score and average over these. In order to calculate the network score for a specific DAG D, in a CG network, we need to know the prior probability and the likelihood of the DAG. For simplicity, we could for example choose to let all DAGs be equally likely, then

$$p(D|d) \propto p(d|D)$$

In a CG network, the likelihood of the DAGD is given by

$$p(d \mid D) = \int_{\theta \in \Theta} p(d \mid \theta, D)p(\theta \mid D)d\theta,$$

To evaluate which DAG or possible several DAGs that represent the conditional independences in a Bayesian network well, we want to find the DAG or D AGs with the highest network scores. To calculate these scores, we must specify the local probability distributions and the local prior distributions for the parameters for each network under evaluation. We see in the above equation that it, besides the likelihood of the parameters, also involves the prior distribution over the parameters, $p(\theta \mid D)$. This means that we for each possible DAG have to specify a prior distribution for the parameters. In [1] this method is extended to the mixed case. With this method, the parameter priors for all possible networks can be deduced from one joint parameter prior, called master *prior*. To specify this master prior, we only have to specify a prior Bayesian network, i.e. a prior DAG and a prior probability distribution, together with a measure of how confident we are in the prior network.

2.5 Ethical Considerations

Ethical clearance was obtained from the Hospital.

3. RESULTS AND DISCUSSION

For this study, the data of heart failure patients which was taken from Asella Referral Hospital is used and analyzed using Bayesian Networks. The data of size 263 were obtained from record reviews of all in patient heart failure patients admitted to Medical ward from February, 2009 to March, 2012. In this analysis, nine variables are considered each containing 263 observations as presented in Table 2.

Table 2. Variables used in this analysis

Node index	Variables
1	Age
2	Hypertension
3	HIV
4	Diabetes
5	TB
6	anemia
7	Sinus
8	Renal inefficiency
9	Death

Here we consider Bayesian networks with both discrete and continuous random variables. We use the deal package of R Statistical Software to analyze the data of heart failure patients obtained from Asella Referral Hospital.

The purpose of analyzing data under this section is to find dependency relations between the variables where the main interest lies in finding out which variables influence the death status of heart failure patients.

Age is continuous variable which may cause the death of heart failure patients. However, in deal continuous parents of discrete nodes are not allowed. Thus, describing such a relation is impossible. A remedial measure is handle death as a continuous variable, even though this is clearly not.

3.1 Specification of a Bayesian Network

Here is the R-code for building Bayesian Network for Heart failure Data.

```
> Data<- read.table("mom.dat",header=T) ##
invoke Data from working Directory
> attach(Data)
> Data<-
data.frame(age,hypertension,HIV,diabetes,TB,a
nemia,sinus,renalineffeciency, death)
> Data$death<-as.numeric(Data$death)
> Data$age<-as.numeric(Data$age)
> Data$anemia <-as.factor(Data$anemia)
> Data$diabetes <-as.factor(Data$diabetes)
> Data$hypertension <-
as.factor(Data$hypertension)
> Data$sinus <-as.factor(Data$sinus)
> Data$TB <-as.factor(Data$TB)
> Data$HIV <-as.factor(Data$HIV)
> Data$renalineffeciency <-
as.factor(Data$renalineffeciency)
```

Hereafter, we are in position to specify a prior Bayesian network. We use the empty DAG as the prior DAG since we have no prior knowledge about specific dependency relations and let the probability distribution of the discrete variables be uniform. The assessment of the probability distribution for the continuous variables is based on data.

```
> library(deal) ## call deal package
> Data.nw<-network(Data) ## specify prior
network
> Data.prior <- jointprior(Data.nw) ## create
joint prior distribution
Imaginary sample size: 256
# banlist for age and HIV as none of
#the other variables can influence these
variables.
> from1<-c(2,3,4,5,6,7,8,9)
> to1<-rep(1,8)
> from2<-c(1,2,4,5,6,7,8,9)
> to2<-rep(3,8)
> from3<-rep(9,6)
> to3<-c(2,4,5,6,7,8)
> banlist<-
matrix(c(from1,from2,from3,to1,to2,to3),ncol=2)
> banlist(Data.nw) <- banlist
```

The ban list is a matrix with two columns. Each row contains the directed edge that is not allowed. The final stage is to learn the parameters in the network and initiate the structural learning using *auto search ()* and *heuristic ()*.

```
> Data.nw <-
getnetwork(learn(Data.nw,Data,Data.prior))
> Data.search <-
autosearch(Data.nw,Data,Data.prior,trace=TRU
E)
> Data.heuristic <-
heuristic(getnetwork(Data.search),Data,Data.pr
ior,restart=2,

degree=10,trace=TRUE,trylist=gettrylist(Data.se
arch))
```

NB: The banlist forces:

- Death to be a leaf node (death can only receive arcs) (in our dataset death is variable number 9)
- Age and HIV cannot receive arcs (in our dataset age is variable number1 & HIV is variable number 3).

As can be seen from the Bayesian network plot, Fig. 1, death depends directly on Human Immune deficiency Virus (HIV), hypertension, diabetes, anemia, renal inefficiency and sinus. Hence, given these variables, death is conditionally independent on TB and age.

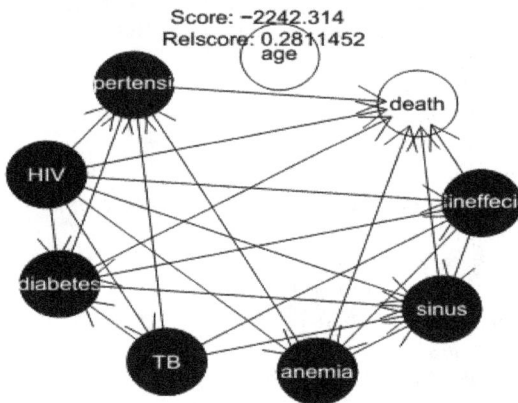

Fig. 1. Bayesian network plot for heart failure data

Death is conditionally independent on TB, given all other variables. We also see that age is independent from all other variables. How can we explain these findings? TB has an impact on death but only indirectly through complications like HIV, hypertension, diabetes, anemia, renal inefficiency and sinus. TB does not provoke death directly but only through these events, which absolutely seems very reasonable. Anemia is one of the important variables that can lead to death directly, but also indirectly: through

hypertension and sinus. This shows that anemia has some- how three ways to impact death: directly or indirectly, because it increase the possibility to importance of hypertension and sinus.

As a comparison, we see that HIV has a direct effect and also an indirect effect through all other variables. There are many further interesting indirect effects in this network.

Age seems independent from all other variables. This is an interesting finding of the Bayesian network. Age is clearly associated with death in the other studies (like GAM), but here, when focus is on conditional independence, we estimated that all other variables have an impact on death, direct or indirect, but age has not. We can understand this in the following way: age is in some sense a surrogate variable for health status, in itself age is not a danger, but through events that become more lively with age, like hypertension. Indirect effects are therefore possible, but not direct ones. Apparently there is not enough support in our data to estimate age as a master node that from the top regulates all other variables which then point to death even though age is known as main cause of cardiology.

We build up another separated network that includes age and other causes of heart failure (HIV, hypertension, diabetes, etc) but excludes death in order to discover relationships between age and other causes (HIV, hypertension, diabetes, etc). For brevity, we prefer to determine which variables influence the presence or absence of hypertension. From a medical viewpoint, it is possible that hypertension is among the classical variables related to heart failure and influenced by some of the variables listed in this research.

R-code for new network for presence or absence of hypertension

```
> Data<- read.table("mom.dat",header=T) ##
invoke Data from working Directory
> attach(Data)
> Data2<-
data.frame(age,hypertension,HIV,diabetes,TB,a
nemia,sinus,renalineffeciency)
> Data2$age<-as.numeric(Data$age)
> Data2$anemia <-as.factor(Data2$anemia)
> Data2$diabetes <-as.factor(Data2$diabetes)
> Data$hypertension <-
as.numeric(Data2$hypertension)
```

```
> Data2$sinus <-as.factor(Data2$sinus)
> Data2$TB <-as.factor(Data2$TB)
> Data2$HIV <-as.factor(Data2$HIV)
> Data2$renalineffeciency <-
as.factor(Data2$renalineffeciency)
> library(deal) ## call deal package
> Data.nw2<- network(Data2) ## specify prior
network
> Data.prior2<- jointprior(Data.nw2)
Imaginary sample size: 128
> from1<- c(2,3,4,5,6,7,8)
> to1<- rep(1,7)
> from2<- c(1,2,4,5,6,7,8)
> to2<- rep(3,7)
> from3<- rep(2,5)
> to3<- c(4,5,6,7,8)
> banlist2<- matrix(
c(from1,from2,from3,to1,to2,to3),ncol=2)
> banlist(Data.nw2)<- banlist2
> Data.nw2 <-
getnetwork(learn(Data.nw2,Data2,Data.prior2))
> Data.search2 <-
autosearch(Data.nw2,Data2,Data.prior2,trace=T
RUE)
> Data.heuristic2<-
heuristic(getnetwork(Data.search2),Data2,Data
.prior2,
restart=2,
degree=10,trace=TRUE,trylist=gettrylist(
Data.search2))
```

The network is displayed in Fig. 2. On the contrary to Fig. 1, Fig. 2 implies age is directly related to hypertension which justifies our assumption of indirect impact of age on death status of heart failure patients through hypertension.

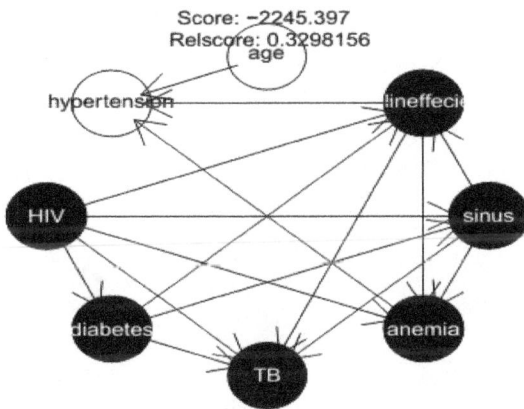

Fig. 2. Network for absence/presence of hypertension

We can build up another separated network that includes age and other causes of heart failure (HIV, hypertension, diabetes, etc) but excludes death status in order to discover dependency relationships between age and other causes (HIV, hypertension, diabetes, etc) in similar manner.

3.2 Discussion

In this paper we have established a nice way of determining the the impact of several variable on death status of heart failure patients. We have given an introduction to Bayesian networks with both discrete and continuous random variables. Several literatures were done on mixed variables (Discrete and continuous). For instance [4,5] and [11]. We also applied Bayesian Networks to clinical data obtained from Asella Referral Hospital. Different literatures have been done on the use of Bayesian Networks in clinical studies one of which is [12].

4. CONCLUSIONS

In this paper we described a powerful technique for analyzing Heart Failure data based on the theory and algorithms for learning Bayesian networks. We explained how to apply these techniques to Heart Failure data. The result of this analysis showed that death of a patient can be determined by HIV, hypertension, diabetes, TB, anemia, renal inefficiency and sinus directly or indirectly. The finding revealed that age does not have direct impact on death of a patient but it has an impact indirectly through complications like hypertension.

CONSENT

It is not applicable.

ACKNOWLEDGEMENTS

The authors would like to express their special gratitude to Professor Arnoldo Frigessi for his useful comments while conducting this study. They also acknowledge Asella Referral Hospital for its cooperation during the time of data collection.

COMPETING INTERESTS

Authors have declared that no competing interests exist.

REFERENCES

1. Calvin FS. Handbook of graphic presentation. 2nd ed. A Ronald Press Publication, New York: Wiley. 1954.
2. Cowell RG, Dawid AP, Lauritzen SL, Spiegelhalter DJ. Probabilistic networks and expert systems. Springer-Verlag, Berlin-Heidelberg-New York. 1999.
3. Hastie T, Tibshirani R, Friedman J. The elements of statistical learning: Data mining, inference, and prediction. Springer Series in Statistics. 2nd ed. Stanford, California. 2008.
4. Bøttcher SG. Learning bayesian networks with mixed variables. Artificial Intelligence and Statistics 2001, Morgan Kaufmann, San Francisco, CA, USA. 2001;149-156.
5. Bøttcher SG. Learning bayesian networks with mixed variables. Aalborg University. 2003.
    Available: http://www.math.auc.dk/ãlma
6. Koch KR. Introduction to Bayesian statistics. 2nd ed. Springer. 2007.
7. Neapolitan RE. Probabilistic reasoning in expert systems: Theory and algorithms. A Wiley-Interscience Publication. John Wiley & Sons, Inc., New York. 1989.
8. Pearl J. Probabilistic reasoning in intelligent systems: Networks of plausible inference. Morgan Kaufmann Publishers, Inc., San Mateo, California. 1988.
9. Bøttcher SG, Dethlefsen C. Learning Bayesian networks with R, In K. Hornik, F. Leisch and A. Zeileis (eds), Proceedings of the 3rd International Workshop on Distributed Statistical Computing. ISSN 1609-395X. 2003b.
10. Heckerman D, Geiger D, Chickering D. Learning Bayesian networks: The combination of knowledge and statistical data. Machine Learning. 1995;20:197-243.
11. Bøttcher SG, Dethlefsen C. Deal: A package for learning Bayesian networks. Journal of Statistical Software. 2003a; 8(20):1-40.
12. Bøttcher SG, Dethlefsen C. Prediction of the insulin sensitivity index using Bayesian network. Department of Mathematical Sciences, Aalborg University Denmark. 2004.

25

A Tough Pill to Swallow- Spontaneous Retropharyngeal Hematoma: A Rare and Unusual Complication of Rivaroxaban Therapy

Ali Naqvi[1*], Dalia Hawwass[1] and Arnold Seto[2]

[1]*UC Irvine Health, 101 City Drive South, Orange CA 92868, USA.*
[2]*VA Long Beach Healthcare systems, 5901 E 7th Street, Long Beach, CA 90822, USA.*

Authors' contributions

This work was carried out in collaboration between all authors. Author AN managed the literature search and manuscript preparation. Author DH assisted in data collection. Author AS edited and revised the manuscript. All authors read and approved the final manuscript.

Editor(s):
(1) Francesco Pelliccia, Department of Heart and Great Vessels University La Sapienza, Rome, Italy.
Reviewers:
(1) Hugo R. Ramos, National University of Cordoba, Cordoba, Argentina.
(2) Kazuo Higa, Fukuoka University, Fukuoka, Japan.
(3) Iana Simova, National Cardiology Hospital, Sofia, Bulgaria.

ABSTRACT

Aims: We present the first case of a patient that developed a spontaneous retropharyngeal hematoma as a complication of rivaroxaban therapy.
Case Presentation: A 49-year-old Caucasian male with chronic atrial fibrillation on rivaroxaban presented to the hospital with a rapidly expanding spontaneous retropharyngeal hematoma. He required emergent intubation for airway protection and subsequently was treated with catheter-directed embolization and surgical evacuation.
Discussion: Our report presents a case of a spontaneous retropharyngeal hematoma on rivaroxaban therapy. Unfortunately, most patients with this complication typically present with insidious symptoms including mild neck pain and ear ache, and as a result the diagnosis can easily be overlooked. Therefore, it is of utmost importance that physicians maintain a high index of suspicion, as early recognition and appropriate therapy can reduce morbidity and mortality.
Conclusion: This case highlights a rare but life-threatening hemorrhagic complication of rivaroxaban therapy.

Corresponding author: E-mail: naqvia@uci.edu

Keywords: Retropharyngeal hematoma; rivaroxaban; atrial fibrillation.

ABBREVIATIONS

INR- international normalized ratio, PT- prothrombin time, GFR- glomerular filtration rate, BMI- Body Mass Index, mmHg – millimeter of mercury

1. INTRODUCTION

Multiple new agents have recently become available for anticoagulation and stroke prevention in patients with atrial fibrillation. These novel medications have alleviated significant burdens associated with standard warfarin therapy by providing predictable anticoagulation without the need for frequent dose adjustments or routine laboratory monitoring. Rivaroxaban (Xarelto, Janssen Pharmaceuticals) has gained tremendous popularity as a result of its once a day dosing and minimal drug-to-drug interactions. Rivaroxaban is an oxazolidinone derivative optimized to inhibit Factor Xa bound to prothrombinase complex, and ultimately functions to disrupt both the extrinsic and intrinsic pathway of the coagulation cascade [1]. As clinical indications for rivaroxaban continue to expand, complications such as major bleeding events will also rise. We describe a case of spontaneous retropharyngeal hematoma as a complication of rivaroxaban therapy.

2. PRESENTATION OF CASE

A 49-year-old male with permanent atrial fibrillation with a CHADS2-VASc score of 1 for hypertension and multiple failed attempts at cardioversion presented to an urgent care clinic with right-sided otalgia. The patient received otic drops and was discharged home but returned the following day with progressively worsened ear pain, dysphagia, and severe hoarseness that was quickly evolving. No notable abnormalities were seen on physical examination. Given the severity and progression of symptoms, urgent imaging was performed. Computed tomography with contrast of the neck revealed a 4x3x3 cm right-sided hypopharyngeal hematoma. There was no history of any preceding trauma. The patient was sent directly to the emergency department. On initial evaluation, patient's vitals were heart rate of 98 beats per minute, blood pressure of 108/74 mmHg, respiratory rate of 22 breaths per minute, and oxygen saturation of 95% on room air. BMI notable for 27 kg/m^2. Laboratory studies revealed hemoglobin of 11.9 g/dL, platelets of 186 x 10^3/μL, INR 1.0, PTT 28.5 sec, creatinine of 0.9 mg/dL, estimated GFR 100 mL/min/1.73 m^2 and normal liver function testing.

His home medications were reviewed and included the following: Lisinopril 40mg daily, hydrochlorothiazide 25 mg daily, and rivaroxaban 20 mg daily. All medications were last taken one-day prior to his arrival. Interval imaging was performed and confirmed a rapidly enlarging retropharyngeal hematoma measuring 9x3x3 cm. The hematoma extended from the right lateral oropharynx and expanded anteriorly into the nasopharyngeal region with evidence of submucosal bleed involving the uvula and soft palate, concerning for impending airway compromise. He underwent emergent nasal fiberoptic intubation that was challenging requiring nearly 2 hours. Diagnostic angiography was subsequently performed, which demonstrated active extravasation from multiple branches of the right external carotid artery for which patient underwent fibered coil embolization of unspecified vessels.

A multi-disciplinary approach was taken to manage the patient including the assistance of otolaryngology, interventional radiology, cardiology, and the critical care team. Given the patient's severe presentation and clinical status, the patient was transferred to our facility for higher level of care. He was evaluated by otolaryngology and underwent an open tracheostomy with transoral incision, drainage, and evacuation of the hematoma under laryngoscopic guidance. Patient's post-operative course was complicated by atrial fibrillation with rapid ventricular response, which was controlled with intravenous rate-control agents. He improved clinically and his tracheostomy was downsized, capped, and decannulated. After eleven days of hospitalization, the patient was discharged home without any further complications. The decision was made to hold anticoagulation following his recent bleed with close outpatient follow-up with cardiology.

3. DISCUSSION

This is the first documented case report of a spontaneous retropharyngeal bleed associated with rivaroxaban therapy. A report published earlier this year presented a case of a ruptured parathyroid adenoma leading to anterior neck

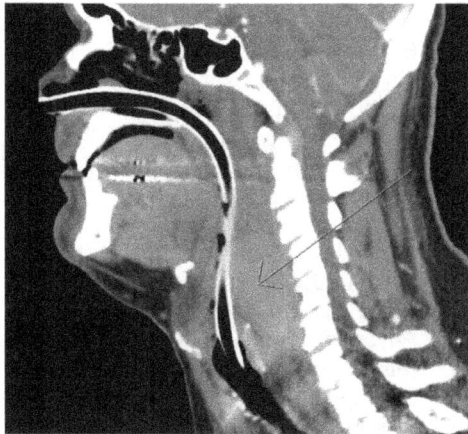

Fig. 1. (Left) Sagittal view on computed tomography of the neck revealing a retropharyngeal hematoma partially compressing the nasopharyngeal tube

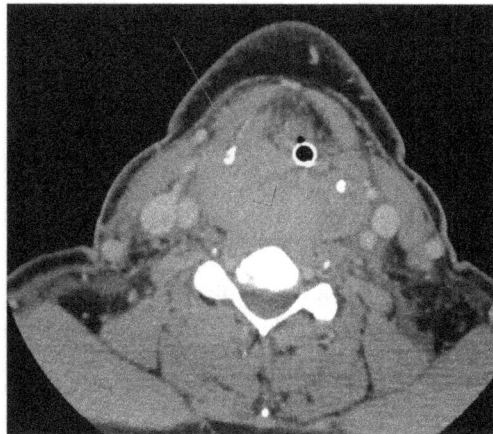

Fig. 2. (Right) Cross-sectional view of the enlarging hematoma with evidence of left-sided tracheal deviation

hematoma on rivaroxaban [2]. As previously mentioned, rivaroxaban has many benefits in comparison to warfarin including rapid onset of action, less drug-to-drug interactions, wider therapeutic window, and fewer serious bleeding events. Reported complications of rivaroxaban include intracranial, retroperitoneal, and gastrointestinal bleeds, but the case documented here highlights an extremely rare but life-threatening complication that can occur in patients on chronic anticoagulation [3]. Retropharyngeal hematomas typically occur in the setting of cervical trauma, infection, surgery, carotid aneurysm, or internal jugular vein rupture, but can also occur spontaneously. Majority of medication-associated cases of retropharyngeal hematomas are as a result of warfarin therapy, but we present a case herein of a young otherwise healthy male that experienced a spontaneous retropharyngeal hematoma as a complication of rivaroxaban [4].

Clinical diagnosis of a retropharyngeal bleed can be challenging. Patients may present with nonspecific symptoms of dyspnea and cough that can prematurely be attributed to other causes. Thus, providers caring for patients on anticoagulants including rivaroxaban should have a high index of suspicion for diagnosis for a retropharyngeal hematoma, and any patient with stridor, dysphonia, and dysphagia should invariably have an urgent airway evaluation as these are ominous signs for impending airway obstruction. Prompt imaging should include lateral soft tissue radiograph of the neck which can reveal widening of the retropharyngeal or

prevertebral space or computed tomography studies as described above. Health-care providers need to be judicious about starting these novel anticoagulation agents and understand that they are not without risk. Unfortunately, in contrast to bleeding with warfarin, which has a clear protocol for reversal with Vitamin K and fresh-frozen plasma [5], rivaroxaban lacks any guidelines regarding direct reversal. Interventions such as fresh-frozen plasma (FFP) and recombinant activated factor VII have been studied and so far been ineffective. Additionally, the use of recombinant factor Xa and prothrombin complex concentrates (PCC) as reversal agents lack proper prospective trials and are currently not widely available [6]. Thus, any hemorrhagic complication as a result of rivaroxaban will require supportive care and urgent surgical intervention on a case-by-case basis. This report draws attention to an unusual complication of rivaroxaban therapy and brings awareness to the community, as early recognition and appropriate therapy can reduce morbidity and mortality.

4. CONCLUSION

This case highlights a rare but life-threatening complication of rivaroxaban therapy that physicians should consider when prescribing rivaroxaban or other novel anticoagulants.

CONSENT

All authors declare that 'written informed consent was obtained from the patient (or other approved parties) for publication of this case report and accompanying images.

ETHICAL APPROVAL

It is not applicable.

COMPETING INTERESTS

Authors AN and DH have no disclosures. Author AS is a speaker for Janssen Pharmaceuticals.

REFERENCES

1. Abdulsattar Y, Bhambri R, Nogid A. Rivaroxaban (xarelto) for the prevention of thromboembolic disease: An inside look at the oral direct factor Xa inhibitor. Pharmacy and Therapeutics. 2009;34(5): 238. PubMed ID: 19561868

2. Shamban L, Patel B, Forman A, Ahmad N. Spontaneous anterior neck hematoma associated with rivaroxaban leading to primary hyperparathyroidism and hypercalcemia. Journal of Medical Cases. 2015;6(2):87-90.
    DOI: 10.14740/jmc1825w

3. Prins MH, Lensing AW, Bauersachs R, van Bellen B, Bounameaux H, Brighton TA, et al. Oral rivaroxaban versus standard therapy for the treatment of symptomatic venous thromboembolism: A pooled analysis of the EINSTEIN-DVT and PE randomized studies. Thrombosis Journal. 2013;11(1):21.
    DOI: 10.1186/1477-9560-11-21 PubMed ID: 24053656

4. Bloom DC, Haegen T, and Keefe MA. Anticoagulation and spontaneous retropharyngeal hematoma. The Journal of Emergency Medicine. 2003;24(4):389-394. PubMed ID: 12745040

5. Srivastava S, Solanki T. Retropharyngeal haematoma - An unusual bleeding site in an anticoagulated patient: A case report. Cases Journal. 2008;1(1):294.
    DOI: 10.1186/1757-1626-1-294

6. Marlu R, Hodaj E, Paris A, Albaladejo P, Cracowski JL, Pernod G. Effect of non-specific reversal agents on anticoagulant activity of dabigatran and rivaroxaban: A randomised crossover *ex vivo* study in healthy volunteers. Thrombosis and haemostasis. 2012;108(2):217-24.
    DOI: 10.1160/TH12-03-0179

26

Severe Coronary Artery Ectasia with ST Elevation MI: A Challenging Situation

Abid Hussain Laghari[1*], Khwaja Yousuf Hasan[1], Izat Shah[2] and Khawar Abbas Kazmi[1]

[1]*Department of Medicine, Aga Khan University Hospital, Karachi, Pakistan.*
[2]*Cardiac Catheterization Laboratory, Aga Khan University Hospital, Karachi, Pakistan.*

Authors' contributions

This work was carried out in collaboration between all authors. All authors read and approved the final manuscript.

Editor(s):
(1) Federico Quaini, Department of Internal Medicine, University-Hospital of Parma, Italy.
Reviewers:
(1) Dmitry Napalkov, Moscow State Medical University, Russia.
(2) Aşkın Ender Topal, Dicle University, Medicine Faculty, Turkey.

ABSTRACT

Aim: To report a case of huge coronary artery ectasia presenting with acute myocardial infarction; a relatively rare finding encountered during coronary angiography.

Presentation of Case: A young male presented with chest pain and profuse sweating at a local hospital. Electrocardiogram showed Infero-posterior STEMI. Patient received streptokinase. His symptoms settled however the electrocardiogram changes did not resolve. He presented at our hospital after 24 hours with chest discomfort. He was vitally stable and a murmur of MR was audible. His Troponin-I was raised and electrocardiogram showed ST elevations with Q waves. Coronary angiogram showed giant ectasia and occluded right coronary artery (RCA). Percutaneous coronary intervention of RCA was done; with TIMI II flow but still had some residual thrombus. The patient was kept on Tirofiban infusion. His CRP and homocysteine levels were raised. Dual antiplatelet, statin, ACE Inhibitor, beta blocker with vitamin B12 and folic acid supplement were continued.

Discussion: Coronary artery ectasia is a form of atherosclerosis seen in 0.3–4.9% of coronary angiography procedures. It is described as dilation of the coronary arteries >1.5 times compared to adjacent normal vessel. An excessive expansive remodeling with enzymatic degradation of the extracellular matrix is considered to be the major pathophysiologic process. Clinical importance

---

Corresponding author: E-mail: drabidlaghari@yahoo.com

inclines on its association with acute coronary syndrome.

Conclusion: A case of huge coronary artery ectasia presenting with acute myocardial infarction and successfully treated with PCI.

Keywords: ST elevation myocardial infarction (STEMI); coronary artery ectasia (CAE); percutaneous coronary intervention (PCI).

1. INTRODUCTION

Coronary artery ectasia (CAE) is a well-recognized but relatively rare finding faced during diagnostic coronary angiography [1–3]. It is commonly described as inappropriate dilation of the coronary arteries exceeding more than 1.5 times the largest diameter of an adjacent normal vessel [1]. Although several mechanisms are proposed; the pathophysiology of CAE is still underrecognized. Similarly no consensus stands about the natural history and management of this condition due to scarcity of data.

2. PRESENTATION OF CASE

A 37 year old man; presented with history of chest pain, vomiting and profuse sweating at a local hospital. Chest discomfort lasted for four hours. ECG was done that revealed Infero-posterior wall ST-Elevation MI. He received streptokinase at the local hospital and his symptoms settled, however ECG changes did not resolve. He was referred to a tertiary care hospital after 24 hours with mild chest discomfort. He had a sedentary life style and history of 20 pack year smoking and tobacco chewing. He denied any other addiction. His family history was negative for premature ischemic heart disease. He was not taking any regular medicines before this event.

Clinical examination of this young overweight man (BMI-29) revealed pulse of 110 beats/minute, blood pressure of 130/70 mmHg. Jugular veins were not distended. Cardiac auscultation revealed 2/6 pansystolic murmur at apex radiating to axilla and chest examination was normal.

Blood tests showed normal complete blood count, urea, creatinine and electrolytes. His Troponin-I was raised (106 ng/ml) and electrocardiogram (ECG) showed ST elevations in inferior leads along with Q waves (Fig. 1). Patient received antiplatelets, statin and heparin in emergency department. We decided to proceed with coronary angiogram and

revascularisation due to recurrence of symptoms and persistant ST elevations. Coronary angiogram showed giant ectasia of left anterior descending (LAD) artery and right coronary artery (RCA) (Figs. 2 and 3). The left circumflex artery (LCx) was normal. The ectatic right coronary artery was full of thrombus and totally occluded from distal segment before dividing into posterior descending artery (PDA) and posterior left ventricular branch (PLV) (Fig. 3). RCA was engaged with Judkins Right 4 (JR4) 6 French guiding catheter. PDA was wired with Runthrough Intermediate wire. Manual aspiration was done with thrombuster catheter. Large amount of thrombus was extracted. After thrombus extraction, PLV was faintly visible. The PLV branch was wired with another Runthrough Intermediate wire, manual aspiration of thrombus was done and the thrombus was extracted. After extracting large amount of thrombus the blood flow in distal RCA improved however there was still some residual thrombus (Fig. 4). Patient was kept on glycoprotein IIb/IIIa inhibitor (Tirofiban) infusion for 48 hours and remained asymptomatic post procedure. The patient was worked up for cause of coronary artery ectasia. He was found to have raised CRP and homocysteine levels; 20 mg/dl and 45.2 micromoles/dl respectively. His vitamin B12 level was within normal range. Autoimmune profile and syphilis serology were negative. Dual antiplatelet therapy, statin, ACE Inhibitor and beta blocker were continued. Vitamin B12 and folic acid were added to his treatment. He underwent an echocardiogram that revealed mild left ventricular dysfunction with ejection fraction of 45% and segmental wall motion abnormalities correlating to the right coronary artery territory. Moderate mitral regurgitation with regurgitant fraction 41% and structurally normal valve was observed. The patient was subsequently discharged from the hospital in stable condition. He was counseled with regards to smoking cessation and life style modification. At follow-up clinic visit (after two weeks) he is stable and asymptomatic.

3. DISCUSSION

Coronary artery ectasia (CAE) is defined as localized or diffuse dilatation of coronary artery lumen exceeding the largest diameter of an adjacent normal vessel >1.5 times [1]. The reported incidence of CAE varies between 0.3–4.9% of patients undergoing coronary angiography procedure [1,3]. CAE detection rate may rise with the use of modern non-invasive imaging technologies like computed tomography and magnetic resonance coronary angiography [4].

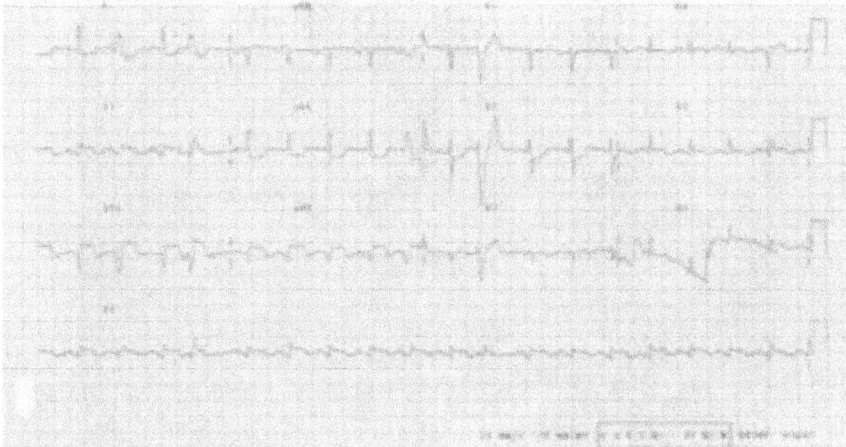

Fig. 1. Electrocardiogram showing ST segment elevations in inferior leads along with Q waves and reciprocal changes in lateral leads

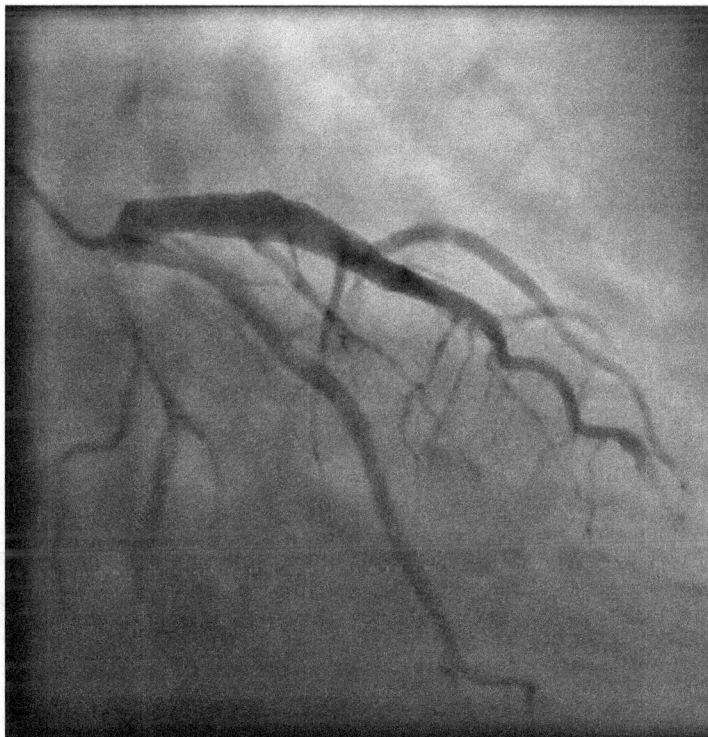

Fig. 2. Coronary angiogram showing ectatic left anterior descending artery

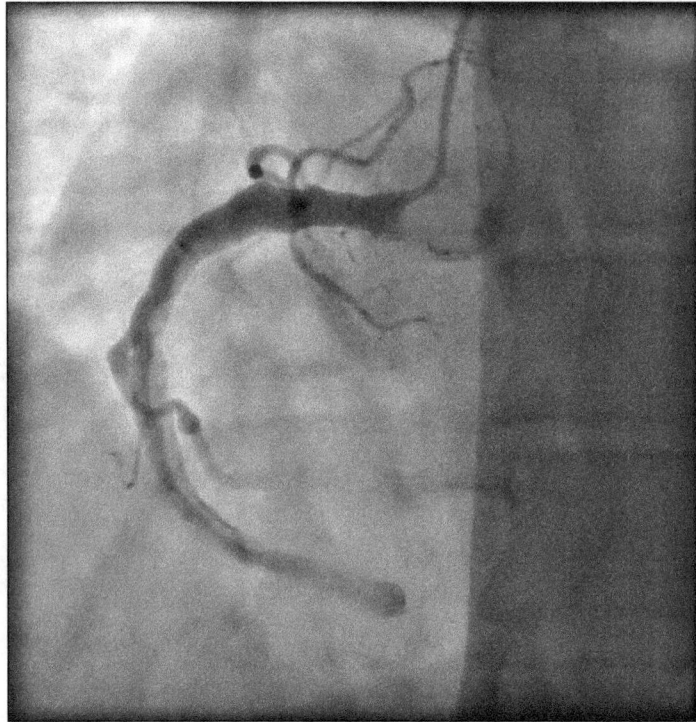

Fig. 3. Coronary angiogram showing ectatic right coronary artery filled with thrombus and totally occluded

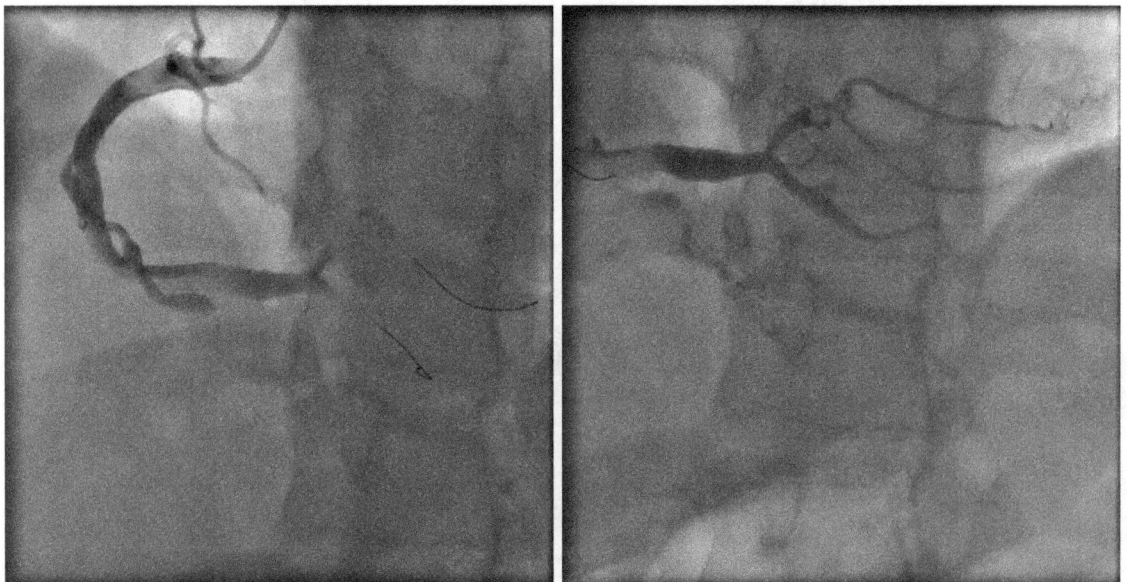

Fig. 4. Coronary angiogram: ectatic right coronary artery after thrombus aspiration showing flow in PDA and PLV branches and some residual thrombus

The incidence of CAE is higher in men (2.2%) than in women (0.5%) [3]. In the CASS registry postmortem incidence is reported 1.4%. Atherosclerosis is considered to be the main etiologic factor responsible for >50% of cases in adults [1,3]. Kawasaki disease is the most frequent etiology in children. Coronary artery ectasia is considered to be a result of excessive expansive remodeling, which happens as a result of enzymatic degradation of the extracellular matrix and thinning of the vessel tunica media. Patients with CAE without obstructive coronary artery disease may present with positive stress tests, angina pectoris or acute coronary syndromes (ACS). Ectatic artery may be a source of thrombus formation with distal embolization, vasospasm or spontaneous artery rupture as the most catastrophic sequela. CAE is classified according to the coronary artery diameter as small (5mm), medium (5–8 mm) and giant (more than 8mm). There are significant histopathological similarities between ectasia and atherosclerosis. The vessel lumen may be narrowed, retained or dilated with advancement of atherosclerosis process. Some atherosclerotic plaques, as a consequence of a phenomenon called 'positive arterial remodeling, do not decrease luminal size, probably due to expansion of the tunica media and external elastic membrane. This finding may be the reason of ectasia or aneurysms of coronary arteries. Positive remodeling is basically a compensatory mechanism to retain luminal size during the progression of atherosclerosis. Significantly raised levels of C-reactive protein (CRP) and vascular endothelial growth factor (VEGF) were isolated in patients with CAE, which suggests extensive inflammation and neovascularization in ectatic vessel wall [5,6]. CAE is associated with angiotensin-converting enzyme DD genotype and familial hypercholesterolemia suggesting a genetic preponderance [7,8]. There is controversial association between hypertension and CAE [3]. CAE is linked to apical hypertrophic cardiomyopathy with high wall tension during ventricular systole. Right coronary artery is the most commonly involved vessel in the coronary tree (40–61%) which is followed by left anterior descending artery (15–32%) and left circumflex artery (15–23%) [1,3,4]. Solitary left main trunk ectasia is almost an exception. CAE may coexist with aneurysms of additional arterial beds, mainly abdominal aorta, even with venous varicosities. Coronary angiogram is gold standard for diagnosing coronary ectasia. Extent of CAE and corrected TIMI frame count are associated with severity of angina in patients with CAE [9]. CAE in patients younger than 50 years may be suggestive of connective tissue disorders or vasculitis. In such situations further workup to identify the cause should be considered, as was done in this case. The clinical features suggesting coronary aneurysms secondary to Kawasaki disease are the history of Kawasaki disease, matching symptoms, Asian race, proximal location of coronary artery aneurysms, giant aneurysms (more than 8 mm), young age and lack of significant coronary stenosis (>50%). Accurate diagnosis of Kawasaki disease is crucial because the treatment strategies differ from conventional atherosclerotic ectasias [10]. According to Markis classification of CAE, typeI and type II CAE have a worse prognosis than type III and IV. Mortality rate of CAE at 2 years is reported up to 15%. There is still no consensus for management of CAE amongst the experts. Risk factor modification and administration of aspirin to all CAE patients is logical due to the high coincidence with coronary artery disease and acute coronary syndrome. Statins may have an important role by inhibiting the enzyme matrix metalloproteinase [11]. Nitrates may cause steal phenomenon by dilating epicardial coronary arteries, and increase anginal symptoms [12]. Treatment of CAE with angina or myocardial ischemia includes aspirin, statin and anti-ischemic medications (calcium channel blocker, beta blocker and trimetazidine) [12]. Acute coronary syndrome (ACS) associated with CAE must be managed on an individual basis. The presence of thrombus may warrant to implement extra therapeutic decisions, like thrombolysis, heparin infusion or glycoprotein IIb/IIIa receptor inhibitors and thrombus aspiration during primary percutaneous coronary intervention (PCI) [13]. Long term anticoagulation is suggested by many authors however no randomized trial demonstrated its benefit. Percutaneous or surgical revascularization may be an option in patients with coexisting obstructive lesions and significant ischemia despite medical therapy [14]. Coronary intervention of stenosis adjacent to ectasia is in itself challenging with regards to optimal stent sizing, misplacement of stent, early stent thrombosis and restenosis. Additional care should be taken during stenting because adequate stent expansion and wall apposition is needed [15]. Covered stents offer superior angiographic results compared to the bare metal stents, but long term advantage has not been proven. The use of large sized peripheral stents in ectatic coronary arteries is also an option. In patients with evidence of enlargement of saccular aneurysms with high risk of rupture, surgical resection may be considered.

4. CONCLUSION

CAE is mostly a form of atherosclerosis seen in 0.3 4.9% of diagnostic coronary angiography procedures. An excessive expansive remodeling with enzymatic degradation of the extracellular matrix and thinning of the vessel media as a result of chronic inflammation is considered to be a major pathophysiologic process. Clinical importance inclines on its association with acute coronary syndrome as was the case in our patient. Management options include risk factor modifications for coronary artery disease, anti-ischemic therapy, antithrombotic management and percutaneous or surgical revascularization.

CONSENT

Patient himself gave the written informed consent for case report.

ETHICAL APPROVAL

It is not applicable.

COMPETING INTERESTS

Authors have declared that no competing interests exist.

REFERENCES

1. Hartnell GG, Parnell BM, Pridie RB. Coronary artery ectasia. Its prevalence and clinical significance in 4993 patients. British Heart Journal. 1985;54(4):392–5.

2. Sorrell VL, Davis MJ, Bove AA. Current knowledge and significance of coronary artery ectasia: A chronologic review of the literature, recommendations for treatment, possible etiologies, and future considerations. Clinical Cardiology. 1998; 21(3):157–60.

3. Swaye PS, Fisher LD, Litwin P, Vignola PA, Judkins MP, Kemp HG, et al. Aneurysmal coronary artery disease. Circulation. 1983;67(1):134–8.

4. Diaz-Zamudio M, Bacilio-Perez U, Herrera-Zarza MC, Meave-González A, Alexanderson-Rosas E, Zambrana-Balta GF, et al. Coronary artery aneurysms and ectasia: Role of coronary CT angiography. Radiographics. 2009;29(7):1939–54.

5. Turhan H, Erbay AR, Yasar AS,Balci M, Bicer A, Yetkin E. Comparison of C-reactive protein levels in patients with coronary artery ectasia versus patients with obstructive coronary artery disease. The American Journal of Cardiology 2004;94(10):1303–6.

6. Savino M, Parisi Q, Biondi-Zoccai GG, Pristipino C, Cianflone D, Crea F. New insights into molecular mechanisms of diffuse coronary ectasiae: A possible role for VEGF. International Journal of Cardiology. 2006;106(3):307–12.

7. Gulec S, Aras O, Atmaca Y, Akyürek O, Hanson NQ, Sayin T, et al. Deletion polymorphism of the angiotensin I converting enzyme gene is a potent risk factor for coronary artery ectasia. Heart. 2003;89(2):213–4.

8. Sudhir K, Ports TA, Amidon TM, Goldberger JJ, Bhushan V, Kane JP, et al. Increased prevalence of coronary ectasia in heterozygous familial hypercholes-terolemia. Circulation. 1995;91(5):1375–80.

9. Zografos TA, Korovesis S, Giazitzoglou E, Maria Kokladi, Ioannis Venetsanakos, George Paxinos, et al. Clinical and angiographic characteristics of patients with coronary artery ectasia. International Journal of Cardiology; 2012.

10. Daniels LB, Tjajadi MS, Walford HH, Jimenez-Fernandez S, Trofimenko V, Fick DB Jr, et al. Prevalence of Kawasaki disease in young adults with suspected myocardial ischemia. Circulation. 2012;125(20):2447–53.

11. Massaro M, Zampolli A, Scoditti E, Carluccio MA, Storelli C, Distante A, et al. Statins inhibit cyclooxygenase-2 and matrix metalloproteinase-9 in human endothelial cells: Anti-angiogenic actions possibly contributing to plaque stability. Cardiovascular Research. 2010;86(2): 311–20.

12. Kruger D, Stierle U, Herrmann G, Simon R, Sheikhzadeh A. Exercise-induced myocardial ischemia in isolated coronary artery ectasias and aneurysms (dilated coronopathy). Journal of the American College of Cardiology. 1999:34(5):1461–70.

13. Steg PG, James SK, Atar D, Badano LP, Blömstrom-Lundqvist C, Borger MA, et al. ESC guidelines for the management of acute myocardial infarction in patients presenting with ST-segment elevation. European Heart Journal. 2012;33(20): 2569–2619.

14. Ochiai M, Yamaguchi T, Taguchi J, Ohno M, Yoshimura H, Kashida M, et al. Angioplasty of stenoses adjacent to

aneurysmal coronary artery disease. Japanese Heart Journal. 1990;31(6):749–757.

15. Manginas A, Cokkinos DV. Coronary artery ectasias: Imaging, functional assessment and clinical implications. European Heart Journal. 2006;27(9):1026–31.

Permissions

All chapters in this book were first published in CAIJ, by SCIENCE DOMAIN international; hereby published with permission under the Creative Commons Attribution License or equivalent. Every chapter published in this book has been scrutinized by our experts. Their significance has been extensively debated. The topics covered herein carry significant findings which will fuel the growth of the discipline. They may even be implemented as practical applications or may be referred to as a beginning point for another development.

The contributors of this book come from diverse backgrounds, making this book a truly international effort. This book will bring forth new frontiers with its revolutionizing research information and detailed analysis of the nascent developments around the world.

We would like to thank all the contributing authors for lending their expertise to make the book truly unique. They have played a crucial role in the development of this book. Without their invaluable contributions this book wouldn't have been possible. They have made vital efforts to compile up to date information on the varied aspects of this subject to make this book a valuable addition to the collection of many professionals and students.

This book was conceptualized with the vision of imparting up-to-date information and advanced data in this field. To ensure the same, a matchless editorial board was set up. Every individual on the board went through rigorous rounds of assessment to prove their worth. After which they invested a large part of their time researching and compiling the most relevant data for our readers.

The editorial board has been involved in producing this book since its inception. They have spent rigorous hours researching and exploring the diverse topics which have resulted in the successful publishing of this book. They have passed on their knowledge of decades through this book. To expedite this challenging task, the publisher supported the team at every step. A small team of assistant editors was also appointed to further simplify the editing procedure and attain best results for the readers.

Apart from the editorial board, the designing team has also invested a significant amount of their time in understanding the subject and creating the most relevant covers. They scrutinized every image to scout for the most suitable representation of the subject and create an appropriate cover for the book.

The publishing team has been an ardent support to the editorial, designing and production team. Their endless efforts to recruit the best for this project, has resulted in the accomplishment of this book. They are a veteran in the field of academics and their pool of knowledge is as vast as their experience in printing. Their expertise and guidance has proved useful at every step. Their uncompromising quality standards have made this book an exceptional effort. Their encouragement from time to time has been an inspiration for everyone.

The publisher and the editorial board hope that this book will prove to be a valuable piece of knowledge for researchers, students, practitioners and scholars across the globe.

List of Contributors

Puneet Aggarwal and Tilak Raj Khurana
Department of Internal Medicine, PGIMER & Dr RML Hospital, Baba Kharag Singh Marg, New Delhi, India

Ranjeet Nath
Department of Cardiology, PGIMER & Dr RML Hospital, Baba Kharag Singh Marg, New Delhi, India

Swati Yadav
Department of Pathology, AIMSR, Bhathinda, Punjab, India

Prem Krishna Anandan, Basavaraj Baligar, J. S. Patel and Prabhavathi Bhatt
Resident in Cardiology, Sri Jayadeva Institute of Cardiovascular Science and Research, Bengaluru, Karnataka, India

Cholenahally Nanjappa Manjunath
Department of Cardiology, Sri Jayadeva Institute of Cardiovascular Science and Research, Bengaluru, Karnataka, India

C. Dhanalakshmi
Department of Echocardiography, Sri Jayadeva Institute of Cardiovascular Science and Research, Bengaluru, Karnataka, India

U. A. Fabian, M. A. Charles-Davies, K. S. Akinlade, O. G. Arinola and E. O Agbedana
Department of Chemical Pathology, College of Medicine, University of Ibadan, Ibadan 200284, Nigeria

A. A. Fasanmade and M. O. Owolabi
Department of Medicine, College of Medicine, University of Ibadan, Ibadan 200284, Nigeria

J. A. Olaniyi
Department of Haematology, College of Medicine, University of Ibadan, Ibadan 200284, Nigeria

O. E. Oyewole
Department of Health Promotion and Education, College of Medicine, University of Ibadan, Ibadan 200284, Nigeria

J. R. Adebusuyi and O. Hassan
Medical Social Services Department, University College Hospital, Ibadan 200212, Nigeria

B.M. Ajobo
Dietetics Department, University College Hospital, Ibadan 200212, Nigeria

M. O. Ebesunun
Department of Chemical Pathology, College of Health Sciences, Olabisi Onabanjo University, Ago-Iwoye 120005, Nigeria

K. Adigun
General Out Patient Unit, University College Hospital, Ibadan 200212, Nigeria

Prem Krishna Anandan, Subramanyam K, Shivananda Patil, R. Rangaraj and Cholenahally Nanjappa Manjunath
Department of cardiology, Sri Jayadeva Institute of Caridovascular Science & Research, Bengaluru, Karnataka, India

Maciej Chojnicki, Konrad Paczkowski, Radosław Jaworski and Mariusz Steffens
Department of Pediatric Cardiac Surgery, Mikolaj Kopernik Hospital in Gdańsk, Poland

Ireneusz Haponiuk,
Department of Pediatric Cardiac Surgery, Mikolaj Kopernik Hospital in Gdańsk, Poland

Department of Physiotherapy, Gdańsk University of Physical Education and Sport, Poland

Katarzyna Gierat-Haponiuk
Department of Rehabilitation, Medical University of Gdańsk, Poland

Hadi A. R. Hadi Khafaji
Department of Cardiology, Saint Michael's Hospital, Toronto University, Canada

Jassim M. Al-Suwaidi
Qatar Cardiovascular Research Center and Adult Cardiology, Heart Hospital, Hamad Medical Corporation, Doha, Qatar

Andrea Engelhardt, Pinar Bambul Heck, Peter Ewert and Alfred Hager
Department of Paediatric Cardiology and Congenital Heart Disease, Deutsches Herzzentrum München, Technische Universität München, Germany

Renate Oberhoffer
Department of Paediatric Cardiology and Congenital Heart Disease, Deutsches Herzzentrum München, Technische Universität München, Germany
Institute of Preventive Pediatrics, Technische Universität München, Germany

Ali Moukadem and Alain Dieterlen
MIPS Laboratory, University of Haute Alsace, 68093 Mulhouse, France

Christian Brandt
Center of Clinical Investigations, University Hospital of Strasbourg, Inserm, BP 426, 67091 Strasbourg, France

Emmanuel Andrès
Department of Internal Medicine, University Hospital of Strasbourg, BP 426, 67091 Strasbourg, France

Samy Talha
Laboratory of Physiology and Functional Explorations, University Hospital of Strasbourg, BP 426, 67091 Strasbourg, France

Methuselah Jere, Fastone M. Goma, Longa Kaluba and Charity Kapenda
Department of Physiological Sciences, School of Medicine, University of Zambia, Lusaka, Zambia

Ben Andrews
Department of Internal Medicine, School of Medicine, University of Zambia, Lusaka, Zambia

Ahlam Kadhim Al Hamdany
Department of Physiology, College of Medicine, Babylon University, Iraq

David J. Cornforth
Applied Informatics Research Group, University of Newcastle, Callaghan NSW 2308, Australia
School of Engineering and Information Technology, University of New South Wales, Australian Defence Force Academy, Canberra, Australia

Herbert F. Jelinek
Centre for Research in Complex Systems, School of Community Health, Charles Sturt University, Albury, Australia
Australian School of Advanced Medicine, Macquarie University, Sydney, Australia

Silanath Terpenning and Loren H. Ketai
Department of Radiology, University of New Mexico, Albuquerque, NM, 87131, USA

Stacy M. Rissing and Shawn D. Teague
Department of Radiology, Indiana University, School of Medicine, 550 N University Blvd, Indianapolis, IN 46202, USA

Mohamed Kaled A. Shambesh, Taher Mohamed Emahbes and Zeinab Elmehdi Saleh
Department of Community Medicine, Faculty of Medicine, University of Tripoli, Libya

Iman Mohamed Shambesh
Department of English, Faculty of Education, University of Tripoli, Libya

Malik Abdurrazag A. Elosta
CELTA, American Star Books, Headquartered in Frederick, Maryland, USA

Jorge A. Brenes-Salazar and Paul A. Friedman
Department of Medicine, Division of Cardiovascular Diseases, 200 First St SW, Rochester, MN 55901, Mayo Clinic Rochester, USA

Haliah Z. Al Shehri
Adult Cardiology Department, Prince Salman Heart Center, King Fahad Medical City, Riyadh, Saudi Arabia

Yahya S. Al Hebaishi and Abdulrahman M. Al Moghairi
Adult Cardiology Department, Prince Sultan Cardiac Centre (PSCC), Prince Sultan Military Medical City, Riyadh, Saudi Arabia

Mohammed Al-Biltagi
Department of Pediatric, Faculty of Medicine, Tanta University, Egypt

Amjad Al-Kouatli
Department of Cardiology, King Faisal Specialist Hospital and Research Center, Jeddah, Saudi Arabia

Jameel Al-Ata
Department of Cardiology, King Abdulaziz University Hospital, Jeddah, Saudi Arabia

Ahmad Jamjoom
Department of Cardiovascular, Cardiothoracic Surgery Section, King Faisal Specialist Hospital and Research Center, Jeddah, Saudi Arabia

Heba Abouzeid
Department of Pediatrics and Cardiovascular, Pediatric Cardiology Section, King Faisal Specialist Hospital and Research Center – Jeddah, Saudi Arabia and Faculty of Medicine, Zagazig University, Egypt

Shivakumar Bhairappa, Prakash Sadashivappa Surhonne, Shankar Somanna, Rohit Chopra and Cholenhally Nanjappa Manjunath
Department of Cardiology, Sri Jayadeva Institute of Cardiovascular Sciences and Research, Rajiv Gandhi University of Health Sciences, Jayanagar 9th Block, BG Road, Bangalore 560069, India

Gabriele Giacomo Schiattarella, Fabio Magliulo, Vito Di Palma, Giovanni Esposito and Plinio Cirillo
Department of Advanced Biomedical Sciences, School of Medicine, University of Naples Federico II, Naples, Italy

Donatella Brisinda, Francesco Fioravanti, Emilia Iantorno, Anna Rita Sorbo, Angela Venuti, Claudia Cataldi, Kristian Efremov and Riccardo Fenici
Clinical Physiology-Biomagnetism Center, Catholic University of Sacred Heart, Rome, Italy

Pietro Scicchitano, Michele Gesualdo, Santa Carbonara, Annapaola Zito, Gabriella Ricci,
Francesca Cortese and Marco Matteo Ciccone
Department of Emergency and Organ Transplantation (DETO), Cardiovascular Diseases Section, University of Bari, Piazza G. Cesare 11–70124, Bari, Italy

Pasquale Palmiero
Department of Cardiology, Local Health Service-Brindisi, Italy

Pietro Nazzaro
Department of Basic Medical Sciences, Neurosciences and Sense Organs, Division of Neurology- Stroke Unit, Hypertension, University of Bari, Bari, Italy

Pasquale Caldarola and Luisa de Gennaro
Department of Cardiovascular Disease, "San Paolo" Hospital, Bari, Italy

William D. Lynn and Omar J. Escalona
University of Ulster, School of Engineering, Engineering Research Institute, Newtownabbey, BT37 0QB, UK

David J. McEneaney
Craigavon Area Hospital, Southern Health and Social Care Trust, Cardiac Unit, SHSCT, Portadown, BT63 5QQ, UK

B. Uday Kiran, M. Sushma, V. Uma Maheshwara Rao and D. Jhansi Laxmi Bai
Department of Pharmacology, CMR College of Pharmacy, Kandlakoya, Medchal, R R Dist, Hyderabad, 501 401, India

K. V. S. R. G. Prasad
Department of Pharmacology, Institute of Pharmaceutical Technology, SPMVV, Tirupathi, Andhra Pradesh, India

V. Nisheetha
Department of Pharmacology, Sri Sai Jyothi College of Pharmacy, Vattinagula pally, Gandipet, Ranga Reddy Dist, Hyderabad-500 075, India

Muzeyin Ahmed Berarti
Department of Statistics, Wolaita Sodo University, Ethiopia

Ayele Taye Goshu
Department of Statistics, School of Mathematical and Statistical Sciences, Hawassa University, Ethiopia

Muzeyin Ahmed Berarti
Department of Statistics, Wolaita Sodo University, P.O.Box 138, Ethiopia

Ayele Taye Goshu
Department of Statistics, School of Mathematical and Statistical Sciences, Hawassa University, P.O.Box 05, Ethiopia

Ali Naqvi and Dalia Hawwass
UC Irvine Health, 101 City Drive South, Orange CA 92868, USA

Arnold Seto
VA Long Beach Healthcare systems, 5901 E 7th Street, Long Beach, CA 90822, USA

Abid Hussain Laghari, Khwaja Yousuf Hasan and Khawar Abbas Kazmi
Department of Medicine, Aga Khan University Hospital, Karachi, Pakistan

Izat Shah
Cardiac Catheterization Laboratory, Aga Khan University Hospital, Karachi, Pakistan

www.ingramcontent.com/pod-product-compliance
Lightning Source LLC
Chambersburg PA
CBHW080459200326
41458CB00012B/4030